Understanding and Preventing

SUDDEN DEATH

Understanding and Preventing

SUDDEN DEATH

Your Life Matters

Koon-Hou Mak

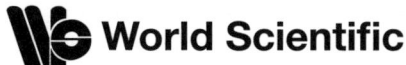

World Scientific

NEW JERSEY · LONDON · SINGAPORE · BEIJING · SHANGHAI · HONG KONG · TAIPEI · CHENNAI

Published by

World Scientific Publishing Co. Pte. Ltd.

5 Toh Tuck Link, Singapore 596224

USA office: 27 Warren Street, Suite 401-402, Hackensack, NJ 07601

UK office: 57 Shelton Street, Covent Garden, London WC2H 9HE

Library of Congress Cataloging-in-Publication Data
Mak, Koon Hou.
　Understanding and preventing sudden death / Koon-Hou Mak, Mak Heart Clinic, Singapore.
　　pages cm
　Includes bibliographical references and index.
　ISBN 978-9814641142 (hardcover : alk. paper) -- ISBN 978-9814641159 (pbk. : alk. paper)
　1. Sudden death. 2. Sudden death--Prevention. I. Title.
　RB150.S84M35 2015
　618.92'026--dc23

　　　　　　　　　　　　　　2014046091
　ISBN 978-9814678568 (pbk. alk. paper) -- Singapore Heart Foundation edition

British Library Cataloguing-in-Publication Data
A catalogue record for this book is available from the British Library.

DISCLAIMER
This book serves as a general guide for readers to understand sudden death syndromes. However, the material in this book is not intended to replace professional medical care or attention provided by a qualified practitioner. It cannot and should not be used as a basis for diagnosis or choice of treatment for an individual. The mention of any product, service or treatment should not be considered as an endorsement by the author or publisher. Readers are advised to consult their respective doctors and healthcare professionals regarding specific management approaches for their own medical conditions. The publisher, author or any other person involved in the production of this book is not responsible for any adverse consequence caused by any person reading or following the material in this book.

The names and identifying details of some of the individuals in this book have been changed to protect their privacy.

Reflections on *Sudden Death*

"Our world, an overcrowded world, she is full and even overfilled with creative minds. You can recognize their talent everywhere: Painters, musicians, sportsmen and women. Recognizing talent in Science is a different issue, a sport on itself. Dr Mak is not only a physician, but someone with the qualities of an artist, a musician, a sportsman and with a brain that brings together art, sport, science and the very essence of life and simple intelligence together.

This is a book supposedly meant for beginners. But, this is not a book for idiots. In some way, it is a book for intellectual masochists: People willing to enjoy the pain of learning. This is a real intellectual experience that you will love or hate. I do love this book!"

Professor Dr Pedro Brugada
Chairman, Cardiovascular Division
UZ Brussel — VUB
Brussels, Belgium

"An excellent book on the hard truths about heart matters. It provides deep insights into the complexities and realities of sudden death and the enormous impact it may have on the individual and the family and offers useful tips on prevention."

Adjunct Associate Professor Chew Suok Kai
Deputy Director Medical Services
Ministry of Health Singapore
Saw Swee Hock School of Public Health
National Univeristy of Singapore

"There is almost no one in the world that has not been affected by cardiovascular death. For anyone, from the interested layperson to the heart care specialist, who wants to understand everything that is currently known about the heart disease, this is the resource for you. Chalk full of case studies, historical perspectives, and most importantly, a truly expert synthesis of the available data, this surprisingly easy-to-read book provides everything you ever wanted to know about the causes, mechanisms, and preventive strategies of cardiovascular death."

Steven Steinhubl, MD
Digital Medicine Director
Scripps Translational Science Institute
Cardiologist
Scripps Clinic
La Jolla, California

"To the layman, heart disease and sudden cardiac death can be very heavy and difficult topics to digest, but Dr Mak has taken on a light hearted approach and made it accessible to all. Prevention of heart disease starts with the basics of education, and the Singapore Heart Foundation is proud to support Dr Mak's new book on sudden cardiac death as a valuable resource, in carrying out the work that we do."

Vernon Kang
Chief Executive Officer
Singapore Heart Foundation

"Sudden cardiac death is responsible for nearly 20% of all deaths in developed countries. Although there is a plethora of books on sudden cardiac death targeted at doctors and nurses, there are only a handful of books, if any, on this subject for the general public. Therefore, Dr Mak should be congratulated for this book that provides valuable and practical information on this subject for the layperson. His book covers the major aspects of sudden death from cardiac causes including genetics and familial arrhythmic conditions and chronic cardiac conditions that put patients at risk of sudden death and means of prevention and treatment with drugs and devices. Identifying patients who are at risk of sudden death is not well covered but it should be noted that this is a complex area especially in the screening of young people participating in sports to prevent sudden cardiac death and is probably beyond the scope of this book. A major strength of this book is the recommendation of CPR training and encouragement of 'empowering the rescuer' with practical information on first aid in the treatment in cardiac arrest in the out-of-hospital setting. Dr Mak is the author of the highly successful '*Your Heart Matters: Answers to a Healthier Heart*' and this new book adds to the excellent work that he is doing in educating the public on important cardiovascular matters. I recommend this book strongly."

Professor Chim C. Lang
Professor of Cardiology
Medical Research Institute
Division of Cardiovascular and Diabetes Medicine
University of Dundee

"A clear, easy to understand book that comes with interesting anecdotes and illustrations. Recommended for anyone with an interest in health."

Chang Ai-Lien
Senior Correspondent
The Straits Times

"This is an excellent book and it should help to raise awareness in the local legal community of the need to look more closely into the real underlying cause in sudden death cases."

Lek Siang Pheng
Medico-legal lawyer
Partner
Rodyk & Davidson LLP

"Much has been changed in the field of cardiac arrhythmia and sudden cardiac death (SCD) since I did my 6-month cardiology rotation as a medical officer almost 30 years ago. Successful innovative catheter therapies and protective devices have been determinant in enhancing treatment and prevention strategies of individuals at risk. However, despite the advances, SCD still remains a major contributor to mortality in our society. While most deaths occur in adult cases are associated with ischemic heart disease, heart failure or have had a prior heart attack, occasionally the youngest and the fittest, even those who have become our role models for their athletic abilities may also die suddenly. Many of these young potential victims do not know they are at risk. When SCD claims their life during their most productive years, unprepared families become devastated. There is a real need for all lay publics to understand various causes of SCD and measures which could prevent these from happening. Those with known cardiac disease should make an effort to educate themselves on their risk for SCD. This book is very educational not only for lay publics but also for medical, nursing and allied health professionals who are not in the field of cardiology but want to learn more about SCD."

Professor Lim Shih Hui
Master, Academay of Medicine, Singapore
Senior Consultant
Neurology at SGH
National Neuroscience Institute

"Hearing of yet another case of sudden cardiac death in the news is always disturbing, but often little further information is available. This book reflects the enormous task undertaken by Dr Mak and his co-authors in distilling the most important information from the vast minefield of scientific literature on this topic and presenting it in a straightforward and easy-to-read format. There is also excellent advice on early detection, diagnosis, appropriate treatment and prevention. Both patients and health professionals will find this a useful and comprehensive reference."

Dr Hsu Li Fern
Cardiologist and Electrophysiologist
Novena Heart Centre
Visiting Consultant
National Heart Centre of Singapore

"As I read this book, I was amazed at the depth and wealth of information on the complex subject of sudden cardiac death SCD. The author initially approached the different aetiologies of SCD, with detailed analysis of the aetiology, prevalence, presentation (with some unusual presentation), recognition and diagnosis and treatment, with documentation of cases and case histories. It was the detailed and comprehensive coverage of the difficult subject that struck me most. The approach is interesting, as he likened the different conditions to something that can be more easily understood, the quotations are captivating, and the case histories were at times simply like reading a mystery thriller. As I continued to read, it gets more and more interesting, like reading a thriller. Part II on whether SCD can be prevented, continued in the same interesting vein, covering the role of screening, issues on physical activity and exercise, control of risk factors, certain foods and nutrients and medications, along an evidence-based approach. The different medications — betablockers, angiotensin converting enzyme inhibitors, angiotensin receptor blockers, aldosterone antagonists, statins and antiarrhythmics, were addressed. Other modalities, including cardiopulmonary resuscitation CPR training, defibrillators, the importance of time (in seconds) when SCD occurs, implantable defibrillators (who should receive them) and the practical aspect of living with ICD, ending on the new option of subcutaneous defibrillator. To cap it all, there were 926 references! Simply amazing!

This book is very informative, addressing the subject of SCD in a very interesting manner and certainly makes good reading and referencing. I wish to congratulate Dr Mak Koon-Hou for this outstanding book on the difficult subject of sudden cardiac death."

Tan Sri Dato' Seri Dr Robaayah Zambahari
PSM, DSA, PJN, SPMJ, SPMP, DPMS, DPMP, DSAP,
DIMP, DPCM, DPMK, DSNS, JSD, KMN
Senior Consultant Cardiologist & Head of Department
Institut Jantung Negara
Kuala Lumpur, Malaysia

"Sudden unexpected death syndrome (SUDS) is not a common condition. However, an unexpected death is not only a great tragedy to family and friends, but also equally a significant loss to society, especially if it occurs in young individuals. Doctors and the public naturally want to know how to recognize and treat the underlying causes, so that it can be prevented or at least delayed. Dr Mak Koon-Hou's book aims just to answer these two important questions.

The book is divided into two major parts. Part one deals with the epidemiology, diagnosis and descriptions of the underlying aetiology, including most of the causes of sudden cardiac death (SCD) and other important non-cardiac causes such as intracranial haemorrage and epilepsy. These are described in great details covering prevalence, clinical presentation, modalities of investigation and risk stratification. Part two deals with preventive measures and treatment strategies largely on coronary artery disease, which is the most common cause of SCD in older individuals. No effort is spared in the exposition of the role of diet, exercise, medications and various devices to prevent SCD. Emphasis is also given to hypertrophic cardiomyopathy, which is the most common cause of SCD in younger individuals. Important practical advice is given to individuals after preventive treatments such as insertion of pacemaker and intracardiac defibrillator."

"This book is well written primarily for general readership. However, the contents are comprehensiveand references full-bodied and up to date to rival scientific text for the medical profession. This reviewer, as a paediatric cardiologist dealing with problems of SUDS in children and adolescents, finds it educational and a joy to read, especially the historical records of discovery of diseases, drugs and devices and relevant case history of patients. I strongly recommend this valuable book to the public and doctors."

Professor William C.L. Yip
Adjunct Professor,
National University of Singapore

Visiting Consultant,
National University Hospital

Consultant Paediatric Cardiologist,
Gleneagles Hospital

"This is certainly not your run of the mill medical textbook. Dr Mak's painstaking research gives us a glimpse of the rare and unusual in medicine. An interesting read for the layman and a useful reference for doctors."

Salma Khalik
Senior Health Correspondent
The Straits Times

"Sudden cardiac death has been in the spotlight of public interest for many years. It is timely that the myths and fears about this condition are explained to the public. Dr Mak's latest book is a well-researched and comprehensive, yet highly readable and enlightening account of this important medical challenge. Filled with brief vignettes which bring to life the personal impact of sudden cardiac death, coupled with detailed explanations of their underlying causes, it is suitable for any layman who is keen to understand more about sudden death, as well as medical professionals. A highly recommended book for anyone with an interest in this area, as well as doctors who need to update themselves."

Professor Terrance Chua
Medical Director
National Heart Centre of Singapore
Chairman, Board of Directors
Singapore Heart Foundation

"Dr Mak is a renowned cardiologist and has previously written several books. This is yet another one which is written with excellent expertise, inundated with appropriate quotes and wise advices. The first part of the book is on both common and less common but nevertheless important causes of sudden death, while the second section deals with ways of prevention. The entire book is well-referenced, reflecting Dr Mak's high academic standards. At the same time, the anecdotal stories will certainly touch the heart of all readers. They come from his huge volume of clinical experiences. This is a book which can keep me awake all night long, at the edge of my bed, reading and enjoying every part of it. I strongly recommend it for both professionals and the public."

Associate Professor Poh Kian Keong
President, Singapore Cardiac Society
Editor-in-Chief, Singapore Medical Journal
Senior Consultant
Cardiac Department
National University Hospital

"Dr Mak Koon-Hou's stories of sudden death offer many perspectives covering the multiple aetiologies, presentations, preventive measures and treatments that have been used over the ages. These perspectives are not told as cold scientific information, but presented as interesting anecdotes that hold the attention of the reader who yearns for the next story and the next and so on. It is also a history of the development of the understanding of the art and science of sudden death. For practitioners of emergency cardiac care, this should offer an opportunity for a reflective insight into so many of these perspectives.

While the examples and statistics provided by Koon-Hou are principally from the American, European and larger Asian societies, the stories are equally relevant to Singapore. The examples quoted by Koon-Hou should serve as a stimulus to interested readers to understand better the local perspectives for sudden cardiac death and create the environment that would be optimal for the prevention of SCD, where possible, the risk reduction of this condition, where feasible and treatment as prompt as possible.

This production should challenge our practitioners into considering the various perspectives of sudden cardiac death and lead to earlier identification of causes and better outcomes for those who encounter sudden cardiac death."

Professor V. Anantharaman

Chairman, National Resuscitation Council, Singapore

Senior Consultant, Department of Emergency Medicine, Singapore General Hospital

Clinical Professor, National University of Singapore

Adjunct Professor, Duke-NUS Graduate Medical School

Dedication

This book is dedicated to my wife, Li-Hwei, and children, Joshua and Esther, for their love, support and patience.

About the Author

Dr Koon-Hou Mak is a cardiologist with clinical interest in interventional cardiology. He has published extensively in several top-tier cadiology and medical journals. Dr Mak is a member of the International Editorial Board of the *European Heart Journal* for more than 10 years. Currently, he is in private practice at Gleneagles Medical Centre. Dr Mak is actively involved in educating the public on heart diseases by speaking in symposia, on the radio and television. For more than 10 years, he has served as Director of the Singapore Heart Foundation and has launched the "Healthier Choice" symbol. He has also written a well-received book, *Your Heart Matters*, which has been translated to Bahasa Indonesian. Due to its popular demand, an expanded and updated version was published.

Preface by ESM Goh Chok Tong

Emeritus Senior Minister
Singapore

Sudden Cardiac Death (SCD) is becoming increasingly common in Singapore society; it can happen to seemingly healthy people. Thankfully, we are not powerless, and can do something about it. We can start by developing greater awareness of this health issue and by educating ourselves.

With better knowledge, we will be better prepared and equipped to deal with SCD when it happens. We may even be able to prevent it from occurring, through routine check-ups, and lifestyle changes.

Dr Mak Koon-Hou's book fills an important gap for the layman and will help him attain better heart health. I congratulate Dr Mak for his contribution to the community on this important subject, and recommend the book for its easy read and practical usefulness.

GOH CHOK TONG
Emeritus Senior Minister
Republic of Singapore

Preface

During one of my medical meetings in Europe, I visited the Städel Museum in Frankfurt, Germany, and saw a sculpture entitled "The Kiss of the Sphinx" (Figure 1). It was created by Christian Behrens in 1879 and is owned by the Letter Foundation in Cologne. This figurine captures the essence of sudden death. The unsuspecting victim holds onto his 7-string lyre while a winged creature grasps his chest and, with its sharp claws, pierces his heart. In doing so, the creature sucks out the essence of life.

Certainly, the syndrome of sudden death is not new. However, we may not be familiar with the Parable of the Rich Fool in the Bible (Luke 12:13-21). It is about a wealthy man who was proud of his possessions and boasted about his plan to expand his warehouse. In the meantime, he just wanted to "… relax, eat, drink, be merry."[1] Although the morale of this story was not to measure one's worth according to worldly riches, this man faced an unexpected outcome. Shortly after, he died suddenly in the middle of the night. Besides spiritual truths, Jesus also expounded on one of the most common presentation of coronary artery disease — sudden death. Lack of physical activity, indulgence in food and alcohol, and a lack of a genuine purpose in life were the three key factors mentioned — "relax, eat, drink (and) be merry." This condition is more relevant in today's world of affluence. Over-eating and a relatively sedentary lifestyle predispose to several chronic illnesses, and in particular coronary heart disease. So it is not surprising that many of us have known someone who had died suddenly, especially an older person, because when we age, we will die eventually. But when it occurs in a younger individual, the event is sensationalised by the media. Young people are not supposed

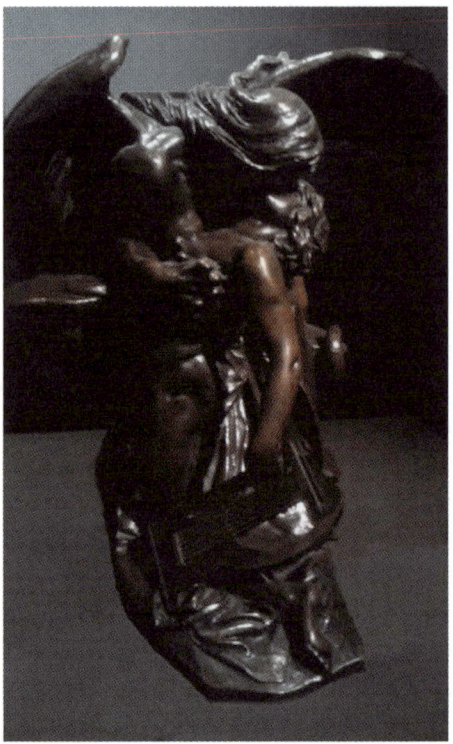

Figure 1.   The Kiss of the Sphinx.

The Kiss of the Sphinx was created by Christian Behrens (1852–1905) in 1879. It is a sculpture from era of "Schwarze Romantik" and is currently owned by the Letter Foundation in Cologne, Germany. The Foundation was established in 1993 and aims to promote art and culture. It collects, preserves and maintains the works of artists. Currently, the sculpture is housed in the Clemens-Sels-Musuem in Neuss, Germany.

to die and they should not die especially when they are doing exercises, something that we are taught to do as part of healthy living. Sudden death in the young is uncommon and when it happens, the event receives substantial news coverage. In today's world of social networking, the information generates wide ranging public responses and outcry regarding prevention and accountability.

While there are several other reasons for death, as a cardiologist, my patients frequently ask me if they or their children are at risk. Indeed, the shroud of ignorance on the subject instils much fear.

Fortunately, in the past several years, our knowledge on sudden death has increased substantially. However, we are unable to echo Sir Winston Churchill's words, "I always avoid prophesying beforehand because it is much better to prophesy after the event has already taken place." Although whatever we know is never sufficient, it provides a framework for each of us to work on. Time will further improve our understanding on the subject so that new courses can be charted.

Sudden death does not respect any person. I happened to be with a group of doctors and each started to share how the child of one of their colleagues died suddenly; from cardiomyopathy, myocarditis, and the list goes on. One of them walked away, remarking how the conversation has degenerated into a morbid discussion. As the public becomes more aware of the condition, it is timely to consolidate this information. If there are terms and procedures that are unfamiliar, my previous book, *Your Heart Matters,* will provide you with the basic concepts of heart diseases and the management. Although there are still several gaps in our understanding of this condition, I sincerely hope that this book is helpful. If you find the several statistics and references confusing, boring and distracting, skim over them first. Refer to them later.

I would like to thank ESM Goh Chok Tong, Professor Eric J. Topol, Professor Pedro Brugada, my friends and colleagues for their kind words. In particular, the editorial assistance by Mr Chua Hong Koon and Ms Darilyn Yap from World Scientific is greatly appreciated.

Koon-Hou Mak
Singapore

Foreword

How frequently do we hear someone lamenting: "He was such a healthy active young man... He did not smoke... He did not drink... He ate healthily and even exercised regularly... But he just died suddenly... Some of them died in their sleep... Others died while exercising...?" The cases that frequently appear in newspaper and social media headlines are those occurring during sporting events, which is even more puzzling and ironic. At that time, their deaths were shrouded in mystery. With limited information, these reports struggled in their attempt to clarify the situation. The public remained baffled and the medical community had to answer pertinent questions raised by concerned patients: How did they die? Why are the young dying suddenly? Who is at risk? Am I at risk?

Sudden death is a growing phenomenon in recent years. While the occurrence of sudden death is not new, its growing occurrence in younger individuals in recent years has instilled much fear in the general public. The trepidation is further fuelled by the lack of information. There is a real need for everyone to understand sudden death, and to dispel both misinformation and unwarranted apprehensions surrounding this condition.

In his latest book, Dr Mak covers extensively on the topic of sudden cardiac death from the various causes of sudden cardiac death — which includes genetics and familial rhythm disorder and chronic heart conditions. Several historical accounts and captivating anecdotes, which are used to illustrate less common diseases, will certainly help the general public recognize these diseases better. Written in lay language, the ways to treat these illnesses and prevent sudden death are discussed. I believe that this book is also beneficial for the medical, nursing and allied health professionals as well.

I highly commend Dr Mak for making such an important and substantial effort to educate us on this somewhat taboo subject. You will find a wealth of information solidly backed by scientific literature that has been translated to practical steps which could save a life!

Professor Eric J Topol
Director, Scripps Translational Science Institute
Chief Academic Officer, Scripps Heatlh
The Gary and Mary West Chair of Innovative Medicine
Professor of Genomics, The Scripps Research Institute
Editor-in-Chief
Medscape

Abbreviations

ACC	American College of Cardiology
ACE	Angiotensin converting enzyme
AHA	American Heart Association
ARVC	Arrhythmogenic right ventricular cardiomyopathy
BBC	British Broadcasting Corporation
CAST	Cardiac Arrhythmia Suppression Trial
CMR	Cardiac Magnetic Resonance
CPR	Cardiopulmonary Resuscitation
CRT	Cardiac resynchronization therapy
CRT-D	Cardiac resynchronization therapy with defibrillator
CRY	Cardiac Risk in the Young
DART	Diet And Reinfarction Trial
DHA	Docosahexaneoic acid
DNA	Deoxyribonucleic acid
ECG	Electrocardiogram
ECMO	Extracorporeal membrane oxygenation
EPA	Eicosapentaenoic acid
ESC	European Society of Cardiology
FDA	Food and Drug Administration
GISSI	Gruppo Italiano per lo Studio della Sopravivivenza nell'Infarto miocardico
GPS	Global Positioning System
HRS	Heart Rhythm Society
IABP	Intra-aortic Balloon Pumping
ICD	Intra-cardiac defibrillator
LDL	Low-density lipoprotein
LQTS	Long QT-interval Syndrome

MADIT-CRT	Multicenter Automatic Defibrillator Implantation Trial with Cardiac Resynchronisation Therapy
MRI	Magnetic Resonance Imaging
NYHA	New York Heart Association
PVC	Polyvinyl chloride
ROC	The Resuscitation Outcomes Consortium
SADS	Sudden arrhythmic death syndrome
SPECT	Single Photon Emission Computed Tomography
SUDEP	Sudden and unexpected death occurring in epilepsy
SUNDS	Sudden unexplained death syndrome
vs.	Versus
VTE	Venous thromboembolism
WHO	World Health Organization
WPW	Wolff-Parkinson-White

Contents

PART I

Introduction

It Just Did Not Happen Suddenly, or Did It?

"Νενικήκαμεν"
"We have won!"

Pheidippides, 490 BCE

Sudden death is supposed to occur suddenly: it is to have taken place unexpectedly and without warning; whereby heart function ceases abruptly resulting in death. The first thing that comes to our mind regarding sudden death is that the cause is a heart attack. While a heart attack (acute myocardial infarction) may result in sudden cardiac death, there are several other causes. Furthermore, the sudden onset is a matter for debate. Traditionally, the individual was previously well but died within an hour of onset of symptom.[2] When there are no witnesses, death occurring within 24 hours may also be considered sudden. Indeed, about 30% to 40% of cardiac arrest was unwitnessed.[3] Other known causes, such as multiple injuries due to a road traffic accident or suicide, should be excluded. But again, the issue of accidents is complicated. Did the driver or person have an acute medical event that caused the unfortunate incident? Or was it the "shock" of the accident that resulted in the death of the victim?

3

How Common is Sudden Death?

We often read or hear about people dying suddenly. In the United States, there are approximately 295,000 out-of-hospital cardiac arrests yearly.[4] Of note, sudden death accounted for approximately two-thirds of the total deaths from cardiovascular disease.[5] However, there was wide regional variation within the country, and the incidence of sudden death ranged from 180,000 to >450,000 yearly.[6] Such surveys have been conducted in several countries. Overall, the incidence of sudden death in the population ranges from 50 to 100 per 100,000.[3,4,7–9] As expected, the incidence of sudden death increases with age. For men, it was about 100 per 100,000 for 50 years old and 800 per 100,000 for 75 years old.[10] The rate of sudden death is generally lower for women, about 30% of that of men and lags behind by at least 10 years.[11] But this trend tends to reverse after the age of 65.[12] Most sudden cardiac arrests occur in the community and less than 5% to 10% survive even when they are attended to by emergency medical services.[4] Therefore, the occurrence of sudden death in various reports may be influenced by how each case is identified and counted.

Gender Differences

Although the causes of sudden death varies according to age and sex; overall, coronary artery disease is the most common cause, accounting for 80% among men and 45% among women.[13] In the United Kingdom, coronary artery disease accounted for 59% to 86% of sudden deaths.[14,15] So, sudden death does not only refer to heart attack although individuals with heart attack may die suddenly. In about 5% of them, a cause cannot be determined in some reports.[13,16,17] Similar to men, coronary risk factors contributed to sudden death in women.[18,19] However, about two-thirds of women do not have a known history of heart disease compared to half in men.[3,11,18] Furthermore, they were less likely to have previously known reduced left ventricular function or coronary artery disease.[19] These differences may account, at least in part, for the variation in temporal trends. In the United States, from 1989 to 1998, while the occurrence of sudden death increased by about 21% for women who were 35 to 44 years of age, it fell by 2.8% for men in the same age group.[20]

Incidence and outcomes following an out-of-hospital cardiac arrest event differed between the two sexes. From 1998 to 2007, the pattern of occurrence cardiac arrest for 15,701 men and 11,179 women was studied in the population of Osaka prefecture.[22] For girls whose age is 12 years or younger, the likelihood for an out-of-hospital event was three-quarters that of boys. Between the ages of 13 and 49 years, this risk further reduced to two-fifths. When they are 50 years or older, women were about half as likely as men to suffer from an out-of-hospital cardiac arrest event. Not only that, out-of-hospital events occurred less frequently among female and the chances for good neurological recovery was twice that of male between the ages of 13 and 49 years. The investigators attributed the favourable outcome among women with out-of-hospital cardiac arrest to the protective effect of oestrogens.

No Easy Answers

When considering those who died suddenly without previous illnesses, the causes of unexpected sudden death were different. In the United Kingdom, the proportion of unexplained sudden deaths was estimated to be 3.8% in 1988[14] and 4.1% in the 1990s,[15] despite intensive evaluation by three cardiac pathologists. In a later study involving all coroners in the United Kingdom, no abnormality was detected in the heart for 269 (59%) of 453 individuals who died suddenly during post-mortem examination.[21] A new name, sudden adult death syndrome, was coined. Since abnormal rhythm was the mechanism of death, it was re-named as sudden arrhythmic death syndrome (SADS). The potentially lethal rhythm disorder is largely due to abnormal proteins on the surfaces of the heart muscle that result in disturbances in electrical discharge.

In Times of Ages Past

Throughout history, sudden death has been recorded. More than 4,000 years ago, it has been found in the archives of ancient Egypt.[23] Ebers Papyrus (c. 1550 BC) recorded, "When thou examines a person with a suffering in his abdomen, he is ill in his arm, in his breasts, and in the stomach-region; and it is told him that it is the uat-illness ... then thou sayest: 'It is Death that has penentrated his mouth and take up its abode.'"[24] In China, when "an intermittent pulse" is detected, it is "a predictor of imminent death."[23] Even Hippocrates recognised that "intense chest pain that radiates to the clavicle (collar bone) and back is a sign of poor prognosis ... (and) ... obese individuals are more likely to die suddenly ..." Perhaps the most famous story of sudden death is based on the origins of the word "Marathon." After winning an exigent battle between the Persians and the Greeks, Pheidippides, a messenger ran about 26 miles (about 42 kilometres) from Marathon, the site of the fighting, to Athens to break news of the victory. On arrival, he announced "Νενικήκαμεν" (or "Nenikékamen", which may translate to "We have won") before collapsing and died (Figure 2). This was the story believed to mark the origin of this arduous event. But it was not so straight-forward.

It was in 492 BCE when Darius I, King of Persia, with a large military force — consisting of a fleet of 600 ships, was to invade Greece. During the journey, the fleet faced attacks and a sudden severe storm which wrecked half its fleet. Although weakened, the Persians attacked Greece initially in 490 BCE with 25,000 men and 600 triremes. King Darius chose the Bay of Marathon to be the place for landing because of a broad plain of a mile wide and six miles long, which would be suitable for the Persian cavalry. On the other hand, the Greeks being democratic, opinions were divided as to how the invading force should be dealt. But time was not on their side. So about 11,000 men from Athens and Platanos were hastily gathered and led by General Miltiades to face the Persians. Soon the Greeks realised that they were greatly outnumbered, Pheidippides was sent to Sparta to seek assistance. As much as they would like to, the Spartans were celebrating a

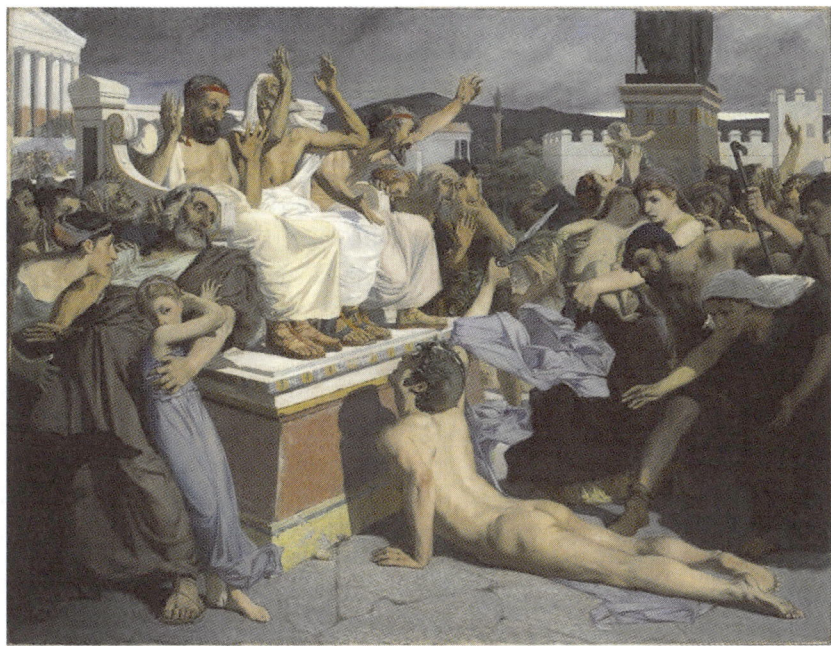

Figure 2. Le soldat de Marathon (The Soldier of Marathon) by *Luc-Olivier Merson, 1869.*

Pheidippides giving word of victory after the Battle of Marathon.
Photograph obtained from http://commons.wikimedia.org/wiki/File:Phidippides.jpg

religious festival and were unable to participate in that war. During the 9-day Karneia, military activites were suspended. So, Pheidippides ran back with the disappointing news in about 48 hours, and the entire trip was estimated to be 150 miles (about 241 kilometres). He then fought the battle valiantly in full armour. This event was thought to have taken place during the months of August or September, right in the heat of summer. After this exhausting battle, Pheidippides ran his final race, from Marathon to Athens (Figure 2).

Sudden Death in the Uniformed Services

Although death is not an uncommon occurrence during war, soldiers may also die during peacetime. Some of these unfortunate incidents were sudden. The uniformed services tend to keep excellent records of their personnel as part of their routine and accountability. In the United States Armed Forces, there were 6.3 million 18-year-old recruits undergoing intense military training for 8 weeks over a 25-year period.[25] There were 277 deaths that were not related to injuries. So, the estimated rate of occurrence of sudden death was 4.4 per 100,000 recruits. Another study was conducted by the United States Armed Forces on mortality trend from 1998 to 2008,[26] with a mean annual population of 1.39 ± 0.02 million, which provided additional insight into the causes of sudden death among relatively young adults. Over this period, 14,771 service personnel passed away. After excluding those who died from wars, homicides, accidents and illnesses, records for review was available for 902 of them. Only about 40% of the witnessed deaths (slightly more than two-thirds of all sudden deaths) were deemed to be associated with some form of exertion. Majority of them were engaged in recreational sporting activities, particularly running. Overall, an abnormality of the heart was detected in approximately 80% of this group of deceased soldiers. However of those who were younger than 35 years, more than 40% did not have any structural heart abnormalities. Indeed, the differing causes of sudden death among older and younger individuals have been documented by other researchers.[27,28] Generally, blockage of heart arteries (atherosclerotic heart disease) is the most common cause of sudden death for those older than 30 to 40 years. Although less than a third of them had symptoms, chest pain was the most frequent complaint, occurring a week prior to their demise. Regardless of age, about 56% of the soldiers who died from atherosclerotic heart disease were symptomatic.

Despite the limitations of these studies, the information provides guidance on the understanding and evaluation of patients. Among individuals older than 35 to 40 years, the principal strategy for the prevention of sudden unexpected death is to adopt a healthy lifestyle. This approach will reduce the likelihood of atherosclerotic heart disease, which is the major cause of sudden death in this group of individuals. Although sudden cardiac death is not always due to a heart attack, patients with a heart attack can certainly die suddenly. For younger individuals, congenital abnormalities and uncommon rhythm disorder have to be sought after. Although there are several structural heart conditions and electrical abnormalities that have been discovered as causes of sudden cardiac death, they are not always easy to detect. Also, there are still many more that we do not know and other challenges that we must face. We may be able to identify individuals who are at high risk of sudden cardiac death, most deaths have occurred among patients with lower risk.[29] While the occurrence of sudden death increases with age, the corresponding relative risk diminishes.[10] This public health paradox arises from the lack of specific markers in identifying the larger number of individuals who are at low risk and yet succumb to sudden cardiac death (Figure 3).[30]

In the Sporting Arena

In 1972, Dr Tom Bassler, a cardiologist and a member of the American Medical Joggers Associated claimed that there was not a "single ischemic heart disease death among marathon finishers of any age."[31] The naivety was short-lived and deaths among young sportspersons have been increasingly recognised. From 1 January 2000 to 31 May 2010, there were 10.9 million individuals who participated in marathon and half-marathon events.[32] Since there were 59 subjects with cardiac arrests, with mean age of 42 years, the overall incidence rate was 0.54 per 100,000 participants. Understandably the rate was higher among marathoners (1.01 per 100,000) than half-marathoners (0.27 per 100,000). Of these 59 cases, 47 (71%) died and so the rate of fatal cardiac arrest was 0.39 per 100,000 runners. When sudden death occurs in a young athlete, it generates substantial media attention. This is because participating in sports is supposed to be a healthy activity. Thus, the fact that the individual, especially those who are young, dies as a result of sports paricipation is devastating to both the family and society. Data have shown that young competitive athletes are 2.8 times more likely to suffer from sudden death than non-competitive individuals.[33]

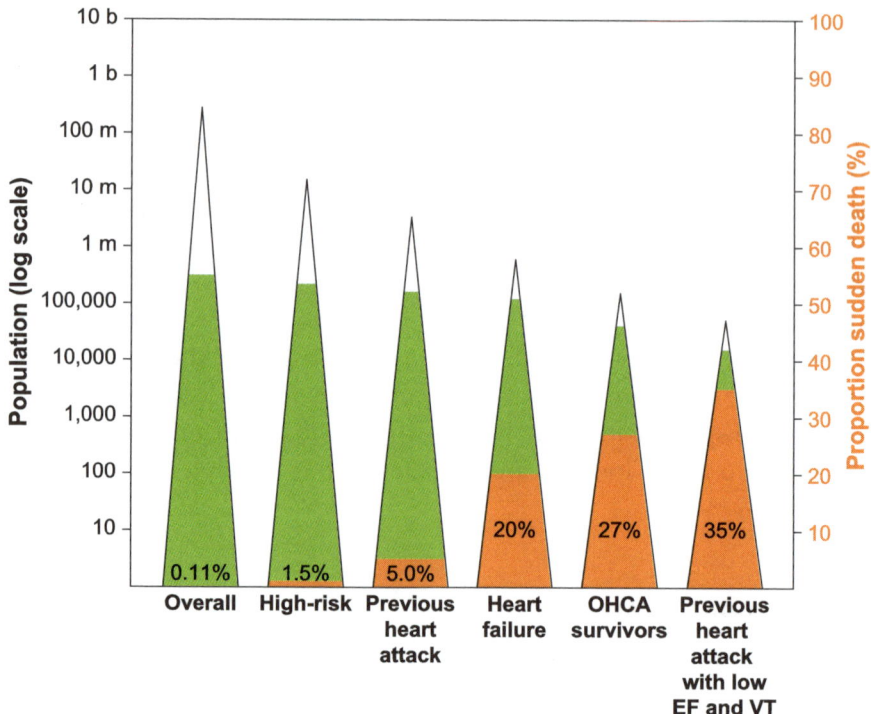

Figure 3.   The sudden death public health paradox.

m = million ($\times 10^6$); b = billion ($\times 10^9$); OHCA, out-of-hospital cardiac arrest; EF, ejection fraction; VT, ventricular tachycardia. The estimates for the rates of sudden death based on the risk of the population group. The first column represents the overall population of the United States (white). Although the risk for sudden death is about 0.1%, the absolute number is high (green). While the risk for sudden death was higher among individuals (red and the figure indicated in each triangle) with high-risk characteristics (~1.5%), the *absolute* number is considerably smaller because of the total number. This trend persists because of the smaller *absolute* number but are at *greater* risk for sudden death. So those with previous heart attack and abnormal heart rhythm has the *highest* risk for sudden death (~35%) but the absolute number was the lowest. (Adapted from Myerburg RJ, Mitrani R, Interian A Jr, Castellanos A. Interpretation of outcomes of antiarrhythmic clinical trials: design features and population impact. *Circulation* 1998; **97**:1514–1521).[30]

Realising this challenge, some of these conditions associated with sudden death are to be explained subsequently so that they may be recognised more readily and professional advice could be sought. In general, since coronary artery disease is a principal cause for sudden death, its associated risk factors such as high blood pressure, diabetes mellitus, high cholesterol level, cigarette smoking, obesity and physical inactivity should be addressed. Indeed, information on symptoms before an out-of-hospital cardiac arrest event was obtained from 1,042 individuals whose collapse of cardiac origin was witnessed by bystanders or emergency medical service provides in Osaka, Japan, from 2003 to 2004.[34] Of the 644 (62%) with symptoms, 259 (40%) of them presented several minutes before the collapse. The most common symptom is breathlessness followed by chest pain and then fainting. Therefore, a doctor should also be consulted when there are certain symptoms such as chest pain on physical exertion, fainting spells and palpitation, in particular when the heart is beating rapidly and is associated with giddiness.

The common causes of unexpected sudden death syndromes are continously being elucidated. Improvement in medical technologies has clarified our understanding of these conditions. In particular, there have been substantial advances in cardiovascular medicine in the past decade. Of these, the genetic basis for diseases has become an attractive approach in the clinical management of patients in modern medicine. Increasingly, associations have been discovered between certain medical conditions and various proteins which are linked to specific genes. In the context of unexpected sudden death, the quest to unravel defects in the various components of the heart and the related genes has broadened the horizon of genomic medicine. Genetic studies have helped to clarify several underlying mechanisms of disease and provide an additional tool to assist doctors in making diagnosis of the disease and scientists to develop new treatment modalities.

PART II

Sudden Unexpected Death Syndromes

Surprise! Happy ... Birthday?

Heart Attacks and ... Heart Attacks

"She smiled, and there it was again, that aching pressure in his chest. Love, or a heart attack. Kind of the same thing."

Somebody to Love
Kristan Higgins

In the United States, about 1 in 3 persons die from heart disease.[5] On the other hand, in Singapore, the ratio was about 1 in 4 in 2010.[35] Of the various types of heart disease, coronary heart disease has become the most common form of heart disease. This is due to narrowing of the blood vessel supplying the heart. Heart attack, or myocardial infarction, is the most dramatic of the range of presentations. It occurs when the blood vessel is blocked suddenly and completely. Heart attack carries a relatively high mortality rate and approximately 50% of the victims die suddenly, before reaching a healthcare facility.[36] What is even more surprising is that as many as half of the patients with their first heart attack did not have preceding symptoms.[37] In other words, the symptoms might have been ignored, at least initially, because the victim did not have prior experience. Naturally, this may lead to a delay in diagnosis and treatment,[38] and may also partly account for individuals who die suddenly without pre-existing symptoms. The suddenness and unexpectedness of the event adds to the drama and suspense of the

15

condition. Over a 10-year period in Israel, there were 130 persons who died suddenly between the ages of 20 to 40 years.[39] Coronary artery disease accounted for 46% of the deaths. However, there are several less commonly known conditions that cause heart attacks. These diseases are not always associated with the usual risk factors of heart attack, such as high blood pressure, diabetes mellitus, cigarette smoking and high cholesterol level.

Broken Walls and Obstructed Passages: Non-Atherosclerotic Coronary Occlusion

Saruman: If the wall is breached, Helm's Deep will fall.

The Two Towers,
The Lord of the Rings,
J.R.R. Tolkien

Sally Bee was a busy mother with three young children. While attending another child's birthday party with her 9-month-old baby, she felt sick and had severe crushing chest pain with shortness of breath and sweatiness. Her friends thought that Sally had a hyperventilation attack, brought her ice, water and a bag to breathe into. Nonetheless, an ambulance was summoned and brought her to the hospital. Tests were performed, including electrocardiography, and she was observed for a couple of hours. As heart attack in a 36-year-old woman was highly unlikely, not surprisingly, Sally was discharged home with medicines for indigestion. Although she felt better initially, the symptoms recurred a few days later. Their intensity was more severe than the first episode. Her husband called for an ambulance and brought her to the hospital. Despite the severity of the symptoms, Sally was left alone in a cubicle with a sense of impending doom. She felt like she was going to die and her breathing became laboured. Sally attributed the lack of attention to her young age, being a female without any of the traditional risk factors such as hypertension, diabetes mellitus, abnormally high cholesterol level or cigarette smoking. Further information regarding risk factors, tests and treatment may be obtained from my previous book, *Your Heart Matters* (Revised and Expanded Edition, Armour Publishing, 2011).

Highly unlikely but not impossible, it was a student nurse who stumbled into her cubicle and recognised the abnormality in her electrocardiogram. Subsequently, Sally was told by the doctors that she had suffered from a major heart attack. This triggered a series of events leading to a transfer to another hospital so that coronary angiography could be performed. She was found to have "spontaneous coronary artery dissection" which is a rare medical condition characterised by a tear in the vessel wall. The cause for the tear is unknown but blood leaks into the wall. This results in narrowing of the channel where blood flows and eventually obstructing it, leading to the heart attack. Miraculously, Sally survived and was discharged from the hospital two weeks later. Her recovery was slow but certain, largely driven by her will to live and positive attitude towards living.

In the Olmested County in Minnesota, the annual incidence of spontaneous coronary artery dissection was estimated to be 0.26 per 100,000 persons (0.33 for women and 0.18 for men).[40] Over a 32-year period, there were 87 cases and the majority (82%) were women. Although mortality was low in this series, recurrence occurred in 17% after about 4 years, and by 10 years, it was almost 30%. This is an uncommon condition and affects young women more frequently.

There are diseases that occur less frequently in the general population but tend to affect female more commonly, such as systemic lupus erythromatosus, Takayasu's disease and other autoimmune disorders. One such case was Lucy Low, who was celebrating her friend's birthday. She was happily dining and drinking with her friends at Boat Quay. Later in the night, Lucy developed chest pain and was brought to a public hospital. Not unlike Sally, the symptoms were considered to be less ominous than a middle-aged man with the same complaints, especially after partying and drinking. So, the diagnosis of a heart attack took a longer time because she is a young woman. In treating individuals with acute heart attack, time is of the essence. The key strategy is to re-open a blocked artery, usually with coronary angioplasty, as soon as possible. Therefore, the longer the duration to treatment, the greater the amount of damage to the heart muscle. Correspondingly, the outcome is poorer.[41] For Lucy, it was unfortunate that another 7 hours passed before the diagnosis was made. The delay has resulted in considerable damage to the heart. So, we must stay vigilant when evaluating a young woman with chest pain and not dismiss it summarily. The public health challenge today is how to make this a cost-efficient strategy.

Importantly, the risk of sudden death declines with time after a heart attack. The timing of sudden death or cardiac arrest was studied in a large clinical trial of 14,609 patients after a heart attack and impaired heart function.[42] As such, these patients were at increased risk because they either suffer from heart failure or reduced heart function, or both. The investigators found that the risk was highest in the first 30 days, about 1.4% per month, in particular, the first week. Subsequently, the risk fell rapidly and the risk was lowered to 0.14% per month after 2 years. However the study was conducted between 1998 and 2001, and the management of patients has improved substantially since then. Importantly, less than half of the patients were treated with medicines or coronary angioplasty to re-open the blocked vessel. Furthermore, the majority of the patients received clot-dissolving medicines instead of contemporary superior treatment with coronary angioplasty.[43] Understandably, outcomes have improved with current therapies and so the results of this study may not be entirely applicable today.

From Heart Attack to Heart Failure

Over the past decade, treatment for patients with heart attack has improved substantially. Correspondingly, the number of heart attack survivors has increased significantly. Like Lucy Low, the damaged heart has resulted in reduction of its pump function in some patients. These individuals may have heart failure, characterised by being tired easily, poor effort tolerance, ankle swelling and breathlessness. They are unable to do the things that they used to. When the heart pump is unable to meet the demands of the body for daily living, the patient is in heart failure.

The pump function is measured by several indices and the most common parameter used is the ejection fraction. It is expressed as a fraction, proportion or percentage. Briefly, ejection fraction is a measure of the volume of blood that is pumped out of the heart divided by the total volume of blood in the heart just before it contracts. Generally, a normal value is at least 50% or 0.5. The index can be measured by ultrasound (echocardiogram), nuclear methods, cardiac magnetic resonance (CMR) and cine left ventriculography. Several of these techniques look at the heart in two-dimension. But the heart is a three-dimensional object and mathematical formulae have to be applied to obtain the value. As such, the calculated value may vary with different modalities and observers. Although ejection fraction may not always correspond to symptoms of heart failure,[44] it has been shown to be a predictor for outcome after a heart attack.[45,46] Among patients with heart failure, for every 10% (or 0.1) fall in ejection fraction below 45%, all-cause mortality increased by 39%.[47]

To simplify the grading of severity of heart failure in a patient, the New York Heart Association (NYHA) functional classification is commonly used. This is based on the ability of the individual to perform daily activities, and ranges from I to IV[48] (Table) and is useful in guiding treatment and prognosis. In this classification, higher classes are associated with the lower the effort tolerance. When a patient is in NYHA class IV, breathlessness occurs even at rest.

Although the information provided by Table appears to be straight-forward, it is frequently a challenge to doctors to categorise patients as class II or class III in daily practice. Despite its limitation, the functional status is useful in determining the prognosis of a patient. Indeed, for every increase in the functional class, the risk of dying increases by about 1.6 times.[49] In addition, sudden death may

Table   New York Heart Association (NYHA) Classification of Heart Failure.

Class	Description
I	No limitation in daily activities. Ordinary activities do not cause undue fatigue, shortness of breath, palpitation or chest pain.
II	Slight limitation in daily activities. Comfortable at rest but ordinary activities result in fatigue, shortness of breath, palpitation or chest pain.
III	Marked limitation in daily activities. Comfortable at rest but less than ordinary activities results in fatigue, shortness of breath, palpitation or chest pain.
IV	Symptom at rest. Breathless at rest and discomfort is aggravated by any physical activity.

occur more frequently among patients with mild to moderate symptoms of heart failure. Pump failure may be the more common mode of death for those with more severe symptoms.[50] Importantly, several medicines that have been shown to improve survival among patients with heart failure also increase ejection fraction and achieve a better NYHA functional status.[51,52] Likely, these beneficial effects correspond to the reduction of death. Indeed, sudden death may account for as many as half of the patients with heart failure (either from heart attack or other causes) and low ejection fraction,[53] particularly among those who were in NYHA functional class II.[54]

However, using left ventricular ejection fraction as the key determinant for sudden death has not been consistently shown to be accurate.[55] Together with the somewhat subjective assessment of functional status, other techniques have been investigated if they are able to ascertain risk more accurately. One of the underlying mechanisms for generation of fatal abnormal heart rhythm is the electrical instability of the heart muscle after the electrical stimulations, which causes the heart muscle to contract.[56] These changes are reflected on *highly sensitive* (that is, not routine) surface electrocardiographic technique as T-wave alternans.[57] Thus, it is able to detect beat-to-beat variation of the amplitude of the T-wave. When reviewing various studies with different populations, the presence of T-wave alternans was associated with a four-fold greater risk of potentially fatal abnormal heart rhythm compared to those without T-wave alternans.[58] Nonetheless, the occurrence of seriously abnormal heart rhythm among patients without T-wave alternans was 3% over a 21-month period. When using this parameter alone, its predictive value may be comparable to other techniques, such as ejection fraction. But when used together with other determinants, T-wave alternans was able to provide a significantly better assessment in refining the risk for sudden death.

Different Origins, Dangerous Routes

"...*which way I ought to go from here?*" "*That depends on a good deal on where you want to get to,*" said the Cat.

Alice's Adventures in Wonderland
Lewis Carroll

Coronary artery can be blocked by mechanisms other than cholesterol plaques, dissection flap and clots. In 1992, a review of 150 consecutive Italians, 35 years and younger, who died suddenly, 16 cases (10.7%) were not related to the thickening of blood vessels.[59] Of the twelve with abnormalities of the coronary artery, the origin of three deceased was not from the usual position. All three died during exertion. Indeed, not everybody's coronary arteries arise from the same places and go through similar courses.

On Sunday, 4 December 2011, the Standard Chartered Marathon started at 6:30 am at the Sentosa Gateway in Singapore. It was a cool and cloudy morning. One of the participants, Malcolm Sng Wei Ren, completed the 21-kilometre run in 1 hour 53 minutes and 20 seconds. He was a first year student at the Singapore Management University and had completed his active National Service (a mandatory period for a young man to serve the government in the military, paramilitary or police services). Shortly after crossing the finish line at about 8:30 am, Malcolm collapsed. Despite deploying 26 doctors, 127 nurses, 820 first-aiders and 32 ambulances, he could not be saved. Malcolm died an hour later. Subsequently, he was found to have a malignant form of coronary artery anomaly which caused his death (Figure 4). Indeed, this group of abnormalities was the second most common cause of sudden death among young American athletes; accounting for about 17% of those who died suddenly.[60] In another review of 6.3 million 18-year-old recruits undergoing 8 weeks of intensive military training in the United States, there were 277 deaths that were not related to injuries.[25] Of these, anomalous coronary artery accounted for 21 (33%) of those who died. But in the general population, coronary artery anomalies account for only a small proportion of sudden deaths. Over a 10-year period, from 1976 to 1985, in Israel there were 162 individuals not older than 40 years who died suddenly.[39] But only one of the deaths (0.6%) was attributed to coronary artery anomaly. These data suggested that high-impact physical activity played a critical role in sudden death for this condition.

Coronary artery anomaly is a congenital condition in which the coronary artery does not originate from the normal position. In a prospective evaluation of 2,388 children and adolescents using echocardiography, the incidence of anomalous origin of coronary

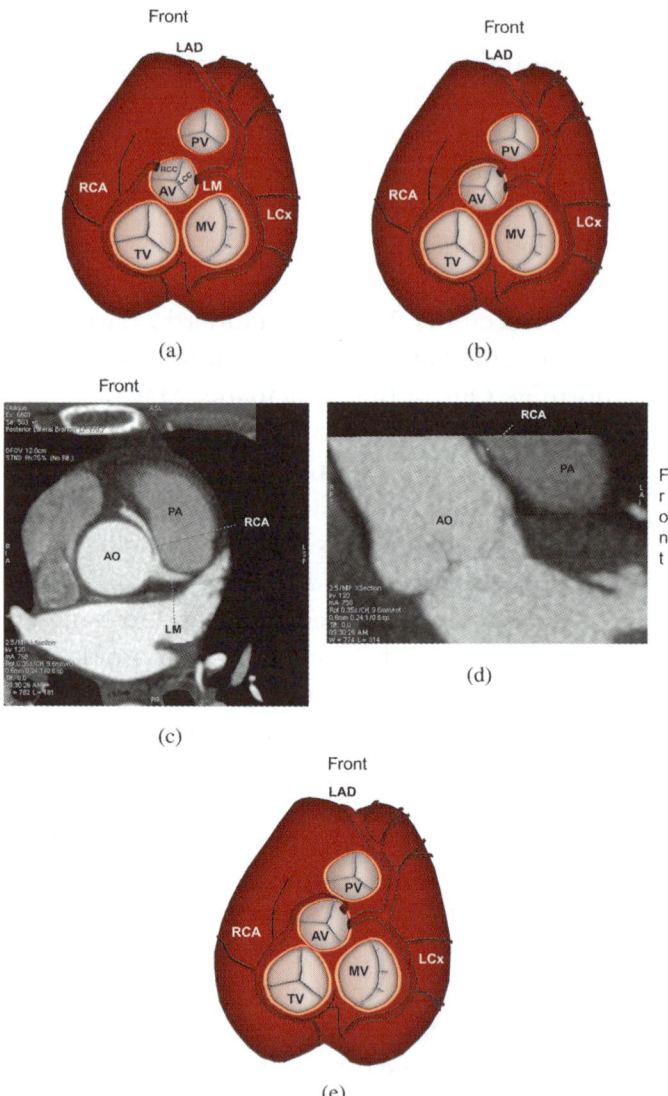

Figure 4.   Anomalous right coronary artery.

This is a cross-section of the heart showing the relationship between the pulmonary valve (PV), aortic valve (AV), mitral valve (MV) and tricuspid valve (TV). The normal position of the coronary arteries is shown in panel A. After the left main (LM) trunk originates from the left coronary cusp (LCC), it divides into the left anterior descending artery (LAD), which runs at the front of the heart, and the left circumflex artery (LCx), which curves around to the back of the heart. The right coronary arteries was 0.17%.[61] However, in an earlier post-mortem study, the rate was estimated to be about 2.85 per 1,000 in Los Angeles County in the United States over a 10-year period.[62] This diagnosis accounted for 5% to 35% of sudden cardiac death among adolescents.[63] In the malignant form, the course of the vessel traverses between the major blood vessels, as in the case of Malcolm. The right coronary artery originates from the left coronary cusp and runs between the aorta and pulmonary artery to continue with the usual course. During physical exertion, flow increases and the major blood vessels expands correspondingly. One of the causes for sudden death in this condition is believed to be the expansion of major vessels, which compress on the coronary artery causing lack of blood sup-ply.[64] In severe instances, particularly when the channel is slit-like and maybe occluded when the heart contracts,[65,66] resulting in a heart attack or abnormal heart rhythm.[65–67] Another feature which is associated with increased risk for sudden death is when the artery enters and traverses within the heart muscle, instead of running on the surface of the heart.[68] With the advent of more sophisticated imaging techniques, intravascular ultrasonic examination provided new insight to the functional abnormality.[69] Intravascular ultrasonic examination is a procedure performed to examine the blood vessel from the channel. A small device that emits ultrasonic waves is inserted into the coronary artery and the structure of the vessel can be visualised. As such, it is able to provide more information than coronary angiography which only shows the channel. Intravascular ultrasound examination not only shows that the vessel does not originate from its usual site, it is under-developed. These changes are likely to account for the lack of blood supply. However, resting and stress

---

Figure 4. (*Continued*) artery (RCA) originates from the right coronary cusp (RCC). In the case of anomalous right coronary artery, the vessel originates from the left coronary cusp. It traverses between the two great vessels (pulmonary artery (PA) and aorta (AO)) before continuing in its usual course (Panel B). Computed tomographic coronary angiography shows in the cross-sectional view of the anomalous right coronary artery (Panel C). In the long section view, the lumen (channel) of the right coronary artery is ovoid or slit-like in shape instead of circular in shape. During exercise, blood flow increases and the great vessels expand. It compresses on the right coronary artery and obstructs blood flow (Panel E).

electrocardiography were not sensitive to identify these abnorma-
lies[61,70] and only about 22% of them have abnormal functional testing.[70] There are several other variants of coronary artery anomaly.[62]

Redundant Bridges and Treacherous Tunnels

Willy Wonka:	There's no earthly way of knowing
	Which direction they are going…
	There's no knowing where they're rowing…
Mr. Salt [*weakly echoing*]:	Rowing…
Willy Wonka:	Or which way the river's flowing…
	Is it raining, is it snowing?
	Is a hurricane a-blowing?
[*sharp gasp*]	
Willy Wonka:	Not a speck of light is showing
	So the danger must be growing…
	Are the fires of Hell a-glowing?
	Is the grisly Reaper mowing?
	Yes! The danger must be growing
	'Cause the rowers keep on rowing
[*practically screaming*]	
Willy Wonka:	And they're certainly not showing
	Any sign that they are slowing!

[*lets out a high-pitched, almost unearthly scream*]

> The Psychedelic Boat Trip in the Tunnel of Hell
> Willy Wonka and the Chocolate Factory (1971)
> Adapted from Charlie and the Chocolate Factory
> by Ronad Dahl (1964)

Although there are variations, coronary arteries generally run on
certain fixed routes on the surface of the heart. In 1737, Heinrich
Reyman described a heart with the coronary artery tunnelling in
and out of the heart muscle,[71] a condition known as myocardial
bridging. When the vessel traverses through the heart muscle,

during contraction, the channel whereby blood flows is narrowed. This phenomenon is also known at the "milking" effect. But unlike other organs, blood flows to the heart mainly when the heart relaxes. Therefore, the reduction in flow during contraction does not generally give rise to symptoms. Interest in this condition increased gradually following the publication of autopsy findings in 100 patients in 1951.[72] On average, myocardial bridging is found in about a third of individuals during post-mortem examination.[73] Indeed, sudden death among patients with myocardial bridging occurred during physical activities.[74] However, not all these sudden death incidents were associated with sports. In a study on 16 young Italians who died suddenly from causes not related to thickening of coronary arteries,[59] myocardial bridging was the only anomaly detected in six of the deceased (Figure 5). It occurred during exertion in two and during rest in three victims. One subject, a 19-year-old girl died in her sleep. The risk of heart attack was greater when the buried segment is deeper, longer and located at its beginning.[75] Interestingly, thickening of blood vessels (atherosclerosis) generally do not occur in the embedded artery. On the other hand, the part of the vessel before myocardial bridge is prone to thickening.[76] Nonetheless, the majority of the patients with myocardial bridging have a benign course.[73] With the advent of multi-detector computed tomographic coronary angiography, myocardial bridging is increasingly detected in individuals with little or no symptoms.[77]

Over a 5-year period, 5,250 patients undergoing coronary angiography in the Montreal Heart Institute, 27 (0.5%) were found to have an intra-myocardial course.[78] Of the eleven studied, five patients had narrowing greater than 75% during ventricular contraction. When heart rate increased, there was significant change in the electrocardiogram and changes in blood biochemistry indicating lack of oxygen supply in four of these individuals (80%). During the test, three patients also had chest pain. On the other hand, the narrowing was between 50% to 75% in four patients. When the heart rate was increased, electrocardiographic change, but without biochemical perturbation, was detected in two individuals (50%). Both patients with narrowing of less than 50% did not have any of

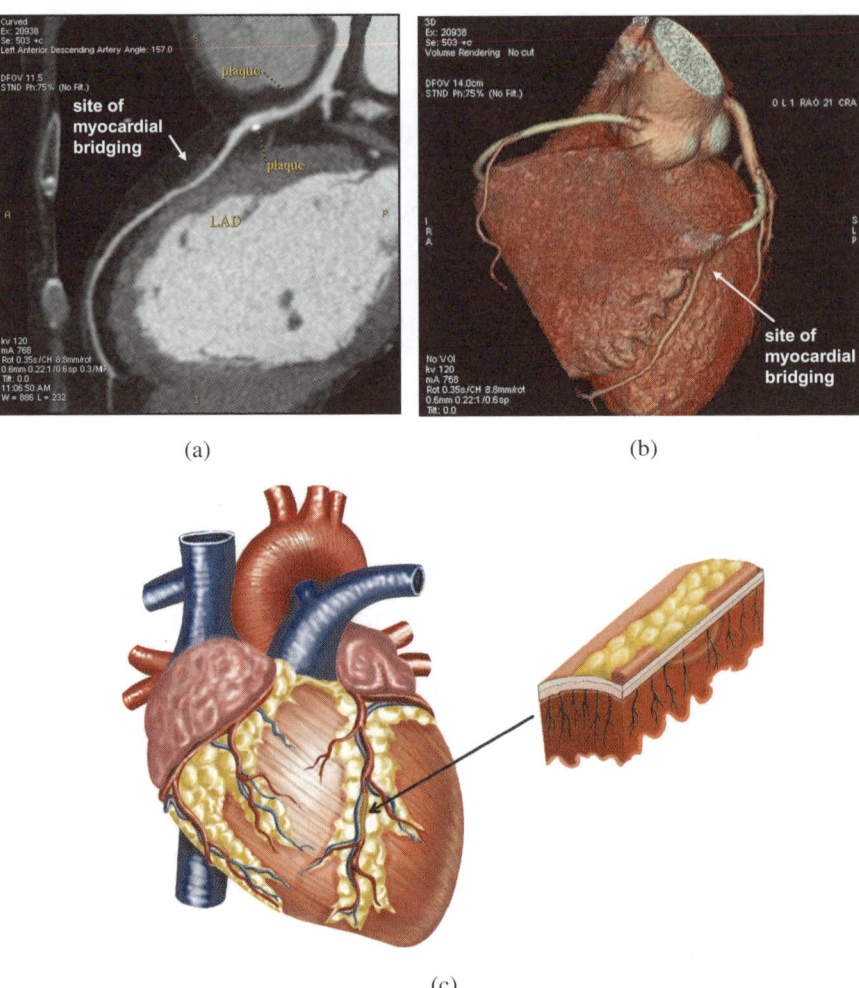

(a)   (b)

(c)

Figure 5. Myocardial bridging.

The blood vessel usually runs on the surface of the heart. In myocardial bridging, the blood vessel dives into the muscle and then re-surfaces to the surface. The white arrow shows the site of the myocardial bridging of the left anterior descending artery (LAD) in the computed tomographic coronary angiography (Panel A) and the reconstructed three-dimensional image (Panel B). There are calcific and non-calcific atherosclerotic plaques before the site of bridging. Panel C shows the illustrated course of the artery. If the course within the muscle is long and deep, the vessel may be "squeezed" when the heart contracts.

these abnormalities. A 48-year-old woman, who exercised regularly, suffered from a heart attack while driving.[79] The only abnormality detected was myocardial bridging. For those with life-threatening rhythm disorder, fainting spells and prolonged uncontrolled symptoms, surgery to "de-roof" or "de-bridge" the intra-myocardial course or bypass procedure may be performed.[80] Although the initial results of coronary stenting was promising,[81] subsequent reports found that its efficacy was limited.[82,83]

A Peculiar Chamber

Thickened Heart Muscle Walls: Hypertrophic Cardiomyopathy

"Just when I think I have learned the way to live, life changes ... "

Hugh Prather
Author, minister and counsellor

He was in a strange room with solid reinforced walls. The cold unfriendly surfaces generated a disquiet and vertiginous sensation. For reasons unknown, the thickened wall protruded into the exit. After being blocked from leaving thrice, his call finally came. Suddenly, the obstruction was cleared. Filled with joy, the 18-year-old left the bright waiting room and entered into eternal peace. "Welcome home, Ben! Welcome!"

His family had been busy getting Christmas dinner ready. After one of the most severe summers with extended period of high temperature and drought in Texas, a record number of more than a million acres was consumed by wildfire in 2011. The wet winter, and even snow, was to bring much cheer and relief to the drained-out heat-exhausted Texans. Ben Breedlove had just opened his Christmas present. An avid contributor to YouTube, with two popular channels, "OurAdvice4You" and the upgraded version, "BreedloveTV", he received a video recorder. Rushing outdoors to try his new equipment in a particularly cold day, he felt unwell suddenly.

29

Ben became breathless and light-headed. So, he went back to the house and lay down on the couch ... but never woke up.

Barely a week earlier, initially known only to his sister, Ally, he posted a candid and moving two-part clip on his illness and described how he had cheated death three times. Like an old silent movie, Ben told his story using hand-written cards with soothing music playing in the background. Unlike any other waiting room with walls filled with impatient people, it was painted white and without walls. With nothing to hold him back, he could move freely. As Ben described the unforgettable peace, he gave his characteristic haunting smile. The first episode occurred when Ben suffered from a seizure at the age of four years and he "... will NEVER forget that feeling or that day." Since then, his journey with hypertrophic cardiomyopathy began. But just as he and everyone else have gotten used to his heart disorder, everything changed.

Characterisation of Hypertrophic Cardiomyopathy

This condition is characterized by thickening of the heart muscle without a known cause; others have called it "chunky heart muscle" disease (Figure 6).[84] It is believed to be the most common illness for sudden death in young people. Other causes of thickened heart muscle include long-standing high blood pressure. The distribution of the thickening tend to be generalized in the left ventricle (the main pump of the heart) among patients with hypertension. Nonetheless, about 10% to 15% of them may have uniform thickening of the heart muscle.[85] However, in hypertrophic cardiomyopathy, the thickening is usually non-uniformed and should be at least 15 mm (the normal left ventricular wall thickness is generally less than 11 mm). However, when the thickness is between 13 mm and 14 mm, the condition is uncertain or borderline and diagnosis can only be made when there are other compelling reasons, such as family members with hypertrophic cardiomyopathy.[86] Among these indeterminate cases, transoesophageal or contrast echocardiography may be useful in establishing the diagnosis.[87] During

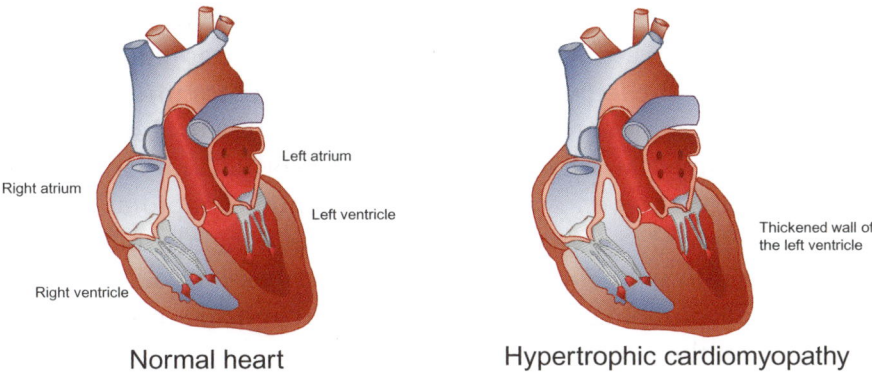

Normal heart   Hypertrophic cardiomyopathy

Figure 6. Hypertrophic cardiomyopathy.

The normal heart consists of four chambers, the right atrium and ventricle and the left atrium and ventricle. Of these, the left ventricle is the pump that propels blood out of the heart to most parts of the body. In hypertrophic cardiomyopathy, the wall is thickened. The site that is frequently affected is the wall between the left and right ventricle. In some cases, the thickened muscle may protrude and obstruct the outflow of the left ventricle. In other patients, the muscle at the tip of the left ventricle may be thickened.

transoesophageal echocardiography, a tube is inserted into the oesophagus (gullet) and stomach to look at the heart. Without the need to penetrate the chest wall, the images obtained are clearer. Newer techniques using cardiac magnetic resonance can provide better imaging quality, especially among those who are less echogenic (ultrasonic waves are not well-transmitted in about 10% to 15% of individuals).[87] It identifies the condition in a minority of patients that echocardiography failed to recognize.[88] With better spatial resolution, cardiac magnetic resonance is likely to determine the presence, severity and extent of hypertrophy more accurately than echocardiogram. However, imaging protocols are more complex and the staff employed to perform this procedure have to be experienced and well-trained. The wall between the two chambers, also called the septum, is the area that is commonly involved.[86] On the other hand, thickening at the apex (tip) of the heart occurs not infrequently (<2% in the Western world).[85] In Japan, and probably other East Asian countries as well, the prevalence of this form of api-cal hypertrophic cardiomyopathy is estimated to be as high as 25%.[89] Other parts of the left ventricle and even the right ventricle may be affected.[90] In addition to thicker muscle, the fibres are also disorgan-ized or arranged in a haphazard manner. Not uncommonly, there may be scarring, even among patients without symptom.[91] These changes can lead to abnormal and sometimes lethal rhythms, which are believed to be the principal cause for a person to die suddenly. The overall pumping function of the heart remains normal until late stage of the condition.[92]

Underlying genetic and structural abnormalities

These changes associated with hypertrophic cardiomyopathy are the result of a gene mutation affecting the various components of the muscle fibre. It is known as the "disease of the sarcomere."[92] The sar-comere is the building block of the contractile component of the muscle cell. Mutation is an alteration of the genetic code which may result in formation of an abnormal protein belonging to a particular part of the sarcomere, and its function may be affected. There are more than 1,400 mutations affecting more than 10 genes in at least 4 chromosomes, which may account for the diversity of presentation[87] and outcome.[85] Although hypertrophic cardiomyopathy is inherited in an autosomal dominant fashion, gene penetrance is variable. When a condition is transmitted in an autosomal dominant manner, it means that the gene may be passed down by one of the parents. Hence, 50% of the siblings and children will suffer from the disease. However, the expression of the gene (penetrance) is incomplete, so the proportion with hypertrophic cardiomyopathy is lower. Likely, the influence of other factors such as exercise, hypertension and other genes[94] could have an impact on the manifestation. Furthermore, there is spontaneous mutation which may account for the reduced likelihood of discovering the disease in other members of the family. About 5% of patients with hypertrophic cardiomyopathy have more than one mutation.[95] So, genetic testing can be useful in determining the type of mutation and counselling.[87] It is also useful in screening first-degree relatives for hypertrophic cardiomyopathy. Since not all mutation cause disease, care has to be exercised when interpreting the results of genetic testing. However, in many instances, a clinical diagnosis is made. The clinical context and results of various imaging techniques have to be taken into consideration.

The Young and the Old

Lisa Salberg is the founder and chief executive officer of the Hypertrophic Cardiomyopathy Association based in the United States. Since the age of 12, she was found to suffer from this condition. Several of her relatives have died from hypertrophic cardiomyopathy (http://www.4hcm.org/hcma-the-organization/about-the-hcma/3084.html, accessed 1 May 2012). However, Lisa continues to live an active life, helping others with the disease and establishing programmes to prevent sudden cardiac death. Diagnosis of hypertrophic cardiomyopathy can also be made in an elderly person. Bernyce was 79 years old when she was found to have hypertrophic cardiomyopathy. Although Bernyce had palpitation in her fifties, she became short of breath at the age of about 72 years. She visited various doctors and several tests were performed in the next five years before establishing the diagnosis. Thus, the condition may be detected from infancy to the elderly and is heterogenous.[96] The majority would have normal lifespan without need for medications or major therapeutic procedures. Infrequently, hypertrophic cardiomyopathy may be associated with congenital syndromes, inherited metabolic disorders and neuromuscular diseases.[97] So when it is discovered in a young individual, the doctor may need to look out for these other conditions. On the other hand, in a child diagnosed with these diseases, hypertrophic cardiomyopathy may need to be excluded.

Not an Uncommon Condition

The prevalence of hypertrophic cardiomyopathy is estimated to be 1 in 500 globally.[98] Since there are about 5 million people in Singapore in 2014, approximately 10,000 persons would be suffering from this condition. This condition is the most frequent cause of sudden death among young athletes.[33,99] However, the prevalence of hypertrophic cardiomyopathy was lower than among competitive sportspersons. In a study of 3,500 elite British athletes, there were only three with hypertrophic cardiomyopathy.[100] This figure translated to approximately 1 in 1,200. Earlier, hypertrophic cardiomyopathy was estimated to occur in about 1 in 1,500 competitive athletes in Italy.[33] Since these individuals displayed excellent physical performance, those with pre-existing heart diseases were unlikely to qualify to be part of this group of competitive sportsperson. Therefore, it was not surprising that hypertrophic cardiomyopathy occurred less frequently. But there are important ethnic differences in the incidence of the condition. In the United States, a multi-ethnic country, African Americans made up only about 12.7% of the population in 2001 (http://www.census. gov/popest/data/historical/2000s/vintage_2001/index.html, accessed on 21 January 2014). But young African Americans accounted for approximately 50% of deaths among young athletes because of hypertrophic cardiomyopathy.[99,101]

Patient Outcomes

Similar to several medical conditions, the outcomes of patients with hypertrophic cardiomyopathy vary considerably and Ben's case was unique. The age of onset and severity of symptoms vary considerably. Shortness of breath or chest pain on exertion, palpitation, lightheadedness and fainting spells are the most common symptoms experienced by patients with hypertrophic cardiomyopathy. On the other hand, several individuals do not have symptoms and continue to live normal lives. Yet, the clinical course can be unpredictable and hypertrophic cardiomyopathy is widely known to be the principal cause of sudden death for young sportsperson and army recruits. The publicity and attention given to this condition has generated much anxiety and fear to patients and their close relatives. Early information from specialised centres suggested the annual mortality to be as high as 6% annually, ranging from 0.7% to 11%.[85]

Subsequent studies derived from population showed that the rate was less than 1% a year.[102]

Cardiac Abnormalities in Hypertrophic Cardiomyopathy

There are several complex inter-related mechanisms that are responsible for abnormal heart function found in hypertrophic cardiomyopathy. Obstruction at the outlet of the left ventricle, caused by localised thickening of the muscle, is the initial pathognomonic description of the disease.[103] With the narrowing passage, the anterior leaflet of the mitral valve leaflet may be pulled towards the aortic valve, increasing the degree of obstruction. This typical finding can be observed in an ultrasonic examination, otherwise known as echocardiography.[104] In addition to determining the site and the degree of thickness, the pressure gradient across the obstruction can be ascertained. About 40% of patients have significant obstruction at rest (instantaneous peak gradient >30 mmHg).[105] After exercising, the pressure gradient became significant in more than 50% who did not have obstruction at rest. Other routine measurements such as heart and valve function are also obtained.

The thickened muscle may be stiff and may not relax easily. Nowadays, there are complex echocardiographic techniques that can be used to determine the relaxation pattern of the heart more accurately.[106] The filling of the heart chambers may be impaired, which may lead to inadequate output. Consequently, the patient may have shortness of breath, chest discomfort or giddiness, even without obstruction at the left ventricular outflow tract. Blood supply to the heart may be compromised because the muscle is thickened, even without the narrowing of the arteries[107] (demand exceeds supply). As such, patients may complain of chest discomfort with physical or mental exertion, angina-like symptom. When blood is flowing across the obstruction, it disrupts the laminar flow pattern leading to distortion of the mitral valve apparatus resulting in leakage of the valve.[108] Sometimes, the left heart chamber may enlarge and the wall contraction weakens.[109] The patient may then develop heart failure.

Screening of Family Members

Hypertrophic cardiomyopathy is an inheritable disease. When an individual is found to have hypertrophic cardiomyopathy, screening is recommended for first-degree relatives; i.e., siblings, parents and children. However, abnormalities of the heart take time to develop and genetic testing may provide some guidance. So these changes may not be seen in a young person. In an asymptomatic child (<12 years of age), imaging of the heart is not routinely performed unless a family member dies suddenly or has suffered from a serious complication from hypertrophic cardiomyopathy. Screening may be performed if the child is undergoing intensive training for competitive sports.[110] On the other hand, adolescents from the ages of 12 to 18 or 21 years, screening may be carried out every 12 to 18 months. For adults, screening may be performed every 5 years unless symptom develops or the affected individual had a severe course. Besides imaging to help establish the diagnosis, ambulatory electrocardiography may be useful in detecting[87] and ruling out abnormal heart rhythm.[111] A fall in systolic blood pressure during stress electrocardiography was observed in 20% to 40% of patients with hypertrophic cardiomyopathy and was associated with a poorer outcome.[112,113]

Patient Management

Management of patients with hypertrophic cardiomyopathy depends on the presence of symptoms, severity of mechanical dysfunction (obstruction or back-flow of the mitral valve) and left ventricular systolic function (pumping action of the heart).[87] While medication is not needed in several of these patients, some medicines should be avoided because they may make the dysfunction more pronounced. For those with symptoms, beta-blockers are generally the drug of choice. But if patients do not respond to this group of medicines or that there are contraindications, rate-limiting calcium channel blockers may be used instead. Other medicines may be useful and surgical procedures such as myectomy, septal ablation and possibly dual-chamber pacing may be performed to alleviate symptoms when medical treatment fails. The thickened muscle that protrudes into the left ventricular cavity causing obstruction to blood flow and symptoms is cut-off surgically. This operation is known as surgical myectomy.[114] Sometimes, the mitral valve may need to be repaired or replaced. Alcohol septal ablation, introduced in 1994, is a percutaneous catheter-based technique that is used to induce a "controlled heart attack" at the thickened muscle.[115] A small tube is placed into the branch of the coronary artery supplying the thickened heart muscle. Subsequently, a balloon is inserted and alcohol is injected to induce the heart attack. However, in the long-term, the procedure may be more suitable for individuals older than 65 years initially.[116] But more recent data suggest that the two procedures have comparable survival.[117] Nonetheless, surgical myectomy may also provide a more consistent result than using alcohol ablation.[118] There may also be an increased risk of electrical abnormality requiring implantation of a permanent pacemaker.[116]

Individuals who are at high-risk for sudden cardiac death include those who were resuscitated from previous collapse,[119] family members who had died suddenly,[120] presence of lethal abnormal heart rhythm,[121] unexplained fainting episodes[122] and left heart thickness greater than 30 mm.[121] The presence of multiple risk factors further increases the risk of sudden death,[123] and an intra-cardiac defibrillator may need to be implanted. Due to the limitation of using these clinical parameters in predicting sudden death, the performance of new techniques was evaluated. By administering a contrast, gadolinium, cardiac magnetic resonance imaging is able to detect scar tissue in the heart.[124] An international group of researchers found that the extent of scar in the heart muscle was associated with increased risk of sudden death.[125] For every 10% in the amount of scar tissue, the risk of sudden death increased by about 50%. This technique was able to provide comparable risk prediction for both high- and low-risk patients.

The intra-cardiac defibrillator is a complex life-saving device. When it detects a life-threatening abnormal rhythm, a small amount of electrical energy is delivered to the heart to terminate it and normal rhythm may be restored. Indeed, among those with previous cardiac arrest or life-threatening heart rhythm, the device triggers off in about 10% of the patients annually. On the other hand, the rate of discharge was about 4% per year for patients with only risk factors.[126,127] Although intra-cardiac defibrillators save lives, inappropriate discharges may occur as high as 25% of patients with hypertrophic cardiomyopathy, especially for younger patients and those with irregularly heart rhythm.[128,129] Inappropriate shocks can be terrifying and painful, and may result in abnormal psychological sequelae. Risk for dying may be as high as 60%, which is higher for those with inappropriate discharges.[129] About 6% to 13% of them may experience lead complications, such as fracture and dislodgement. Infection of the device and systems can occur in 4% to 5% of the device.[127,128] Infrequently, when the efficiency of the heart pump is severely impaired despite adequate treatment, the patient may require transplantation. These patients have outcomes comparable to those with other types of heart diseases.[130]

Life Following Diagnosis of Hypertrophic Cardiomyopathy

Patients with hypertrophic cardiomyopathy are generally permitted to participate in low-intensity sports and recreational activities. On the other hand, intense competitive sports should be avoided, as recommended by the American College of Cardiology[131] and European Society of Cardiology.[132] Thus activities such as brisk walking, bowling, golf, ergometer, treadmill, jogging at slow to moderate speed, swimming and cycling may be allowed. However, every patient should discuss with his or her doctor regarding specific sports. An uncommon condition whereby the heart muscle is thickened as a result of athletic training may confuse the diagnosis of patients with hypertrophic cardiomyopathy. It occurs in less than 2% of male world-class athletes.[133] The intricacies of using the electrocardiogram as a screening tool for athletes, including differentiating normal variants from disease conditions, have been extensively discussed in a document endorsed by the Sections of

Sports Cardiology of the European Association of Cardiovascular Prevention and Rehabilitation, and the Working Group of Myocardial and Pericardial Disease of the European Society of Cardiology.[134] While electrocardiography performed prior to participation in sports may identify those with hypertrophic cardiomyopathy,[134] a recent evaluation suggested that the false positive rate may be as high as 10%.[135]

The First Kiss of Love ... and Death

Emotional Ups and Downs, Electrical Longs and Shorts: The Long-QT Syndrome

"... [Jessica Caitlyn Barnett] *when I was about 12, ..., I started passing out, especially if something scared me ... Four long years this has been going on* [despite visiting several medical specialists] *... ten months later I died of Long QT syndrome...* [and in her vicarious final reflection]*... My grad photo is supposed to be in the year book, not in an obituary ... I did wear my prom gown ... on my own funeral. My limo, a hearse ... No more birthdays. I'll always be 17.*"

Jess' Story — Do No Harm

Sudden death can occur with any form of activity for men or women. Jemma Benjamin was a healthy 18-year-old active sportswoman.[136] She was a long distance swimmer and a hockey player. Jemma was also a hardworking student and was revising for her French examination at home. After immersing herself in another language, she decided to take a break and went to meet Daniel Ross in the afternoon. She must have looked forward to this well-deserved visit. After their *first* kiss just outside her boyfriend's flat in Treforest, Wales, Jemma sat on a sofa. Minutes later, she suddenly slumped with frothing in her mouth and died in front of Daniel's eyes. Post-mortem examination did not detect any abnormality that could have caused her death. As such, the subsequent coroner's inquiry indicated that Jemma was likely to

41

have died from Sudden Arrhythmic Death Syndrome (SADS), a condition that kills approximately 500 Britons yearly. In fact, as many as 30% of sudden death among previously healthy children, adolescents or young adults are attributed to this condition.[137]

The first kiss could have generated an emotion high of love with an adrenaline rush. Jemma has been described as a shy and timid girl. This apparently innocent incident might have led to an overdrive. Extreme feelings of excitement, fear, sadness or strenuous activities may reveal an underlying rhythm disorder, turning this happy event into a "Kiss of Death!" Despite being an athlete who was likely to be accustomed to physical stress and mental strain, she was overwhelmed by the stimulus brought about by the fatal kiss. In other circumstances, loud noises, such as a baby crying in the middle of the night, cell phone's ring and door slamming, could trigger the abnormal heart rhythm as well. On 28 December 2005, Kasia Ber, a 17-year-old girl from Durham, United Kingdom, set her alarm at 7 am for post-Christmas shopping. On waking up, she was shaky and called her boyfriend's name, Scott. Shortly after, Kasia stopped breathing in his arms, and attempts to resuscitate her were unsuccessful. Two weeks earlier, she saw her general practitioner for palpitation and shortness of breath. An electrocardiogram was performed four days later but no specific treatment was prescribed. Her mother, Diane, was subsequently found to have long-QT syndrome (LQTS).[138] The Chinese old wife saying, "大声吓死人" (which literally translates to "loud noises can kill") may have some truth to it.

Sudden death in an apparently healthy young person is almost always emotionally devastating and absolutely frustrating, especially when no abnormality was detected in the post-mortem examination. The life flame in someone with a bright future and who has not experienced life fully was vanquished in the fleet of a moment during a surge of emotion. Parents, siblings and friends of these young ones want to know the "truth." But the "truth" is out there! Or is it? Days turn to weeks, weeks to months, months to years, and years become a lifetime. The search for what took their beloved away appears endless. Nonetheless, those who are alive must continue living. After the initial grief and dismay, fear creeps into the minds' of family and friends. Would I be the next victim? As such, during the evaluation, it is important to establish if there were other members who had unexplained fainting spells or died suddenly, including sudden infant death, drowning, motor vehicle accident or other apparently accidental death. Such occurrences raise the suspicion of a genetic disorder. Examination and genetic testing of family members may unravel the genetic defect in this unfortunate young woman.

The Archetype of Genetic Heart Disease

Like Jemma and Kasia, routine autopsy examination is generally unhelpful in identifying the cause of death. There are several conditions that may be detected by genetic testing. Of these, the most common is the long-QT syndrome, affecting about 1 in 2,500 white live-births.[139] Others have estimated the prevalence to be 1 in 5,000.[140] The QT-interval is part of the electrocardiogram which represents the recovery of electrical of the ventricles after stimulation. During this period, potassium ions return back into the cell and sodium ions move out of the cells. Specialised channels are used to transport them across the cell membrane. Hence, abnormalities of these channels result in the prolongation of this interval.[141] The cells become unstable electrically and predisposes to abnormal heart rhythm, otherwise known as arrhythmia or dysrrhythmia. Ventricular fibrillation, whereby the electrical activity in the ventricle is totally disorganised, is the principal arrhythmia that causes death. During ventricular fibrillation, the heart is unable to contract in an organised and synchronised manner. As such, the heart is unable to produce any output. This situation is almost similar to the heart which has stopped beating (asystole). The difference is that the muscle is contracted in ventricular fibrillation and in a relaxed state in asystole. After a few seconds, the person loses consciousness and there is no pulse, heart sound or blood pressure. Meanwhile, the brain may send signals to the muscles in the chest and abdomen to attempt to breathe. But the rate is considerably slower than normal and differs from usual breathing pattern. It then looks more like someone gasping for breath. In some instances, the victim may give a shriek at the beginning. If the situation is not reversed in a few minutes, the person dies.

Another potentially fatal rhythm disorder is polymorphic ventricular tachycardia, in which the ventricle beats independent of the atrium and at a high rate. If this rhythm persists, it may degenerate into ventricular fibrillation. In one subtype of long-QT syndrome (LQTS3), the heart rate may be slow instead, and may result in fainting episodes if it beats too slowly. Instead of occurring during periods of emotional disturbances or physical stress, abnormal heart rhythm may occur during sleep for patients with LQTS3. Indeed, the risk and manner of cardiac arrest differs among the various subtypes of long-QT syndrome.[142]

Generally, adverse cardiac events occurring in patients with long-QT syndrome was believed to occur among the young (less than 40 years)[143] because sudden death in an older individual might be attributed to coronary artery disease and other heart or vascular diseases. But the risk of aborted cardiac arrest or sudden death was found to be more than 2.5-fold higher among those with prolonged QT-interval compared with subjects with normal QT-interval between the ages of 41 and 60 years.[144] Even among older individuals with coronary artery disease, the risk for sudden death among patients with unprovoked prolonged QT-interval, but without diabetes, was increased by more than 5-fold.[145] Conversely, among women with a certain type of long-QT (LQTS2) syndrome, the risk for fainting spells, and possibly the risk for sudden death or aborted cardiac arrest, was increased by more than 8 times after menopause.[146] However, they were reduced by about 5 times in another type of long-QT syndrome (LQTS1). Female sex hormones are believed to affect the ion channels and could have accounted for some of the changes following menopause. These findings indicate that older patients should also receive sufficient medical attention when ascertaining the risk for sudden death.

There is no physical abnormality detected among persons with long-QT syndrome. Fainting or seizure may be the only preceding symptom although several of them do not have any. In the extreme situation, the patient may be resuscitated from sudden death. Commonly, relatives of a young person who died suddenly are the ones who seek medical attention to determine if they are at risk for sudden death. In about 10% to 30% of sudden death cases, post-mortem examination sometimes failed to identify the cause.[137] In a study of 49 young individuals in North America who suffered from a fatal event, about 35% of these individuals were found to have an abnormal channel protein and the medical examiner's office requested for genetic studies.[147] Although the study sample was selected by the medical examiner, other populations showed comparable rates.[25,137,148] Of these, almost three out of five of the deceased were due to long-QT syndrome.[147] Together with a thorough medical examination of the surviving family members, molecular autopsy may play an important role in their subsequent management.

Although the genetic transmission appeared to be Mendelian, there is a predisposition for female, with a ratio of 2:1.[149] In the classical Mendelian inheritance, the distribution between the two sexes should be almost equal. For reasons unclear, there is a preferential transmission of the abnormal mutation from mother to daughter.

The QT-Interval

When the electrical activities of the heart muscle are amplified and recorded, they give rise to electrocardiographic tracing (Figure 7). Basically, it consists of stimulatory and recovery signals. In a normal tracing, they are named from the alphabets P to U. The QT-interval represents the changes in electrical activities during the recovery phase, after electrical stimulation (Figure 8). There are guidelines as how it should be measured (Figure 9).[150] Nonetheless, the initial electrocardiographic diagnosis of long-QT syndrome was based on a markedly prolonged QT-interval and bizarre T-waves.[151] But changes in T-waves are less common and the duration of the QT-interval remains to be the key determinant of long-QT syndrome. Genetic variations may also account for the duration of QT-interval.[152] Moreover, the identification of T-wave abnormalities depends on the person reading the electrocardiogram. Normal appearing T-wave

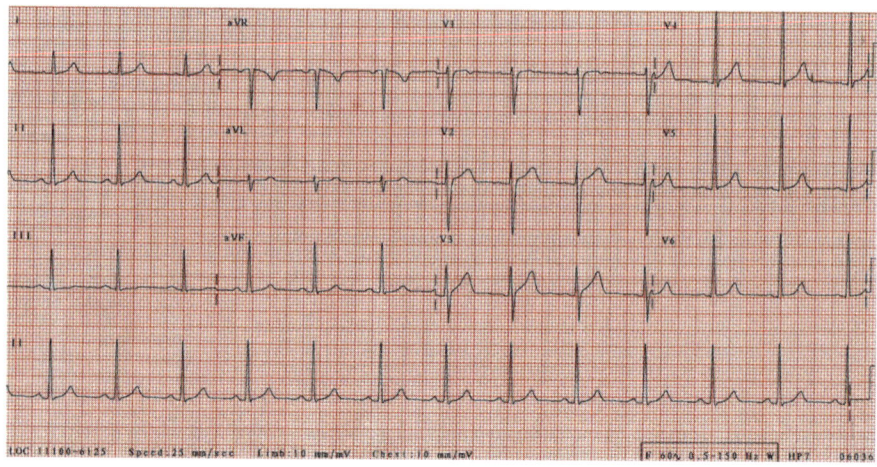

Figure 7. This is a normal 12-lead electrocardiogram showing regular spikes followed by a small "hump".

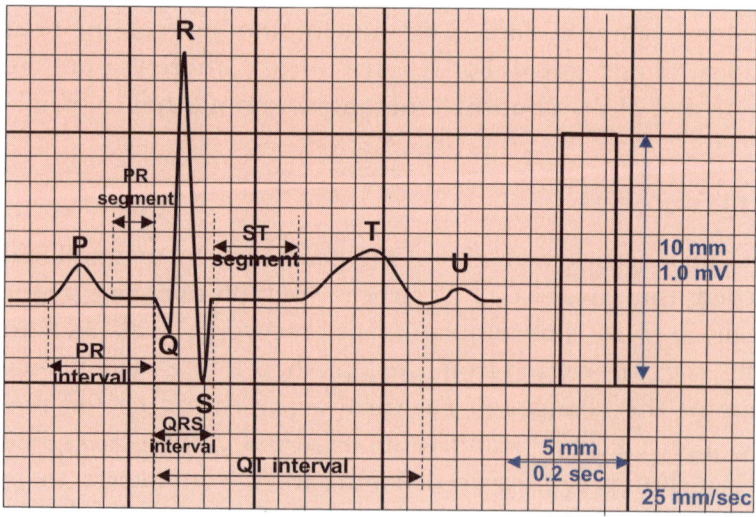

Figure 8. The normal electrocardiogram.

This is a graphical display of the electrical activities of the heart. The patterns form waves and spikes and are named from the alphabets P to U. Several electrodes are placed on the body to visualise the electrical activities from various parts of the body. On one side of the tracing is the calibration marking.

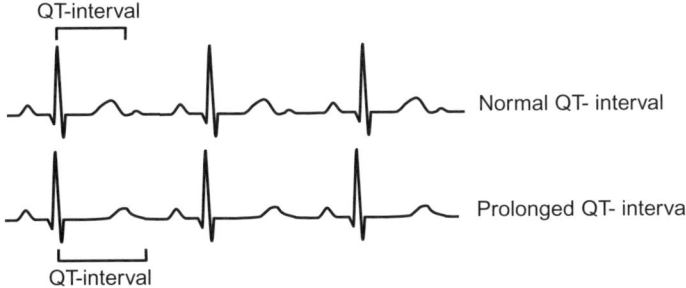

Figure 9. Prolongation of the QT-interval.
Electrocardiographic tracing showing normal and prolonged QT-interval.

was reported in 67% of patients with LQTS1 in one study[153] and 23% in another.[154] Several techniques have been attempted to unmask latent carriers[155,156] or induce changes in the T-wave using adrenaline infusion,[157] exercise[154] and complex mathematical assessment of T-wave morphology based on resting[158,159] or ambulatory[160] electro-cardiographic recordings. Using another drug, adenosine — which slows down the heart rate, a group of Israeli investigators found that the QT-interval increases significantly with abnormal T-wave config-uration in 72% of patients with long-QT syndrome, especially when the heart rate was slow.[161] These ingenious attempts illustrate the challenges in making an accurate diagnosis based on the resting electrocardiogram. Therefore, a standardised procedure for diagno-sis was set up in 1985.[162] It consisted of three major and four minor criteria, including electrocardiographic patterns, symptoms and family history. Of note, only one corrected QT-interval (greater than 440 ms) was used. When the diagnostic criteria were revised in 1993, points were accorded to different QT-interval durations, electrocar-diographic patterns, symptoms and family history.[163,164] Others have used only one *corrected* QT-interval with symptoms to make the diag-nosis.[165] However, the superiority of these diagnostic scores over traditional *corrected* QT-interval in the era of molecular medicine has been questioned by some investigators.[166]

Although the QT-interval appeared to be easily measured from the electrocardiogram, there are important procedures to be adopted.[167] At birth, the QT-interval is not significantly different between the two sexes. Its duration is reduced at puberty for boys.[168,169] As such, QT-interval remains longer in women,[170] and they are more susceptible to adverse cardiac events in adulthood.[143,171,172] Adult female were more than three times likely to suffer from fainting spells or sudden death.[171] Furthermore, it varies with heart rate and so the changes may be subtle and variable.[173]

Several other conditions affecting heart muscle, such as thickening or lack of blood supply, may also lead to longer QT-intervals. Importantly, several medicines, such as those which are used to treat abnormal heart rhythm and psychiatric disorders, and electrolyte abnormalities may also prolong the QT-interval.[167] Indeed, prolongation of the QT-interval has been identified as the single most common cause of withdrawal or restriction of use of marketed drugs.[174] For reasons unclear, women[175] and those starving or dieting[176,177] were more susceptible to prolongation of QT-interval due to drugs. Some of the more common medicines include some types of antibiotics, anti-histamines and anti-psychotic agents. These drugs generally work through the potassium channel which is also responsible for type 2 long-QT syndrome (LQTS2).[178] Therefore, all these factors have to be taken into consideration when determining the QT-interval. As such, others attempted to identify certain patterns of electrocardiographic to assist in making the diagnosis of long-QT syndrome.[179] During follow-up, patients with long-QT syndrome showed considerable variation in the QT-interval.[180] The dynamic change in the duration is independent of age, and risk for subsequent events is raised if the corrected QT-interval, obtained at any time, is 500 ms or greater. Conversely, when the QT-interval shortens, the duration for the recovery of the heart muscle reduces correspondingly so that it becomes less susceptible to lethal cardiac rhythm.[181]

There is overlap of the QT-interval between normal persons and carriers.[182] Indeed, the QT-interval in resting electrocardiogram may be normal[182] and estimated to occur in approximately a quarter of persons carrying the abnormal gene for long-QT syndrome.[184] Specifically, the prevalence for normal QT-interval among those who are carriers for LQTS1, LQTS2 and LQTS3 were 36%, 19% and 10%, respectively.[185] Standing may cause change in heart rate. Due to variation in response to this provocation, the QT-interval may be prolonged differently.[186] In a multinational registry,[184] the genes for long-QT syndrome were determined from 3,386 individuals because a family member has this condition or has suffered from the symptoms. They found that the risk of sudden death or aborted cardiac arrest for those with prolonged QT-interval was approximately 37-fold higher than unaffected family members. In contrast, when the person carries the abnormal gene but the QT-interval was normal, the risk was only 10 times higher. So the risk for sudden death or aborted cardiac arrest was about 4 times lower for individuals carrying the abnormal gene but with normal QT-interval compared with those with prolonged QT-interval. The absolute rates for these adverse events at age 40 years were 0.4%, 4% and 15% for normal family members, persons with long-QT syndrome but normal and prolonged QT-interval, respectively. By 70 years of age, they were 1%, 10% and 24%, respectively. Indeed, the duration of the QT-interval correlated with the occurrence of adverse cardiac events; the longer the period, the greater the risk.[187] Type of long-QT syndrome, female gender and fainting episodes are associated with a greater likelihood for sudden death or aborted cardiac arrest.

Exercise Testing

The diagnostic criteria for long-QT syndrome depend largely on prolongation of the corrected QT-interval, presence of symptoms in the individual and affected relatives.[163] In another large Italian registry of 1,115 family members from 310 individuals with long-QT syndrome, they found that the QT-interval was normal in 40% of the family members.[188] The same group of investigators estimated that the likelihood for an adverse event was 10% by the age of 40 years.[185] As such, other approaches to evaluate these individuals are being developed.

Exercise and recovery following physical activity have been shown to affect the QT-interval.[189] Therefore, it may be a useful tool to identify and stratify the risk of this condition.[190] During exercise, heart rate increases but the degree of shortening of QT-interval varies among patients with different long-QT syndrome. The duration of QT-interval reduction with exercise was greater for patients with LQTS3 than with LQTS2. Their decrease was more than normal controls.[190] Another group of investigators reported that the reduction in the duration of the QT-interval was greater among patients with LQTS2 than LQTS1.[192] Of note, the duration of the QT-interval for those with LQTS1 and LQTS2 lengthened during the recovery period compared with controls. But prolongation of the QT-interval tended to persist longer for patients with LQTS1. The duration of QT-interval may normalise during recovery for those with LQTS2.[193] Others have also detected differences in the manner in which the duration of QT-interval prolonged during exercise and recovered after exertion between LQTS1 and LQTS2 patients.[192,194] Nonetheless, when its absolute value after exercise is at least 460 ms, the diagnosis of long QT-syndrome should be considered.[195] This finding was corroborated by an earlier group of Japanese investigators.[154]

Recently, a group of international researchers attempted to elucidate the changes in QT-interval among first-degree relatives of patients with long-QT syndrome. From the University of Western Ontario, Academic Medical Center in Amsterdam, Tel Aviv University, McMaster University and University of Ottawa, 69 first-degree relatives were recruited from 26 families with a member suffering from long-QT syndrome.[196] The QT-interval was measured at rest while lying down, immediately on standing, at peak exercise, and 1 and 4 minutes after exercising. At rest, the QT-interval was abnormal in approximately half of the carriers of the abnormal gene (females ≥ 480 ms; males ≥ 470 ms). T-wave was also abnormal in about half of them. Conversely, none of the non-carriers had a prolonged QT-interval and T-wave abnormalities were present in less than 10% of them. They found that when the 4-minute QT-interval after exercise was more than or equal to 445 ms, the overall accuracy of detecting long-QT syndrome was greater than 90%. Using these two measurements, the investigators validated their algorithm in another 45 other first-degree relatives of a patient with long-QT syndrome. The investigators attributed their findings to the residual effect of adrenaline produced during exercise. Since the effect of the hormone wears off in 3 to 4 minutes, it is not surprising that the prolongation of the QT-interval persisted until that period. On the other hand, the effect of the para-sympathetic system sets in shortly after exercise, and could have accounted for the differences in the duration of QT-interval between patients with LQTS1 and LQTS2.[197]

Genetic Testing

Genes are inheritable blueprints for our body, and to make proteins in particular. There are several genes that code for various proteins on the heart cell membrane. At least 13 types of proteins, with several hundreds of mutations, have been identified and are associated with long-QT syndrome.[198] These proteins are assembled to form channels across the cell membrane. The channels are specific to certain electrically charged particles, potassium, sodium or calcium ions, which move in or out of the membrane at specific times to stimulate the cell or allow it to recover to baseline. These impulses cause the heart muscle to contract. Mutations may reduce or increase the function of the channels. As a result, the concentration of ions across the cell membrane changes and may or may not result in the contraction of heart muscle. Genetic testing is to identify these alterations. While this technique is crucial in the management of long-QT syndrome, there are several challenges.

Not every change in the genetic code is bad. If a mutation is known to be disease-causing, its identification may be useful in family members with indeterminate or normal QT-interval.[199] However, only about 50% of patients with long-QT syndrome may possess a previously known mutation. There are "private" mutations that are not found in other families. Furthermore, in a normal population, there are natural genetic variation and mutation, part of what is known to be "background noise." So, it may be difficult to distinguish if the mutation is functionally significant or disease causing. The mutation type, location and ethnic background are the other factors which have to be taken in consideration when interpreting the results. Under these circumstances, due to lack of collaborative information, the term "variant of unknown significance" has been used to describe the abnormal gene. Whether this change is normal variant or associated with disease has not been established. As such, the presence of mutation provides a guide to the likelihood of long-QT syndrome rather than a dichotomous indicator for the presence or absence of disease.[200] Furthermore, family history has been shown to be a better predictor for clinical outcomes than genotyping.[183] In the long-QT syndrome, the first three types which are generally due to a point mutation — change in one of the bases in the gene — account for about 75% of the cases.[201] By including other genetic perturbations, such as duplication, deletion and re-arrangment of nucleotide bases, commercially available testing may yield a relevant mutation in 80% of patients.[202,203]

Due to the complexity of mutations and its relevance, the Italian investigators have derived a three-tier approach.[188] The first step involves the identification of previously known mutations and the yield is 58% for five of the more common long QT-syndrome genes. This is followed by complete screening of the coding regions of the two most prevalent types of long QT-syndrome; i.e. LQTS1 and LQTS2. Another 32% of carriers may be identified. The final 10% is ascertained by reading the three affected genes. By adopting this approach, the investigators believed that detection of carriers is rapid and cost-effective.

Even in the attempt to risk-stratify family members of patients with long-QT syndrome, genetic testing is still challenging. Indeed, the usefulness of genetic testing depends on the pretest probability of the disease. As such, routine genetic testing approach for the population at large to identify individuals with long-QT syndrome is unlikely to be fruitful. Furthermore, management of this group of individuals who carry the abnormal gene mutations but without clinical manifestation is unclear. Indeed, realising its presence may generate unnecessary psychological pressure.[204]

Taming the Heart

Beta-blockers are a group of medicines which prevents the action of adrenaline, the hormone that is secreted during physical or mental stress, and probably during emotional events. They have been shown to reduce cardiac risk among patients with long-QT syndrome.[205] In patients with previous fainting spells or aborted cardiac arrest, the use of this medicine reduced the annual recurrence, including sudden death, to a third. On the other hand, the efficacy was lower for asymptomatic family members; in which the risk was reduced by about 40%. However, as high as 14% of patients suffered from another episode of fainting episode, aborted cardiac arrest or death in 5 years.[205] In a study on 375 individuals with long QT-syndrome, use of beta-blocker was associated with a 83% reduction in the occurrence of fainting spells or sudden cardiac arrest among those whose corrected QT-interval exceeded 500 ms.[180] Compliance with beta-blockers and concomitant use of medicine that prolong the QT-interval could have accounted for treatment failure.[206] At the same time, patients are advised against strenuous exercises. Those with type 2 long-QT syndrome should avoid emotional stress and upheavals.

Other modes of treatment using sodium-channel blockers, calcium-channel blockers and potassium-channel opening agents have not been clearly shown to be efficacious in treating patients with long-QT syndrome. Among those with type 2 long-QT syndrome treated with beta-blockers, potassium supplementation plus potassium diuretics may increase the blood level of potassium.[207] The QT-interval and the T-wave morphology improved. However, due to a small number of patients in the clinical trial and brief period of follow-up, the effects on important outcomes such as sudden death or abnormal cardiac rhythm were unclear.

As the cause of sudden death is largely attributed to ventricular fibrillation, the most effective treatment is cardioversion. This is the application of an electrical shock to allow the heart to re-initiate its normal rhythm, somewhat akin to "hard reset" in several of our electronic devices. Numerous medical television dramas have shown how doctors and nurses put paddles on a patient they are resuscitating. After charging, the instruction "stand clear" is given so that none of the healthcare providers are in contact with the patient so that they would not be accidentally electrocuted. In the meantime, the victim receives extra amount of air and the rhythm is checked one more time. If it is still appropriate, the electrical energy is delivered and the body may arch upwards before falling back on the bed. The rhythm normalises and a life is saved! Technology has miniaturised the entire system into an intracardiac defibrillator (ICD). This device incorporates a sophisticated algorithm to analyse the electrocardiogram to determine if an electrical shock should be delivered. If it is necessary, the pulse generator delivers the energy within several seconds. As such, implanting one of these devices in a person who survived a cardiac arrest can save a life. However, not everyone with long-QT syndrome requires an ICD;[208] particularly when there are several complications related to use of this device, such as infection and misfiring. Thus, the decision to implant such a device needs careful consideration. Those implanted at age younger than 20 years, corrected QT-interval greater than 500 milliseconds, prior cardiac arrest or cardiac events despite treatment are more likely to benefit from this treatment.[208]

Since the trigger of abnormal heart rhythm may be related to surges of adrenaline, one therapeutic approach is to remove this stimulus. As such, transecting the nerve providing stimulation has been suggested as a form of treatment for long-QT syndrome in the 1970s.[209] The collections of nerve cells, called ganglia, adjacent to the lower neck and upper thoracic vertebrae are ablated to reduce the release of nor-adrenaline and thereby increase the threshold of ventricular fibrillation and abnormal heart rhythm.[210] Among 174 patients with very long QT-interval treated with this procedure, there was a 91% annual fall in risk of fainting spells, resuscitated sudden death and sudden death for each patient.[211] Interestingly, those with type 1 and type 3 long-QT syndromes were more likely to benefit from this procedure. Although the morbidity associated with surgical sympathetectomy was relatively low, video-assisted thorascopic denervation may further reduce complications.[212,213]

Clues and Red Herrings

The Most Unhearty "Wagyu": Arrhythmogenic Right Ventricular Cardiomyopathy

"The closer you think you are, the less you'll actually see."

J. Daniel Atlas
Now You See Me

Like an intriguing mystery novel, the symptoms of Alexis Katchuk were a series of clues and red herrings to confuse the doctor in making an accurate diagnosis.[214] For more than 10 years, she has been suffering from an eating disorder. Anorexia does not only lead one to grow thin because of severe food restriction for fear of getting fat due to a distorted body image. It has several other adverse health consequences, as a result from malnutrition such as brittle bones, hair loss, kidney and other organ failure. Hence, it was not surprising that doctors attributed the repeated hospitalisation episodes, dizzy spells and palpitation to her eating disorder. The understanding of her symptoms was further clouded by the severe psychological trauma she suffered as a young girl. Alexis was raped and abused by a friend's father. To avoid being violated again, it was certainly not her priority to look attractive by dieting. Instead of doing things other girls do, Alexius participated actively in sports in high school to give her the "high" sensation. So, it was not surprising that doctors thought that the mental scar might have played up her symptoms and tended to take them lightly. In fact, four cardiologists told her that her symptoms were attributed to anorexia. As she began to accept her body, the battle against anorexia was being won. Conversely, the funny sensation over her chest became more severe. Her heart did not feel right and the beats became stronger. Sometimes, she felt dizzy during pounding and suffered from repeated fainting episodes. One day, the symptom was so severe that Alexis landed in the emergency room where she had her cardiac arrest. Her heart stopped beating for 53 seconds! Fortunately, the crash cart was next to her and Alexis was revived. To her dismay, her doctor still attributed the cardiac arrest to anorexia!

After moving to the middle of Missouri, another doctor diagnosed her to have a serious potentially life-threatening irreversible progressive cardiomyopathy, known as Arrhythmogenic Right Ventricular Cardiomyopathy (ARVC), hole-in-the-heart (atrial septal defect) and disorder in one of the heart valves. The funny sensation in her chest was due to abnormal heart rhythm caused by disruption of the heart muscle. Muscle cells were replaced by fat cells changing the size and shape of the heart. So an intra-cardiac defibrillator, which she called Lily, was implanted to treat the potentially lethal arrhythmia. At hindsight, she was extremely upset with the doctors who put the blame on the psychiatric disorders and missed the diagnosis.

So it appears that instead of being a gradual progressive disease, ARVC may be a condition characterised by exacerbations. Patients may be completely well between attacks. Moreover, some of these episodic events may also be asymptomatic. But in other cases, the patient may experience chest pain, palpitation or a cardiac arrest due to a potentially lethal disorder.[215] While the triggers for these attacks are not entirely clear, environmental factors such as physical activity or infection may be likely candidates. But the precise mechanisms as to how these factors bring about the symptoms have not been clearly understood. Nonetheless, with each exacerbation, the disease progresses when the cells begin to pull further apart.

Arrhythmogenic Right Ventricular Cardiomyopathy

This is a relatively "new" uncommon condition which was described more than 30 years ago[84,216] or about two decades after the discovery of hypertrophic cardiomyopathy.[216] As the name implies, it involves the right ventricle predominantly with a progressive loss of heart muscle cells, starting from the outer aspect of the heart muscle wall and extending into the cavity. The front, tip and bottom of the right heart are the common places that are affected, forming the triangle of dysplasia.[217] These cells are replaced by fatty and fibrous tissue.[97] The area may be thinned and bulged out, becoming aneurysmal. This condition is the second common cause of unexpected sudden death in the young and may account for a quarter of victims.[27]

Among fat cells and fibrous tissue (scars) are groups of inflammatory cells, which together, may form the nidus to trigger potentially lethal abnormal rhythms.[218–220] However, the origin of the presence of inflammatory cells may be related to infection or an immunological reaction, or as part of the response to cell death. As part of ARVC, heart muscle cell may eventually die spontaneously.[221,222]

A group of proteins that connects one heart muscle cell to an adjacent cell are known as desmosomes (Figure 10).[223] They are complex structures made up of several sub-units, providing structural integrity of the heart and facilitate a variety of cellular functions. ARVC is likely due to abnormalities in one of these sub-units.[224] Desmosomes not only hold the cells together, they allow signals to transmit efficiently from one cell to another. This important channel for inter-cellular communication enables the heart to contract sequentially and in synchrony. In addition to structural changes of the intercalated discs, the number may be reduced and location may be altered.[225] Disruption of these connecting discs may lead changes in the normal structure and function of the heart muscle. Instead of being tightly bound to one another, the heart muscle cells are pulled apart. Taken together, these adverse modifications may explain the thin or bulging (aneursymal) walls in the regions whereby the right and left heart are more susceptible to mechanical stress.

The prevalence of ARVC ranged from 1 in 1,000 to 1 in 5,000,[33,226–228] with wide regional variation. The peak age of occurrence for this

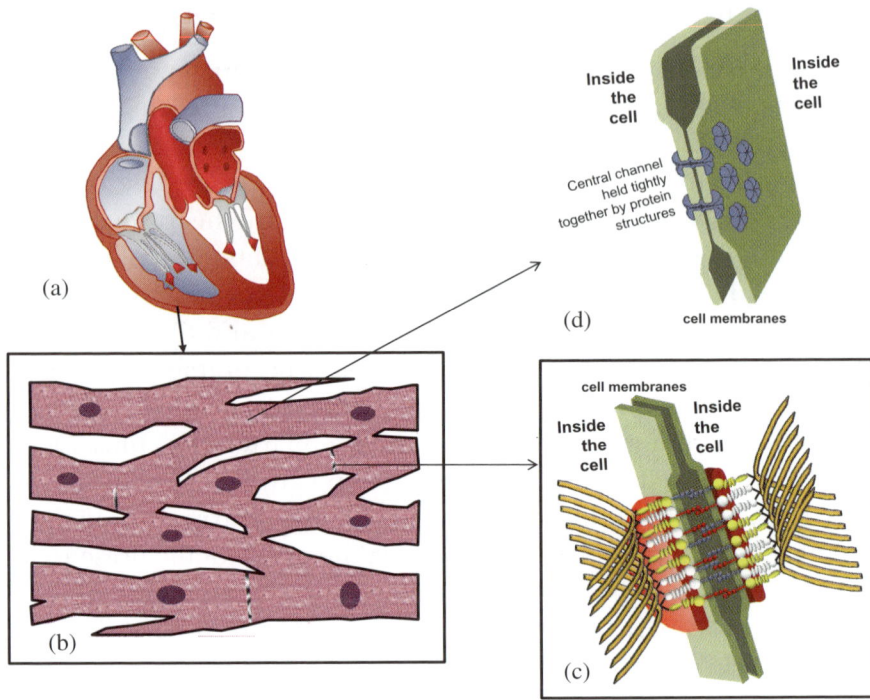

Figure 10.   Heart muscle.

Panel A shows the heart and the microscopic view of the heart muscle is seen in Panel B. The specialised components (desmosomes) (Panel C) hold the muscle fibres together to form a network. When the protein of the different parts of this complex is abnormal, they may not be able to function and may result in the condition, arrhythmogenic right ventricular cardiomyopathy. There are also channels that allow the heart muscle cells to communicate with each other (Panel D).

condition is in the 30s and 40s. With greater awareness and better diagnostic capabilities, patients are likely to be detected at a younger age.[229] Although there was an initial gender disparity, with a ratio of men to women of almost 3:1,[216] recent reports indicated that both sexes were affected with comparable frequency,[227,229] with a marginally higher proportion of male (57%).[230]

Information on a more general population provided some insight into ARVC and sudden unexpected deaths among the young. The Forensic Institutes of Lyon and Saint-Etienne in the southeast of France conducted 14,000 autopsies over a 19-year period.[231] They found 1,930 individuals, between the ages of 1 and 65 years, in which the cause of death could not be attributed to a condition that was not due to heart disease or that the deceased had a previously known heart condition. There were 200 cases of ARVC (10.4%), with 108 male and 92 female, in this series. The average age was 35.5 years for both sexes. Not surprisingly, most of them died at home (63%). Only 7 of the deaths (3.5%) occurred during sporting activity. But the mean age of those who died during physical activities were younger (23 years). Interestingly, about 10% of the deceased were undergoing a surgical procedure. Most of the operations were not extensive or major. This finding suggested that those with abnormal rhythm may be difficult to resuscitate, even in a well-equipped healthcare facility with highly-trained medical personnel. Whether the medicines used for anaesthesia may trigger or complicate the resuscitative procedures were unclear. Another finding of note was that their study revealed that abnormalities in the conduction system were present in about 70% of the patients. Although these changes may not manifest as symptoms initially,[232] the investigators cautioned that doctors should exercise caution when using medicines to treat abnormal heart rhythms. Most of these medicines can further aggravate the delay in conduction.

Patients with ARVC do have symptoms that could suggest its diagnosis. The most common symptoms were palpitation (27%), fainting (26%) and sudden cardiac death (23%) among 100 patients with the condition in the United States.[229] In another 108 newly diagnosed patients with ARVC in North America, the most common symptoms were palpitation (56%) followed by dizziness (27%), fainting (21%) and chest pain (14%).[230] Among young athletes in Italy, ARVC accounted for about 22% of sudden cardiac death. For non-athletes, it was 8%.[233] Of 31 individuals who died and were found to have ARVC at post-mortem examination, 29 died from cardiac arrest.[229] About 62% occurred during routine activity, 31% during exercise and 3.5% during sleep. Interestingly, although the diagnosis of ARVC was not made earlier, 8 (26%) of the 31 patients have other symptoms. Five of the 8 had at least one fainting spell.

The Struggles to Make a Diagnosis

To standardise the diagnosis of ARVC, a group of experts were organised into a Task Force by European Society of Cardiology and International Society and Federation of Cardiology to establish a set of criteria for doctors. They are based on medical and family history, electrocardiographic patterns, structure and function of the right heart.[234] Electrical abnormalities may be revealed in the surface electrocardiogram and rhythm disorders may precede cellular and structural changes in the heart. The pathognomonic change in the electrocardiogram is prolongation of the activation of the right heart and the presence of the epsilon waves (Figure 11),[235] which is a small abnormal spike which may be partially buried in the main electrocardiographic complex. However, it occurred only in the minority of patients (up to 30%) with ARVC.[234,236,237] Other less diagnostic but more common features have been suggested to improve the ability to ascertain the condition.[236,238] There were also missed or skipped beats of a particular morphological pattern in the resting electrocardiogram.[216] A special electrocardiographic technique, known as signal-averaged electrocardiogram, has been developed to detect patterns of electrical instability, or late potentials, as a result of ARVC.[239] Since its presence is not specific for the condition, it was

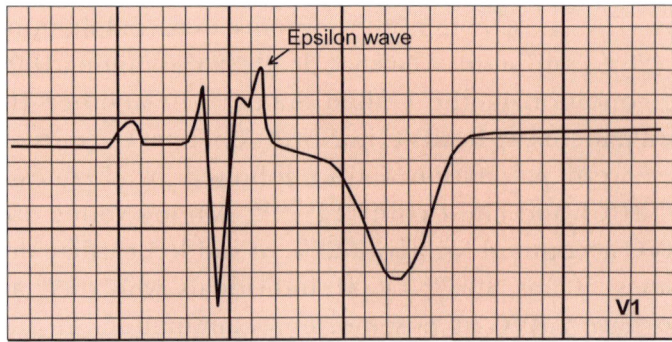

Figure 11.   The epsilon wave.

It consists of a positive deflection at the end of the QRS complex. There are a few patterns of the epsilon wave which is a characteristic finding of patients with arrhythmogenic right ventricular cardiomyopathy.

not able to predict the occurrence of serious rhythm disorders.[240–242] As such, it is considered only as a minor diagnostic criterion.[234,237] Another technique which measures the electrical recovery of the different parts of the heart muscle may also be useful.[243] However, it is not widely adopted because of the need for expertise in interpreting the results especially when the baseline electrocardiogram is not normal.[244] Treadmill stress electrocardiography may also be useful in identifying substrates that are more susceptible to abnormal rhythm disorder during exercise.[245]

Based on patterns in the electrocardiogram, structural changes detected by various imaging techniques such as echocardiography or cardiac magnetic resonance and family history, an International Task Force in 1994 has developed criteria for diagnosis of the condition through.[234] However, imaging techniques are sometimes limited by the quality of the images that can be obtained from the subjects and the cooperation of the patient. In comparison with echocardiography, cardiac magnetic resonance imaging has greater potential to characterise the right heart wall and its dimensions. These features provide a higher confidence in making the diagnosis of ARVC, especially during the earlier phases of the disease, which has a high correlation with the genetic make-up for the condition.[246] Furthermore, there are techniques which can be employed to enhance the qualitative assessment of the heart.[247] However, during cardiac magnetic resonance imaging, the individual must keep relatively still in the scanner for a relatively long duration. As such, it may not be suitable for a person who is unable to tolerate a confined area. The quality of operators is also critical in obtaining discriminating images and the establishment of reference values for right ventricular function.[248] In the normal heart, there may be some fatty tissue in the right ventricular wall, and may be confused with ARVC.[249] Indeed, there may be variability in interpreting the scan by the same observer at different times (intra-operator variability)[246] and different observers (inter-observer variability).[230,250,251] In a study of 108 individuals who were newly-diagnosed with ARVC, echocardiogram and cardiac magnetic resonance imaging were read by two groups of doctors, from the clinic where the patient was first seen and a central coordinating institution.[230] Out of 88 patients who underwent cardiac magnetic resonance imaging, the initial clinic reported 44 subjects to be significantly abnormal while the coordinating centre found that only 24 were significantly abnormal. On the other hand, this trend was reverse for echocardiogram. While the initial clinic reported 26 of them to be abnormal, the coordinating centre found 45. The number found to be abnormal for invasive right ventriculography was similar between the two groups of doctors. These findings illustrated the challenges in cardiac imaging in making an accurate diagnosis of the condition. Overall, cardiac magnetic resonance was able to detect about three-quarters of those with the disease (sensitivity). But when this imaging technique did not show evidence for ARVC, the likelihood that the patient did not have condition was 95% (specificity). Unlike echocardiography and cardiac magnetic resonance, another technique using computed tomography, which exposes the patient to radiation, can also identify some of the changes in the right heart of patients with ARVC.[252,253]

With better understanding of the condition and advanced molecular techniques, the criteria for diagnosis were revised by the Task Force in 2010,[237] probably enhancing the diagnostic capability.[254] Enlargement of the right ventricle and abnormalities in contraction may be detected by various imaging techniques. Structural changes in the right ventricular wall could be observed by using contrast and magnetic resonance imaging.[255] In a contrast study, a substance is injected into the body so that the heart structure could be visualised more clearly. While individual abnormality may be considered as a major criterion in the earlier recommendation,[234] two or more abnormalities are needed in the revised criteria.[237] Unlike what was previously thought, involvement of the left ventricle may not be a late development in the course of the disease.[256]

When other various investigations are inconclusive, those who are suspected of having this condition may be subjected to an invasive procedure to clarify the diagnosis. Since fatty and scarring tissue replaces muscle cells in the hearts of patients with ARVC, one of the initial criteria for diagnosis was to examine small pieces that were removed. This technique is known as endomyocardial biopsy.

A special long catheter is inserted through a vein and positioned in the heart. At the far end of the catheter, there is a small pincer-like knife to "bite" off a tiny specimen. The tissues are then processed and examined under the microscope.[234] However, the initial enthusiasm was dampened by the practicalities of the procedure.[257] Things were not as simple or straight-forward as they seemed. There are several places in the heart that the samples may be obtained, but changes of ARVC may not be seen in all parts of heart. Fat may also be present in normal heart.[249] Furthermore, the investigators were able to define the characteristics quantitatively using an *in vitro* model.[257] Their findings were adopted in the subsequent revision of the criteria.[237] Recently, the use of special staining techniques for specific proteins on the heart muscle specimens have been shown to provide better results in making the diagnosis of ARVC.[258]

Unfortunately, in medicine, everything is not always definitive with the first encounter. Furthermore, several other conditions may mimic ARVC. Congenital abnormalities resulting in an enlarged right heart, such as atrial septal defect (hole in the wall separating the upper chambers or atriae) or blood returning to the heart through anomalous veins, would not be missed by an astute clinician. Other forms of cardiomyopathy may also appear similar. Importantly, adaptations in the heart, particularly on the right side, due to prolonged increased workload that are associated with endurance athletes may lead to changes in the morphological and electrical patterns.[259] These alterations can be confused with the diagnosis of ARVC. In this study, there were three groups, consisting of 40 patients with ARVC, 40 athletes and 40 otherwise normal individuals, known as the control group. The resting electrocardiogram was abnormal in 62% of patients with ARVC, 7.5% for athletes and 2.5% for controls. Notably, the right heart was enlarged for both patients with ARVC and athletes compared with controls. But there were other measurements of the right heart obtained from echocardiography that were different between patients with ARVC and athletes. In addition, the diagnosis is not infrequently uncertain with some individuals. These persons need to be followed-up for symptoms and the various tests may be repeated serially.

New Name, Old Disease?

As early as 1736, a similar condition was described in four generations of a family in Italy by Giovanni Maria Lancisi, the physician to the Pope and a Professor of Anatomy in Rome.[260] In fact, Sir William Osler, a renowned and respected physician in the 19th century, described the heart of a patient who died in his 40s or 50s. Although there was muscle tissue in the heart chambers, the walls of the atriae and ventricles were "parchment-like thinness", Osler reported in 1905.[261] Incidentally, the condition of "parchment-like" heart wall was reported in 1970 when an autopsy was conducted in an 84-year-old woman.[262] She died from pneumonia following surgery for intestinal obstruction.

Subsequently, in 1949, Henry Uhl initially described a congenital malformation of the heart, with almost total absence of heart muscle cells in the right ventricle of an infant who died at the age of 8 months.[263] As Uhl's anomaly was increasingly recognised, some of these patients were found to have enlarged hearts and rhythm disorders. Subsequently, patients with abnormal right ventricle presenting with potentially lethal rhythm disorder were described. Hence, the term "arrhythmogenic" was added to right ventricular dysplasia/cardiomyopathy. This condition was first described by a French physician, Guy Fontaine, in 1977.[216] Whether these two conditions are related is controversial.[264,265] However, others have pointed out the distinct differences between these two anomalies. In Uhl's disease, the right heart muscle did not develop while the foetus was in the womb. In ARVC, there is a progressive loss of heart muscle cells from childhood.

By 1982, the abnormal heart rhythm, left bundle branch block ventricular tachycardia (a distinctive pattern in the electrocardiogram), was comprehensively described in 24 adults with ARVC.[216] Fontaine and his colleagues then correlated the surface electrocardiograms, electrical activity on the surface of the heart and microscopic features of 15 patients with ARVC in 1984.[218] They reported that the delay in electrical activation of the ventricles was due to the abnormal heart cells found in ARVC. These changes resulted in a characteristic electrocardiographic pattern, the epsilon wave. Initially, this condition was thought to congregate in the Veneto Region of Italy[266] where the first patient was encountered in 1977.[267] Subsequently, it was reported as the most common cause of sudden death among young competitive athletes,[268] and parts of Europe.[219] Recently, the prevalence of ARVC has been estimated to be less than 5% of patients who died suddenly and did not have overt heart disease.[269,270] On the other hand, doctors are becoming more aware of the condition and it has been found in other groups as well.

Fortunately, not all of these potentially lethal rhythm disorders are fatal among patients with ARVC. In a recent review,[271] the annual mortality ranged from 0.08%[272] to 3.6%.[273] Patients with only right ventricular involvement may tolerate one of these conditions, ventricular tachycardia.[274] This rhythm disorder may explain why some merely lose consciousness without succumbing to it. However, the patient is unlikely to survive when the heart is contracting in a disorganised fashion, otherwise known as ventricular fibrillation, or at a very rapid rate, otherwise known as ventricular flutter. The more severe form of rhythm disorder is believed to occur when there is a period of active death of heart muscle cells and inflammation, otherwise known as the "hot" phase of the disease. However, patients may not have symptoms during these flare-ups. The series of exacerbations and intersperse with periods of quiescence are believed to be the manner which ARVC progresses. But the presence of an inflammatory response varied widely from 2%[275] to 5.5%[231] to 19%[268] and up to 79%.[219] As such, the precise role of inflammation remains to be clarified. Nonetheless, these activities may be reflected by changes in the electrocardiogram and release of biomarkers that are associated with injury of the heart.[276,277]

Losing Muscle, Gaining Fat

In the early stages of the disease, structural changes may be absent, minimal or subtle.[219] Obviously, the abnormalities occur initially in the right ventricle. The infiltration of fat cells and fibrous (scar) tissue may be localised in the inflow, outflow or apex. In this condition, muscle cells may be transformed to fat cells.[278] Of note, in animal models of

ARVC, the deficiency in some of the desmosomes resulted in transformation of muscle to fat cells due to altered signals from the nucleus.[279] Subsequently, the changes become more diffuse and extend to the posterior (back) and lateral (side) walls of the left ventricle.

The natural history of ARVC has been categorised into four stages and the early phase is "concealed",[266] indicating that there is no clinical sign or symptom of the disease. This period may last several years.[280] Although the individual may be asymptomatic but the risk of sudden death is still heightened, especially during physical exertion. So regardless of symptom or abnormal electrical activity, the individual should avoid strenuous activities once the diagnosis has been made. With hundreds of thousands of beats, the structure of the heart is slowly disrupted by its pumping action. Patients may then start to have symptoms of palpitation, giddiness or fainting spells during the "electrical" phase and the morphological abnormalities become more apparent. If the individual has not died from rhythm disorder, the patient would develop heart failure from diffuse involvement of right ventricle. Eventually in the fourth phase, the left ventricle becomes affected and the individual develops right and left heart failure.[227] When a patient presents at this stage, the diagnosis may be mistaken as dilated cardiomyopathy, another condition which may be associated with sudden death (please refer to *A Large Weak Heart: Dilated Cardiomyopathy* chapter, page 99). However, nowadays, it has been estimated that the left ventricle fails early in the condition[227] and could affect as frequent as 75% of patients.[84]

About half of the patients do not have abnormal physical signs that the doctor can detect on examination.[281] The other half of the patients may have abnormal neck pulsations, heart sounds and murmurs. Thus, these physical signs can be challenging to recognise by a cursory examination and so the doctor has to pay special attention as they can be easily missed.

Managing Patients with ARVC

Since there is weakness of the muscle wall, physical activities which increase the workload of the heart could result in excessive loading and further expansion of the chambers, not unlike blowing up a balloon. Therefore, these adverse responses are likely to worsen the condition and hasten its deterioration. Indeed, this concept has been shown in mice with abnormal proteins involved in linking between heart muscle cells.[282] Furthermore, with exercise, the nervous and hormonal systems stimulate the heart and give rise to potentially lethal rhythms.[283] So, it was not surprising that ARVC has been shown to increase the sudden risk by more than five times among young competitive athletes in the Veneto region of Italy. Therefore, strenuous activities should be avoided for patients with ARVC.

Medicines may be used to prevent the occurrence of such abnormal rhythms. Even among those who had an intra-cardiac defibrillator implanted, medical treatment should also be considered if there is frequent recurrence of these potentially lethal cardiac rhythms requiring repeated discharges. Several drugs have been evaluated to determine their efficacy in treating potentially lethal rhythm disorders.[284] Unlike traditional anti-arrhythmic drugs which were used for treating patients with abnormal rhythms after a heart attack, these investigators found that sotalol (Sotacor) was the most effective, with a 68% overall acute efficacy rate. However, the efficacy in preventing potentially lethal rhythms has not been shown for most other beta-blockers.[230] On the other hand, other medicines such as amiodarone (Cordarone) and verapamil (Isoptin) have also been shown to be efficacious.[284] Although adverse effects from drug treatment did not occur frequently and were generally not serious, these investigators did not recommend the use of amiodarone because of its potentially serious side-effects.

However, for patients who are at high-risk, such as those who have suffered from a potentially lethal rhythm disorder but survived the sudden death event,[274] an intra-cardiac defibrillator may be implanted instead. About two of three individuals with an aborted sudden death event died suddenly.[285] There are other high-risk characteristics, such as fainting,[272,286] in which implantation of an intra-cardiac defibrillator may be beneficial.[274] As a predictor for sudden death, the sensitivity for fainting was only 40%[243] while the specificity was 90%. These figures suggested that fainting was not a frequent symptom before sudden death. However, those who did not faint were less likely to suffer from sudden death. This observation was corroborated by other investigators.[272] Indeed, the rate of shocks delivered to treat abnormal heart rhythm for patients who had fainted before was 9% every year,[287] a figure comparable to those who had suffered from a sudden death event or potentially lethal rhythm disorder. Although the proportion of patients with a history of syncope was lower in a United States study,[288] the appropriate discharge rate for the defibrillator was similar, at 9% annually. Of note, patients who fainted within the previous six months were more likely to receive a shock. The other factors that have been found to be associated with greater risk are young age at diagnosis, severely impaired right heart function, involvement of the left ventricle[242,289,290] and particular abnormalities in the electrocardiogram.[243,291] Although the role of genotyping, establishing the genetic makeup, in guiding the use of an intra-cardiac defibrillator has not been well-established,[292] it may be helpful when certain "malignant" forms of mutation are identified. In Newfoundland, Canada, a group of 11 families with a particular autosomal dominant-type of mutation in chromosome 3, received substantial benefit from implantation of an intra-cardiac defibrillator.[293] Mortality reduction was more evident among men and the 5-year chance of dying for those who received the device was 28% lower. Indeed, patients, in general, treated with this device may improve survival by 24% to 35% over a 3.3-year period. But whether implantation of such a device could be avoided in a lower risk group of patients with ARVC was not clear.[294]

There may be several psychological issues associated with implanting such a device in a young person.[295] In addition to clinical judgment, the decision to implant such an expensive device also depends on the healthcare delivery and financing systems. While an intra-cardiac device saves lives, there are several limitations as well. Similar to any form of treatment, there are complications related to its use. After implantation, the site may be infected and the wound may breakdown. There may be bleeding and clotting of the wires within the blood vessels. Subsequently, the wires may break or dislodge.

When an electric shock is discharged inappropriately, the patient may experience excruciating pain and psychological trauma. Fortunately, these malfunctions have been reduced with better technologies and algorithms. In addition to the cost, patients have to be carefully selected to determine who the most likely individuals to benefit.

The role for invasive treatment?

Among those with ARVC and have received an intra-cardiac defibrillator, discharges are frequently appropriate.[274,294,296,297] To try and reduce the number of discharges, attempts were made to identify the source of the abnormal rhythm and then eliminate it. This approach has been adopted in other individuals with similar rhythm disorder. In some patients with potentially lethal rhythms, a focus can be identified by studying electrical impulse initiation and propagation in the heart.

Catheter ablation is a technique employed to destroy this focus so as to prevent the re-initiation of the abnormal heart rhythm. On locating the site, various types of energy source, such as radiofrequency waves, have been successfully used. In this procedure, catheters are placed into the heart and the site where the abnormal heart rhythm arises is identified. The energy is then applied to eliminate it. Initially, electrical energy was used, a technique known as fulguration, pioneered in France.[298] The experience of the initial 15 patients was reported in 1990.[299] But due to the technical challenges relating to its use, radiofrequency waves have become the dominant energy source for catheter ablation.[300] Initial experiences with this technique have been encouraging, with relatively low recurrence rates of 11%[301] to 20%[302] after an average follow-up period of 17[302] and 27[301] months. However, other investigators have reported much higher rates of recurrence of abnormal rhythms.[303,304] The variation in results may be attributed to operator experience, procedural protocols and techniques. Furthermore, ARVC is a progressive disease and there may be multiple foci for the abnormal heart rhythm. More recently, in the Johns Hopkins Medical Center, 24 patients with ARVC underwent this procedure.[305] At least one focus was found in three-quarters of the procedures performed. Radiofrequency energy was used to ablate the focus in 48 procedures. Only slightly less than half of them (46%) were successful in preventing the initiation of the rhythm disorder. After 32 months, recurrence of the abnormal rhythm disorder was high at 85%. The investigators attributed the lack of durability of the procedure to the progressive nature of the disease. New areas of replacement of muscle by fat cells can give rise to new foci for abnormal rhythm. As such, catheter ablation is not routinely recommended as first-line treatment. A recent pilot study suggested that the failure of this procedure was due to the recurrence of the rhythm disorder as a result of a focus at the outer aspect of the heart.[290,306] Among 13 consecutive patients who had previously undergone the usual catheter ablation procedure but failed, mapping on the outer aspect of the heart was performed.[301] Mapping is the process to locate the size where the abnormal rhythm originates. The doctors found 27 targets and treated them. After a mean follow-up period of 18 months, 10 patients (77%) did not have recurrence of the potentially lethal rhythm. Comparing the various strategies for catheter ablation among 87 patients with ARVC in 80 centres in North America, those who underwent three-dimensional mapping or ablation of the outer aspect of the heart fared better.[307] However, the efficacy of this approach needs to be validated in a greater number of patients in the setting of a controlled randomised clinical trial.

Disconnecting the nerves that supply the heart muscle has been used to treat patients with long-QT syndrome.[213] It has been suggested to treat patients with ARVC. The network of nervous tissues serves to stimulate the heart during physical exertion and mental stress. Preliminary work showed that the procedure was efficacious in preventing recurrence of rhythm disorder in a patient with ARVC.[308] Thus the mode of treatment is still considered as experimental.

Further issues on patient management

Management of patients with an intermediate risk for sudden death has been an issue of frequent contention. This group includes patients with an abnormally rapid heart rate but without a fall in blood pressure or fainting spells and other high risk characteristics. The decision to implant a defibrillator, undergo catheter ablation or receive medicines has to be considered individually. Heart transplantation has also been used as a form of treatment for patients with end-stage ARVC. In the Johns Hopkins Hospital, there were 18 patients with ARVC that received a donor heart.[309] The average age of onset of symptom was relatively young, at 24 years, with a prolonged clinical course. With less than a third having abnormal heart rhythm, heart failure was the most common reason for the procedure. The 1-year survival rate was 94%. After a follow-up period of 6.2 years, 88% were still alive. Indeed, these early results are encouraging. However, obtaining donor hearts has been a challenge. The use of artificial life support system such as left ventricular assist devices in supporting hearts with ARVC has not been established.

Being pregnant also raises the demand on the heart as the heart is sustaining life for two individuals. Its effects are likely to be comparable to performing physical activities. Although the numbers are small, the earlier phases of pregnancy are generally well-tolerated. But as it progresses, the changes become greater and closer follow-up is recommended for the third trimester and puerperium.[310] Of the six women with ARVC who were pregnant and followed up regularly with resting, signal-averaged and ambulatory electrocardiography and echocardiography, two of them complained of palpitation in the last trimester. One of them was found to have sustained ventricular tachycardia following delivery. All the women underwent caesarean section at full-term.

Unwanted Legacy

Approximately 30% to 50% of patients with ARVC are identified because a family member has been diagnosed with the condition,[234,311] depending on the criteria used for diagnosis. Of note, the majority of them (72%) do not have symptoms.[311] Hence, when a patient with ARVC has been determined, family members should be examined to determine if they have the disease as well.

The association between patients and their families is largely attributed to abnormalities of the proteins linking heart muscle cells to one another. Of the proteins involved, plakophilin-2 is the most common protein affected in ARVC.[224] Of these genes, numerous have been identified and the majority of them are inherited in an autosomal dominant fashion. This mode of inheritance means that the disease may manifest if an individual carries one of the abnormal genes and there is a 50% chance of transmitting to an offspring. But only approximately 30% to 60% of patients with ARVC carry the abnormal gene.[312–315] Certain mutations have been shown to be associated with an early age of onset of symptoms and rhythm disorder.[316,317] Unlike other inherited conditions associated with sudden death, expression of the disease may vary even among members of the same family with same gene abnormality,[223] with a propensity for manifestation of the condition among males.[318] The symptoms of individuals carrying certain gene mutation vary substantially,[319] making the diagnosis challenging and management enigmatic. There are other genetic modifiers and environmental effects that result in the variability of the expression of the disease.[320]

Another critical issue in the interpretation of the result of genetic study is the differentiation between an "abnormal" gene and a "causative" gene. Generally, a disease-causing gene should not occur more frequently than 1 in 400 persons. However, in certain populations, genetic mutation that could result in ARVC was found in as frequent as 1 in 200 among Finnish[321] and as high as 6% among Asians.[315]

On the other hand, up to 48% of patients with ARVC have two genetic abnormalities.[322–325] About 10% of relatives of patients with ARVC also carry two abnormal genes. When there were multiple abnormal genes, the risk of manifesting the disease increased by five-fold and may present with more severe signs and symptoms.[314] However, the precise roles of genes in this condition have yet to be clearly defined.

Much less frequently, the condition is inherited in an autosomal recessive fashion and may be accompanied by abnormalities in the hair or skin.[326] Different gene mutations have resulted in Naxos disease and Carvajal syndrome described in patients with ARVC and small nodules in the hands and soles and woolly hair.[84] In these conditions, the patient requires both genes to be abnormal in order for the expression of the disease. Recognising the complexity of the disease and inheritance, a web-based database consisting of the different genetic variants for ARVC has been collated (www.arvcdatabase.info).[327]

Furthermore, not all parents of patients with ARVC have the abnormal gene. New mutation may account for the lower than expected proportion of them with family history of ARVC or of sudden death. As such, a positive family history was present in only 20% to 30% of patients with ARVC. On the other hand, among relatives who were found to have an abnormal gene, less than a third of them met the criteria for diagnosis of the condition.[314] Conversely, a person with a genetic mutation for ARVC may not develop the disease. Other factors, such as viral infection or physical activity, may contribute to the expression of the condition. Therefore, taken together with the complexity of inheritance and background genetic noise, this diagnostic tool cannot be used in isolation. The results must be interpreted with careful and accurate clinical evaluation.[315] Currently, the principal role of genetic testing is to assess the risk of first-degree relatives of a patient with ARVC.[203] So if the patient was found to have a genetic defect that could result in the condition, and the same abnormality is found in the family member, then the likelihood for ARVC is increased. These individuals should be followed up closely. When the mutation is absent in a family member, the chances for developing the disease is less likely. However, there may be another genetic defect that is not identified and can still affect a family member. Due to the intricacies of inheritance and expression of the genetic diseases, a new healthcare profession has emerged. Being trained in medical genetics and their respective conditions together with counselling skills, the genetic counsellor bridges the gap between patients and doctors in coordinating genetic tests and discussion of the test results.[328]

Following Up on Carriers

For otherwise healthy family members who were found to carry the abnormal gene, regular medical examination should be perform, beginning at the age of 10 to 12 years. This condition is uncommon in a younger child. Since there is an initial long pre-clinical phase, the carrier may require regular testing to determine if the individual is at increased risk for sudden death. Clinical history and examination are performed, including a resting electrocardiogram, exercise electrocardiography, signal-averaged electrocardiogram and trans-thoracic echocardiogram. When the echocardiogram is non-diagnostic, cardiac magnetic resonance imaging or even *invasive* right ventriculography — which involves putting tubes into the body to the heart and injecting contrast to visualise the heart chamber through X-ray — may be performed. Fortunately, for a group of patients who have been closely monitored, the risk of dying was relatively small, at 0.08 patient per year.[272]

The role of treadmill exercise stress testing was evaluated among 30 asymptomatic individuals who were carriers of a disease-related mutation for ARVC. The findings were compared with 30 healthy subjects who were matched for age and gender.[245] Matching meant that the age and sex of each healthy subject chosen for the study was comparable to one of the carrier. This technique of obtaining a healthy person was to reduce the chances that the results of the study were due to differences in age or gender. An exercise treadmill stress test was performed in all gene carriers and controls. Specific changes in the electrocardiogram and abnormal beats were clearly defined prior to the study. Of the 30 carriers, these pre-specified abnormalities were detected in 24 of them (80%). Although the findings suggested that exercise electrocardiography may identify a substrate for rhythm disorder, the investigators have not shown that it was associated with an adverse outcome. Nonetheless, they believed that this group of individuals deserved closer monitoring.

Ambulatory electrocardiography may also be useful to ascertain the presence of abnormal heart rhythm. In an international study from the Netherlands and the United States, 69 patients from 40 families who were carriers of a mutation for ARVC were studied.[280] Of these,

54 of them underwent ambulatory electrocardiography. A total of 42 individuals were found to have frequent extra beats (greater than 500 in 24 hours) or at least 3 rapid consecutive extra beats on ambulatory electrocardiography or with abnormal baseline electrocardiography were considered to have an abnormal electrical activity. After a mean period of follow-up for about 6 years, 11 patients (16%) experienced potentially dangerous heart rhythms. By 10 years, it was estimated that a third of these patients would have suffered from a potentially lethal cardiac rhythm. Importantly, all of them had electrical abnormalities. The investigators found that the information provided by cardiac magnetic resonance imaging was able to further discriminate patient risk. When an individual had both abnormal electrical activity and cardiac magnetic resonance imaging, the corresponding rate for sustaining a potentially lethal cardiac rhythm was 64%.

There are means to determine if the abnormal heart rhythm can be artificially induced. This procedure is known as electrophysiological study. Several small long electrodes are inserted and placed in various parts of the heart to measure the electrical activity of specific areas and to determine the flow of electrical activity. By studying the characteristics of the electrical signals and stimulating the heart with abnormal beats, doctors may be able to ascertain areas of abnormal tissues and induce the potentially lethal rhythms. This information may be helpful to guide subsequent treatment.[302] Using a three-dimensional approach to map the electrical and mechanical activities of the heart, the accuracy diagnosis of ARVC could be improved.[329] Despite the potential benefits, the usefulness of routine electrophysiological study remains uncertain.[274,287,330] Nonetheless, after identifying the site of origin of abnormal rhythm disorder, ablation of the focus has been used as a form of treatment for ARVC.[301,304,305]

Despite the fear as a result of the lack of predictability of sudden death in a patient with ARVC, implanting an intra-cardiac defibrillator to all patients is generally not indicated, particularly carriers without symptoms.[287] However, when the function in the right heart is severely affected or when both the left and right heart chambers are affected, the risk of sudden death may be high even though the patient does not have any symptom. Under this circumstance, an intra-cardiac defibrillator may be implanted.[215] Another international study of 106 patients with ARVC and at least one high-risk characteristic with an intra-cardiac defibrillator implanted but without an episode of potentially lethal rhythm disorder shed some light on who else may benefit from the use of such a device.[287] After a period of almost 5 years, about a quarter of the patients, despite receiving anti-arrhythmic agents, were successfully treated by the device because of the occurrence of a life-threatening rhythm disorder. When the investigators evaluated which of the factors predicted the appropriate use of the intra-cardiac defibrillator, they found that those who have fainted before were almost three times more likely to require the device. A family member who had died suddenly was not a determinant for this outcome.

From the age of 10 to 20 years, the examination could be performed once in every 2 years. After 20 years old, it may be performed once every 5 years up to the age of 50 to 60 years. The disease seldom presents in older persons. Since those with two or more mutations are at higher risk,[314] whether an intra-cardiac defibrillator should be implanted with less stringent criteria is uncertain.

Unlike patients with ARVC, information on physical activity for otherwise well individuals who are carriers of the abnormal genes is less clear initially. In general, competitive sporting activities for these persons are usually discouraged,[227,282] particularly when there is a family member who had died suddenly. Recently, a clinical study showed that increasing the amount and intensity of exercise were associated with a greater likelihood of diagnosis, abnormal rhythm disorders and development of heart failure among mutation carriers of ARVC genes.[331] In fact, those who exercised frequently were more likely to suffer from an abnormal heart rhythm. When they reduced their exercise duration, the risk was lowered correspondingly. Therefore, they recommended that patients should lower their frequency and intensity of the exercise regimen. Unfortunately, whether this approach leads to a better outcome needs to be clarified. In addition, the routine use of medicines such as beta-blockers or angiotensin converting enzyme inhibitors to prevent sudden death, abnormal heart rhythm or disease progression among carriers is also unknown.[332]

Slipping into Eternal Rest

Death Creeping into Sleep: The Brugada Syndrome

Forgive me if I sleep until I wake up.

Charles Olson (1910–1970)
American Poet

But sometimes, they don't wake up at all. Thus far, unexplained sudden death has generally occurred during periods of activity. At other times, these events happened during sleep. Indeed, people dying in their sleep have created substantial tension between nations. About 30 years ago, approximately 35,000 Thai people were working in the construction industry in Singapore.[333] After a hard day's work, these young men, who were fit and healthy, went to sleep. In the middle of the night, room-mates heard a loud cry, moaning, groaning, snoring, choking, gasping, gurgling, frothing in the mouth, laboured breathing and other noises. Early the next morning, everyone was waking up and getting ready to work on another day in May 1984. One of them, a 37-year-old man was the first person found dead.[334] After this terrifying first experience, the tragic scene kept replaying night after night. Eventually, from May 1984 to July 1994, a total of 407 apparently well young men died in their sleep.[335] "Who's next" was on everyone's mind and soon fear gripped the entire dormitory. What was disturbing was that doctors and forensic scientists were unable to

77

determine the reason for the death. To the young men, they believed that "widow ghosts (phi am)" may be searching for a husband, and stealing their spirits. So to mislead and avoid being chosen, they painted their finger nails red and masqueraded as women by wearing women's clothes and cosmetics. The deaths of young men had created much tension between the Thai and Singapore governments — issues of poor living conditions and harsh treatment to the workers by some employers were intensely debated. On the other hand, cooking from polyvinyl chloride (PVC) tubes was suggested as the cause of the sudden deaths.[336] Instead of using bamboo tubes, PVC tubes were readily available in construction sites. When heated, these plastic pipes emit toxic hydrogen chloride fumes.

Although the term "sudden unexplained nocturnal death syndrome" or SUNDS was coined, this phenomenon has been reported in several countries. However, not all deaths occurred while sleeping. In Thailand, it is known as "Lai Tai" and has been linked to eating rice cakes or noodles. In rural Northeast Thailand, the estimated annual incidence for men between the ages of 20 to 49 years was 25.9 per 100,000, with seasonal variation, peaking from March to May.[337] More than 40% of their relatives suffered from a similar fate. Ranging from 1 in 5 to 1 in 6 of them also had brothers who had died suddenly.

However, SUNDS has been reported in the Philippines as early as 1917.[338] The condition, known as "bangungut", was brought to attention again in Hawaii in 1948[339] and in 1960 when 11 Filipino sailors died in a similar fashion in the U.S. Naval Base in Guam.[340] "Bangon" means "to rise" and "ungol" means "to groan" during sleep in Tagalog. The perpetrator was believed to be the Batibat, a large female spirit who lived in trees which had been cut down to make beds or houses. As part of her revenge, she would sit on the face or chest of the young men sleeping on those beds or in those houses. From 1948 to 1982, the rate of SUNDS for men between the ages of 25 and 44 years increased from 10.8 to 26.3 per 100,000 person years in Manila.[341] Although these deaths were seasonal, they peaked from December to January. Initially, they were attributed to acute haemorrhagic pancreatitis, voracious eating and excessive drinking.

After the Second World War, there were a series of battles fought in Indochina. In one of the most protracted conflicts, several refugees migrated to various other countries, including the United States. From 15 July 1977 to 30 March 1982, there were at least 51 sudden unexplained deaths among these migrants and the phenomenon of sudden unexplained death re-emerged.[342] What was alarming was that the incidence was approximated to the sum of the five leading causes of death among American men in the same age group. Fortunately, the incidence of these events began to decline after 1982.[343] Majority of refugees were Hmong people from Laos and Vietnam, and they called it "tsob tsuang" due to an assault by an evil spirit.[344] Unlike the others, post-mortem examination showed that the heart was enlarged in 14 out of 18. There were also abnormalities in conduction system.[345] However, the significance of these anomalies was unclear. Majority of these deaths occurred among refugees who had recently arrived in the United States. Since these occurrences decreased with time subsequently, the investigators felt that the improvement in diet could have accounted for the decline of SUNDS. Initially, the underlying cause for sudden deaths was deficiency of vitamin B1 or thiamine[346,347] and abnormal electrolyte levels in the blood.[348] The other observation was the shortening of the QT-interval.[346] This electrocardiographic abnormality may be associated with ventricular fibrillation,[349] which was a disorganised rhythm of the heart and the principal mechanism of causing sudden deaths.

Among different cultures, SUNDS is known by various names. In Japan, it is called "pok-kuri". Even the word "mare" in "nightmare", in old English, refers to a demon torturing those who are sleeping, by riding and trampling on the chest. In the Western world, there is the "Night Hag", which was derived from Polish mythology. "Krisky" or "Plasky" is the shadow with bright red eyes that sits on the chest to torment and draw energy from the sleeper. Eventually, the terror of the night was exposed.

The Brugada Syndrome

In 1987, a man from Poland brought his 3-year-old son to see a cardiologist in the Netherlands because of recurrent fainting episodes and cardiac arrest.[350] His elder sister also suffered from the same symptoms and died at the age of 3 years despite pacemaker implantation and a potent drug used to treat abnormal heart rhythm. Dr Pedro Brugada had not seen that abnormal pattern in the electrocardiogram before — looking like a shark or dolphin fin. The father went back into the Iron Curtain and brought the electrocardiograms of the sister. Indeed, the tracings appeared similar. As more of these cases were identified when doctors began to recognise the unique pattern, the Brugada syndrome was reported in 1992,[351] consisting of a unique electrocardiographic tracing and is associated with increased risk of sudden death. Unlike the other conditions, only about 10% of deaths occur during or after some form of strenuous activities.[352] Majority of them occurred at rest, half of which happened during sleep.

In fact, in one city in Japan, the prevalence of this electrocardiographic abnormality was estimated to be 120 per 100,000 inhabitants.[353] Subsequently, the link between SUNDS and Brugada syndrome was established by Thai investigators,[354] with the same type of abnormal electrocardiographic pattern. Examination of the conduction system in the electrophysiology laboratory of the Thai patients[354] showed changes consistent with the autopsy results of the Southeast Asian immigrants in the United States.[345] Subsequently, these two conditions were shown to be similar phenotypically, genetically and functionally.[355]

From an obscure and esoteric condition, Brugada syndrome has become a common cause of sudden death, accounting for 4% of all sudden deaths.[269] But among those with sudden death and structurally normal hearts, this condition accounted for more than 20% of the deaths.[269] Typically, the condition affects a young man, presenting with a rhythm disorder, usually during sleep, at the age of 40 years.

The reason for normal appearance of the heart is that the abnormality lies in the sodium channel of muscle fibre, which is not visible to the naked eye. There are several types of channels in the lining of the heart muscle which direct the flow of various ions, such as sodium, potassium and calcium, in and out of the cell. The lining is similar to a wall and these channels are like gates to allow substances to move in and out of the cell. In this case, the portals are specific for certain type ion or ions. Movement of these ions generates voltage and electrical activity, resulting in muscle contraction and relaxation. These channels are made from complex protein structures. Like all proteins, its synthesis is regulated by a particular genetic code, deoxyribonucleic acid (DNA). Changes in the blueprint, otherwise known as mutation, would result in the formation of an abnormal ion channel. This condition is inherited in an autosomal dominant fashion, which means that the offspring would have 1 in 2 chance of succumbing to this condition. If the ion channel does not function well, the heart may not pump normally. In the worst case scenario, the heart stops and this is how a person with Brugada syndrome dies. During the period when there is a lack of oxygen in the brain, the victim may groan and has seizure-like activity with frothing of the mouth, as described by several witnesses. But as to the trigger of the lethal rhythm, it remains unknown. To date, there are more than 290 mutations that are linked to a particular sodium ion channel for the Brugada syndrome, which account for more than 75% of patients when there is an abnormal gene. However, these changes were detected in about 21% of the patients with unrelated Brugada syndrome.[356] Since this finding has been subsequently corroborated by a large international collaboration to determine the genetic abnormalities of unrelated patients with Brugada syndrome,[357] using such an approach in identifying patients is unlikely to be useful. On the other hand, it also suggests that there are other ion channels[358] that may be diseased in the condition.

Making the Diagnosis

To make a diagnosis of Brugada syndrome, the individual does not only have the pathognomonic electrocardiographic pattern but should have at least one of the following: life-threatening abnormal heart rhythm (either spontaneous or induced by the doctor in a controlled setting), agonal breathing during sleep, sudden death of a family member younger than 45 years, and family member with similar electrocardiographic findings (Figure 12).[269] Unfortunately, the "diagnostic" pattern in the electrocardiogram, not uncommonly, fluctuates. Sometimes, it may appear by shifting the position of the electrocardiographic leads in the right chest.[269] Importantly, food intake, particularly

Normal electrocardiographic pattern

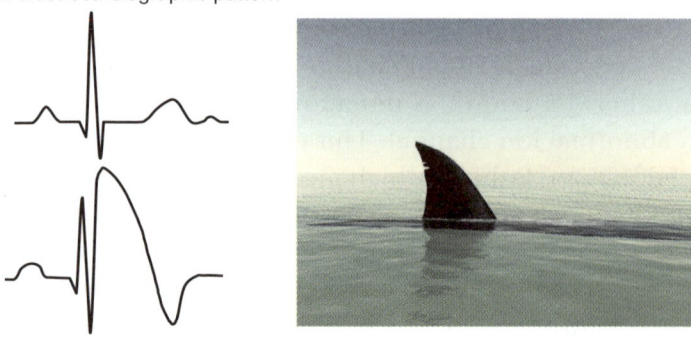

Brugada electrocardiographic pattern
looking like a shark fin

Figure 12. The Brugada electrocardiographic pattern.

The ST-segment is elevated and convex upwards, looking like a shark fin lurking around, seeking someone to devour. There are also changes in the P-wave and T-wave. Image of shark's fin is obtained from Shuttlestock; Image ID: 40797514.

heavy meals, can accentuate the abnormal electrocardiographic pattern.[359,360] In addition, fever[361] and certain types of medicines,[269] in particular those affecting the autonomic system or conduction system of the heart,[362] may unravel this unique tracing. The changes may be further accentuated by modifying the chest leads.[363] With greater awareness of this syndrome, there are an increasing number of medical conditions that could mimic the changes (Figure 13).[269]

Variability in the electrocardiographic pattern has an impact on diagnosis and prognosis. In a study of 43 patients, only one had persistent electrocardiographic changes over a 29-month period.[364] Another 22 of them (51%) had either the Brugada pattern during the initial or subsequent visits. By about 103 days, 13 of the 14 patients (93%) with abnormal baseline electrocardiogram turned into non-diagnostic pattern. The remaining 20 subjects (47%) did not have spontaneous abnormal electrocardiographic pattern. It was only revealed following administration of certain medicines. In a study of family members of an individual with Brugada syndrome, there were 35 of them who were genetic carriers but did not have a diagnostic electrocardiogram. A drug, ajmaline, was administered intravenously

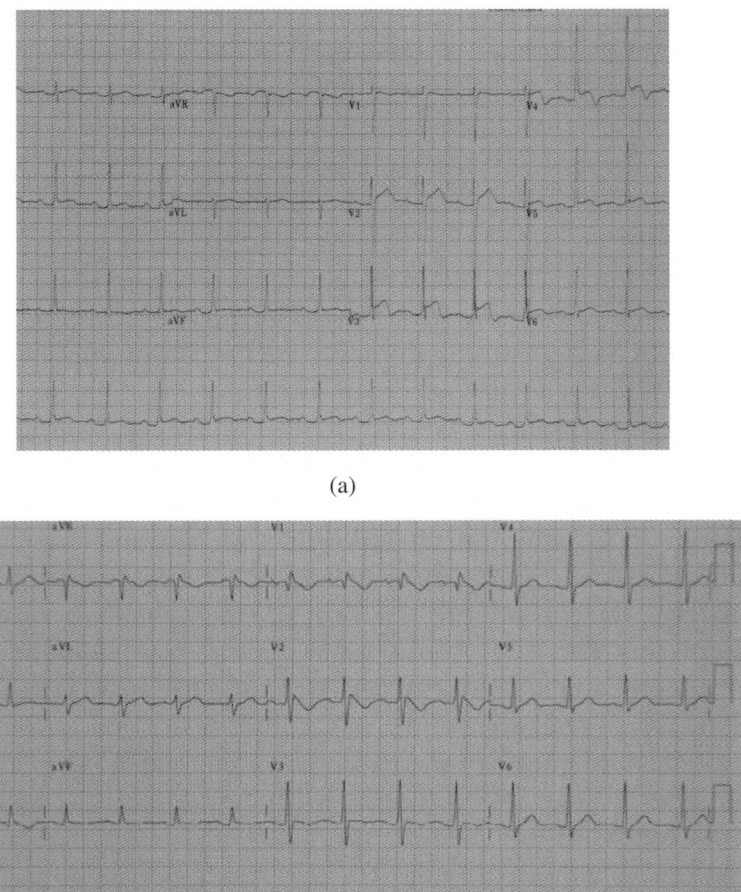

(a)

(b)

Figure 13. Brugada electrocardiographic pattern.

Early repolarisation pattern (panel A) is commonly seen among young individuals and may be mistaken for Brugada syndrome (panel B).

to induce the abnormal electrocardiographic changes and was found to be positive in 80% of them.[365] However, it was also positive in 2 (6%) of 36 other family members who were not carriers and did not have a diagnostic electrocardiogram.

Since 1958, 4,788 Japanese, younger than 50 years, in Nagasaki have been followed up biennially as part of a study of the Radiation Effects Research Foundation.[366] Routine electrocardiography was performed as part of the examination and the incidence of Brugada-like abnormality was 14.2 per 100,000 person-years. Of those with follow-up information, this electrocardiographic change was present consistently in only 11%. Nonetheless, its presence connotes a poorer prognosis. The risk of dying from any cause was slightly more than two times for those with Brugada-like electrocardiogram compared with those without the abnormality. More importantly, the risk of sudden unexpected death was more than 50 times greater over the 40-year period. However, the absolute risk was low, with an annual rate for sudden death of 0.01%. In a different Japanese city, Osaka, the rate of sudden death for those with Brugada-type abnormality in asymptomatic individuals was 0.39% yearly.[353] During routine medical examination of another 3,339 otherwise healthy Japanese, the prevalence of Brugada-like electrocardiographic pattern was 1.22%.[367] About 42% showed normalisation of the abnormality over the 10-year period. In the group of Japanese, the annual risk of fatal arrhythmia was 0.25%.

Genetic diagnosis of Brugada syndrome may be appealing but is limited by several constraints, including costs. Innovative techniques will continue to lower the price of genetic ascertainment. Importantly, abnormal genes for the condition are found in less than 30%. Furthermore, there is always the challenge of differentiating between a mutation and a rare variant. They are describing the same phenomenon of change in the genetic make-up of an individual and mutations believed to occur in patients. On the other hand, genetic variants are known to occur in 2% to 5% of normal individuals.[356] However, genetic testing may be useful in evaluating family members of patients with Brugada syndrome.

Predictors of Outcome

In a follow-up study of 200 patients with Brugada syndrome and their family members, the researchers investigated how electrocardiographic pattern, previous fainting episodes, abnormal genetic markers, family history of sudden death and gender would affect outcome.[368] They found that the occurrence of cardiac arrest was more than six times higher when the patient has a diagnostic electrocardiogram and history of faint. On the other hand, those with only abnormal electrocardiogram, the risk was about two times higher. In contrast, when the electrocardiogram was non-diagnostic with or without fainting spell, the risk was low. In another recent study, the risk for an abnormal rhythm event was more than four times higher when the Brugada type of electrocardiogram was present spontaneously.[369] Recently, history of sudden death in family members was evaluated in 280 individuals with Brugada type of electrocardiogram.[370] They found that even first-degree relatives who were younger than 35 years that had died suddenly did not increase the risk of sudden death. Similar to the earlier study, these investigators reported that the absence of fainting, aborted cardiac arrest, spontaneous abnormal electrocardiographic pattern or abnormal heart rhythm that could be induced by the doctors in the laboratory was associated with a good 5-year outcome.

Initially, prognosis was thought to be poorer for men for this condition.[371] Recently, the prognosis of 1,029 consecutive patients from 11 tertiary centres and four European countries (France, Italy, the Netherlands and Germany) was ascertained.[372] More than a third of them had survived from a cardiac arrest or fainted before. The median duration of follow-up was 32 months, and the average annual rates for the occurrence of a potentially fatal rhythm disorder or sudden death were 7.7% and 1.9% for those who had survived a cardiac arrest and fainted, respectively. For the asymptomatic subjects, this rate was 0.5% yearly. The investigators did not find that family history of sudden death, male gender, presence of the mutated gene and an abnormal heart rhythm which could be induced by the doctors in the laboratory predicted a poor outcome. Only the presence of symptoms and spontaneously Brugada type electrocardiogram were associated with increased risk of abnormal heart rhythm and sudden death. While the majority of these investigations were from the West, the significance of Brugada type electrocardiogram was reported from a Japanese population.[373] Of 13,904 middle-aged men examined in Osaka in 1997, whereby electrocardiogram was routinely performed, Brugada type pattern was detected in 98 (0.7%) of them. After about eight years, the risks of death or dying from heart disease were not significantly different between those with and without Brugada type electrocardiogram, at 4% and 1%, respectively.

As the number of individuals with the Brugada type of electrocardiogram became increasingly recognised, the principal challenge is to identify asymptomatic patients who are at high-risk for sudden death. Electrophysiological studies are invasive tests performed in a controlled environment by trained doctors and technicians to induce the potentially fatal rhythms. It is a series of programmed electrical stimuli applied to the heart. In this procedure, long wires are inserted from the groin, and sometimes from the neck as well, to enter into the various chambers of the heart. Electrical pulses are generated in sequences in prescribed protocols which may result in abnormal rhythms. Previously, it was believed that when the abnormal rhythm is reproduced, the likelihood for sudden death for that person was greater.[269,374] However, subsequent review of the various scientific publications did not establish the usefulness of this approach.[375] Recently, another rigorous evaluation of this technique showed the poor utility in the risk assessment of abnormal heart rhythm.[369] However, these investigators showed that detailed analysis of the electrocardiogram may be helpful in identifying high-risk individuals.[369,376]

Patient Management

Various medicines, including beta-blockers[377] and amiodarone (Cordarone),[378] have not been shown to be effective in preventing sudden death in patients with Brugada syndrome. However, an old medicine, quinidine, may be useful in this case and can prevent laboratory-induced potentially lethal rhythm.[379,380] Cilostazol has also been shown to normalise the Brugada type electrocardiogram in a patient.[381] But overall, only the intra-cardiac defibrillator was useful in preventing sudden death. This is a small device that is implanted into the body and wired to the heart. It can detect abnormal heart rhythms and the micro-computer would analyse and determine if an electrical energy is needed to terminate it. Patients who have survived a cardiac arrest or syncope are likely to benefit from this device.[269,374] Others have evaluated the role of ablation of the right ventricular outflow tract as a therapeutic modality for Brugada syndrome.[382] The rationale was based on the source of the abnormal rhythm, at the outflow tract of the right ventricle. Using sophisticated technology to locus the source, radiofrequency energy was applied to ablate it. Of the nine patients who received this treatment, eight showed normalisation of the Brugada type of electrocardiogram and outcome at 20 months was excellent.

However, its usefulness for asymptomatic individuals is uncertain. As with all interventions in medicine, the potential risk for fatal rhythm disorder must be weighed against risk of implanting the intra-cardiac defibrillator, risk of inappropriate shocks, infection, lead (wire) fracture and quality of life.

"Ah-choo!" "...and you're dead!"
Infection and Inflammation of the Heart: Myocarditis

"Neither rain, nor snow, nor sniffle, nor fever shall keep me from my training schedule."

The Runner's Creed

For the past two days, a 16-year-old has been suffering from a sore-throat and mild fever. There was a flu-bug floating around and his nephews and nieces were sneezing. So, his parents treated him with Panadol Extra and he felt better and continued schooling. Peter was an active boy and liked to play soccer. He was healthy and did not have any pre-existing medical problems. Whenever there was an opportunity, he would gather his friends together and play street soccer. During recess one day, Peter was playing football. A few minutes later, he collapsed suddenly. His friends and teachers tried to revive him. The paramedics arrived shortly and continued cardiopulmonary resuscitation. One of them held a mask over his nose and mouth with her hand and pumped on a bag with the other hand to assist in his breathing. Another paramedic was compressing the chest. Peter was moved quickly into the ambulance and rushed to the hospital. Unfortunately, he passed away soon after arriving at the hospital.

Myocarditis is, in fact, a heterogenous group of conditions and is defined by World Health Organization (WHO) / International Society and Federation of Cardiology (ISFC) as inflammation of the heart muscle that is seen on microscopic examination.[383] It shows white blood cells gathering around the small blood vessels and infiltrating into the heart muscle tissue. In addition, there is evidence of cell death. Using special staining techniques, certain cells can be identi-fied. However, obtaining muscle tissue from a patient suspected of the condition may not be always possible, particularly when there is risk of performing an endomyocardial biopsy. Therefore, the diagnosis is usually made based on the clinical presentation of the individual and excluding other causes. Furthermore, the patient may present with acute heart failure, rhythm disorders and sudden death. On the other hand, it may be a gradual smothering disease. Importantly, the pres-ence of specific cells that is seen under the microscope, such as eosinophilic and giant cell types, may respond to specific treatment.

Although in clinical practice, the cause for the myocarditis epi-sode could not be categorically elucidated in many instances, the majority are attributed to a viral infection and the inflammation induced following a viral infection.[384] It was first described by a French physician, Professor Jean Nicholas Corvisart in 1812.[385] While heart attacks received most of the attention, understanding of inflammation and infectious agents have renewed interest in myo-carditis. For several years, enteroviruses and adenovirus were the common agents that were believed to cause myocarditis.[386] These viruses are known to cause upper respiratory tract infection and gastro-enteritis not infrequently. In fact, about 90% of patients with heart failure and biopsy-proven myocarditis had symptoms of viral respiratory or gastro-intestinal infection prior to the onset of the condition.[387] Other viruses, such as cytomegalovirus, parvovirus B19, human herpesvirus 6, Epstein-Barr virus[388] and even the influenza virus[389,390] are increasingly recognised to be the causative agent for myocarditis. While almost everyone would have acquired an infec-tion from one or more of these viruses, it remains unclear as to why the minority succumb to myocarditis. Although the specific sites of infection were also unknown, parvovirus B19 has been detected in the linings of small blood vessels in the heart but not in the mus-cle.[391] The inflammatory reaction subsequently generated various chemical mediators that could result in the death of the muscle cells. Other viruses could also cause damage to heart muscle cells directly, inducing cell death.[392] Less commonly, microbial agents, including bacteria and parasites, toxins and drugs[393] have also been known to cause myocarditis. There are other specific conditions such as sarcoidosis or autoimmune diseases that are associated with myocarditis. However, these patients may have other signs and symptoms related to the primary disorder.

The understanding of underlying mechanisms causing myocarditis has increased substantially in recent decades. There are special proteins or receptors on the surface of the heart muscle cells that facilitate the entry of the viruses.[394] By designing an animal in which the protein was removed, entry of the virus was prevented. Inflammation of the heart muscle was adverted.[395] Furthermore, some individuals may have a genetic predisposition whereby the body mounts an immunological reaction resulting in inflammation and damage to the heart. Indeed, presence of antibodies to cardiac muscle among relatives of patients with myocarditis may identify those at risk.[396] Genetic mutations giving rise to dysfunctional heart muscle proteins may also increase an individual susceptibility to myocarditis.[397] These characteristics may explain, at least in part, as to why certain individuals succumb to the condition.

Is Myocarditis Common?

Severity of symptoms of patients with myocarditis varies substantially. Since there are those who may suffer from myocarditis without any symptom, the incidence cannot be clearly established. In addition, the proportion of myocarditis causing sudden death ranges widely because of the manner in which the information is collected. When the symptoms are mild, these patients may not be detected. Hence, the true incidence in any community is likely to be unknown. But when a catastrophic sudden death occurs in a young person, it is usually widely publicised which incites fear among parents and the general public. The expectation is high and one death is always one too many.

Nonetheless, information from post-mortem studies provides some insight on the frequency of myocarditis as a cause of sudden death in a population. From January 1994 to April 2003, coroners in the United Kingdom collaborated to record all cases of sudden cardiac deaths in adult.[22] In their study, they excluded patients with coronary artery and other heart disease. There were 453 cases and the age ranged from 15 to 81 years, with median age of 32 years. Myocarditis accounted for 8.6% of the deaths. On the other hand, in Israel, myocarditis is an important cause for sudden death among the young. Over a 10-year period, there were 162 persons less than 40 years of age who died suddenly in Israel.[39] For those less than 30 years old, myocarditis accounted for 22% of the deaths. It was 11% for the deceased who were 30 years and older.

Among 1,606,167 medically screened healthy United States Air Force recruits undergoing a 42-day basic military training from 1965 to 1985, 19 sudden deaths occurred.[398] Importantly, strenuous physical exertion was associated with sudden death in 17 of the 19 deceased. The corresponding rate was estimated to be 0.034 death per 100,000 exercise-hours and myocarditis was the most common underlying cause (42%).

Do I have Myocarditis?

Patients who have myocarditis usually have a recent flu-like illness, and the symptoms may be mild. In other words, the person may not be particularly sick with high fever, incessant runny nose, scorching sore-throat and a hacking cough. Symptoms may be non-specific, ranging from tiredness, muscle ache and just a general feeling of being unwell. There may be accompanying mild fever with respiratory or gastrointestinal symptoms, such as abdominal discomfort and loose stools. The patient may feel that shortness of breath occurred more readily than before. Thus, it was not surprising that only about a third of 174 patients with biopsy-proven myocarditis actually recalled suffering from a viral infection in the previous six months.[399] However, these patients were referred for rhythm disorder and heart transplantation in Italy and the acute episode of myocarditis could have occurred several months or years earlier. On the other hand, for those who were aware of a recent infection, myocarditis occurred after 1 to 4 weeks after the acute episode. Indeed, the peak interval between the infection and onset of myocarditis is about 7 to 10 days.[400] In rare instances, the initial presentation could be fatal. Sudden death is generally the result of a lethal rhythm disorder or fulminant heart failure,[401] and is commonly associated with some form of physical exertion.[398] Although the episode of myocarditis may be asymptomatic (and hence unrecognised), the most common symptom is chest pain as a result of inflammation of the sac around the heart, known as pericarditis.[401] The pain is usually sharp and is aggravated by breathing in, especially when taking a deep breath. Its intensity diminishes on leaning forward. At other times, the patient may present with severe shortness of breath or low blood pressure.[400] These symptoms and signs may be the result of a severely weakened heart. In less severe circumstances, the patient may just have heart failure, particularly for human herpesvirus 6 infection.[402] He or she may feel breathless more readily than before. There are other patients whose presentation is similar to someone with a heart attack,[393] especially when those infected with parvovirus B19.[402]

While the resting electrocardiogram is commonly used as a screening diagnostic tool,[393] it is not a sensitive or specific test for myocarditis.[399] Occasionally, the electrocardiogram may be normal and a high index of suspicion by the attending physician may clinch the diagnosis.[401] Blood tests, such as assays for cardiac enzymes and *high sensitivity* troponins, should be performed to detect damage to the heart muscle. Again, the results merely indicate if there is injury and its extent but do not provide the cause. As expected, markers for inflammation, such as total white cell count, C-reactive protein and erythrocyte sedimentation rate, are raised during the acute phase of the condition. The structure and function of the heart could be readily assessed with ultrasonic examination or echocardiography.[393] However, a normal study does not rule out myocarditis, especially when the clinical presentation, electrocardiography and cardiac biomarkers are consistent with the diagnosis. A more sophisticated form of imaging, cardiac magnetic resonance, is better able to characterise the heart muscle tissue. In particular, it is able to determine swelling and scarring as a result of inflammation and cell death. Using different techniques of magnetic resonance imaging and use of gadolinium contrast, the degree of accuracy for the diagnosis of myocarditis was high.[403]

However, the pattern of presentation has an impact on the ability to make the diagnosis of myocarditis. It is highest for patients who have symptoms of a heart attack.[404] Cardiac magnetic resonance (CMR) imaging may also help to differentiate between reversible and irreversible damage to the heart muscle.[405] It is also useful in following up patients with myocarditis regarding the degree of inflammation in the heart.[406] Nonetheless, criteria have been established based on CMR.[407]

Coronary angiography is generally recommended to rule out narrowing or occlusion of the coronary artery as the cause for injury to the heart. Taking samples of the heart muscle may provide insight on the underlying cause of myocarditis, type and extent of inflammation. The approach of obtaining heart muscle tissue to be examined under the microscope, the procedure known as endomyocardial biopsy, has been adopted to be the "gold standard" for the diagnosis of myocarditis.[383,384,393,408] In addition, other information provided by detailed analysis of the sample may be useful in guiding treatment for the patient.[393] However, the invasive nature and the potential for sampling error[409,410] precluded its broad utilisation. The yield from one specimen was about 25%. When more than five samples were taken, the diagnosis was made in about two-thirds of the patients with myocarditis.

Technological advances in electronics, biosensors and computing power have improved the imaging capability of magnetic resonance imaging. To evaluate the diagnostic capability of CMR in making the diagnosis of myocarditis, the technique was compared with taking muscle tissue for examination. In a study of 132 patients,[411] with acute (n = 70) and sub-acute (n = 62) myocarditis, CMR, using current diagnostic criteria,[407] could only accurately identify about two-thirds (68%) of patients with biopsy-proven myocarditis. Not unexpectedly, the performance of CMR improved to 79% when only patients with symptoms less than 2 weeks, especially among those who presented as if they had a heart attack, were analysed.

One of the current diagnostic strategies in the management of patients with myocarditis is to demonstrate the presence of a recent viral infection. These tests are designed to detect the presence of antibodies against a specific virus in the blood. Although they have been used frequently, they have not been shown to be particularly useful.[412] Another technique is to detect the virus in the heart itself. However, the yield of viral material has also been poor among patients suffering from myocarditis. In an Italian study of 174 patients whose heart muscle tissue was found to be consistent with myocarditis,[399] viral genetic material was only detected in a quarter of them (26%). In a German study involving 124 patients suspected of having myocarditis and undergoing endomyocardial biopsy of the heart muscle, the correlation between the blood levels of antibodies of viral infection and myocarditis was poor.[412] There were only 5 patients (4%) with antibodies detected in the blood had the same virus that was found in the heart muscle. Furthermore, since these viruses are common, the antibodies may be present in a significant proportion of the population. Since there may be reactivation or re-infection of the same virus, interpretation of the blood tests may be difficult. As such, these blood tests are performed less frequently in the context of making a diagnosis of myocarditis. Recently, blood tests have been developed to detect antibodies directed towards various components of the heart muscle.[393]

What Happens after Myocarditis?

When the diagnosis of myocarditis is made, the patient is usually managed symptomatically and closely monitored for the occurrence of abnormal heart rhythms and heart failure. Some of the rhythm disorders can be fatal, and likely to be the cause of sudden death. Although its occurrence is unpredictable, physical exertion is believed to increase the risk of sudden death. Patients with heart failure should be treated according to current guidelines. Less frequently, during the acute phase of myocarditis, the afflicted may present with cardiorespiratory collapse as a result of severe pump failure. In these situations, mortality is high. Although heart-lung machines have been used for open heart surgery for several decades, a less invasive procedure, the intra-aortic balloon pimping (IABP) was available for circulatory support at the bedside. To use the heart-lung machine, large tubes are inserted in the great vessels of the body during the operation and blood is artificially pumped through a set of complex equipment to receive oxygen and remove carbon dioxide. Hence, this system allows surgeons to operate on the beating or non-beating heart. On the other hand, a large balloon catheter is inserted and placed in the large blood vessel in the chest, known as the aorta, during IABP. This balloon inflates and deflates according to the heart cycle to assist in drawing blood out of the less traumatic heart. But the support provided by IABP may not be sufficient, especially in sicker patients. Better tubing which is coated with blood thinner, pumping machinery and more durable equipment for gas exchange have allowed the bypass technique to be performed and maintained by the bedside. The tubes are inserted through the vessels in the groin instead. Known as percutaneous extracorporeal membrane oxygenation (ECMO), this technology has improved the survival in some of these critically ill patients. What this device does is to allow the heart to rest and recover from the acute episode of inflammation. Of 14 patients with fulminant myocarditis receiving this mode of treatment, 10 of them survived (71%). The average time that the device was used was five and a half days. After the acute phase, the long-term outcome of these survivors was comparable to other patients with myocarditis.[413]

In addition to supportive treatment, there are specific approaches that are used to manage patients with myocarditis. A clinical trial was designed to evaluate if the routine use of treatment to suppress inflammation in patients with myocarditis improve outcome.[387] In this study of 111 patients, multi-centre study, heart function and survival were not improved with such treatment. On the other hand, certain specific types of myocarditis can be treated with anti-viral therapies or agents that modulate or suppress inflammation. In a study of 85 patients without viral material in the heart muscle, those treated with the combination of two anti-inflammatory agents have been shown to improve heart function.[414]

Sporting activities should be avoided until the condition is completely resolved. Athletes should defer competitions for at least 6 months after the initial episode.[415] A medical examination should be performed prior to resumption of training and participation of the exercise. Also, non-athletes should also not perform physical activities for 6 months after the onset of myocarditis.[393] All patients with myocarditis should be followed up in the long-term.

Outcome of patients with myocarditis tends to be poorer among men[399,416] and those younger than 40 years old,[416] particularly children.[417] Those who are breathless on minimal physical activity, signs of inflammation and lack beta-blocker therapy fared worse, and were more likely to die or undergo heart transplantation.[418] Mortality is higher for those who present with heart failure, especially when both the right and left heart chambers are involved, compared to patients who had symptoms of heart attack or rhythm disorder.[399] Certain markers in the blood may be useful to predict outcome of patients with myocarditis.[419]

One of the long-term adverse consequences of myocarditis is the development of dilated cardiomyopathy. However, the occurrence is dependent on the method of diagnosis of myocarditis. In a series from the Stanford University Medical Center, 20 patients who were found to have acute myocarditis and had undergone at least two biopsy procedures were followed up for an average of 5 months.[420] The heart became enlarged and weakened in 8 (40%) of them. A report from the King's College Hospital corroborated their findings.[421] From 1980 to 1984, there were 23 patients who were suspected of suffering from acute myocarditis and 12 (52%) of them developed dilated cardiomyopathy after an average follow-up period of 43 months.

Although it is believed that the progression of acute myocarditis to dilated cardiomyopathy is an inflammatory response to an immunological reaction,[422] treatment with anti-inflammatory or immunosuppressive agents did not affect outcome.[387,420] Examining heart muscle tissues repeatedly did not identify specific structures or cell types, including those pertaining to degree of healing or scarring, which could have predicted if the patient will develop dilated cardiomyopathy.[420,421]

Since there is no specific clinical indicator or marker for myocarditis, the key message is to avoid strenuous activities during an acute febrile illness. Even if myocarditis does not develop, temperature rises in the body during exercise. So, the patient may feel hot and sick. Listen to your body. While a person with a runny nose or sneezing may be able to perform light physical activities such as walking or stretching exercises, he or she should rest when tired or experiencing weak or constitutional symptoms such as fever, cough and body ache.

"I Have Just Had a Baby, Not a Cardiac Arrest!"

A Large Weak Heart: Dilated Cardiomyopathy

"Too Big to Fail: The Inside Story of a Cardiac Meltdown"

Adapted from the title of the book by Andrew Ross Sorkin

Deborah Coleman was 32 years old when she was having her second child.[423] After 12 hours of labour, her baby was in distress and an emergency Caesarean section was needed. Instead of regaining consciousness after the operation, Deborah woke up a few days later. To her astonishment, she was told that she had a cardiac arrest. Sceptical of it, Deborah sharply rebutted the doctors, "I'd just had a baby!" Indeed, her baby saved her life. As she was in the operating theatre, her heart stopped. Deborah was promptly resuscitated, and both mother and boy survived. She was placed on life support for 18 hours followed by a medically-induced coma for another two days. Her keen memory and astute mental state were a clear testimony of the excellent treatment Deborah received. However, she could not believe it happened as she maintains a regular exercise regimen and healthy diet. Deborah is a non-smoker and drinks rarely. She did not have coronary heart disease or dissection. Instead, Deborah has a rather uncommon condition known as dilated cardiomyopathy. In many of the cases, the cause is unknown. About 20% to 35% of patients occurred in families and the pattern of inheritance varies.[424] It may be inherited and her son was subsequently found to have this condition. Despite these setbacks, she continued her pursuits and became an accomplished photojournalist, graduating with honours in Photojournalism and Documentary Photography from the University of Gloucestershire, United Kingdom, 17 years later.[425] Her creativity and passion for images continued to fill her work in various exhibitions in Swindon, Wiltshire, in the United Kingdom.

A Huge Flopsy Heart

This condition is characterised by an enlarged heart chamber with weak contraction and is a disease of the heart muscle.[84] It becomes flabby and is unable to pump normally (Figure 14). As a result, the heart chamber becomes progressively larger. Traditionally, there is no other cause for the weak heart muscle such as narrowing of the blood vessel, high blood pressure or abnormal heart valves.[97] Previous episodes of myocarditis could have accounted for 30% to 50% of patients with this condition.[426,427] Dilated cardiomyopathy may also be the result of damage from toxic substances, such as alcohol or drugs, other infectious agents, including parasites, prolonged

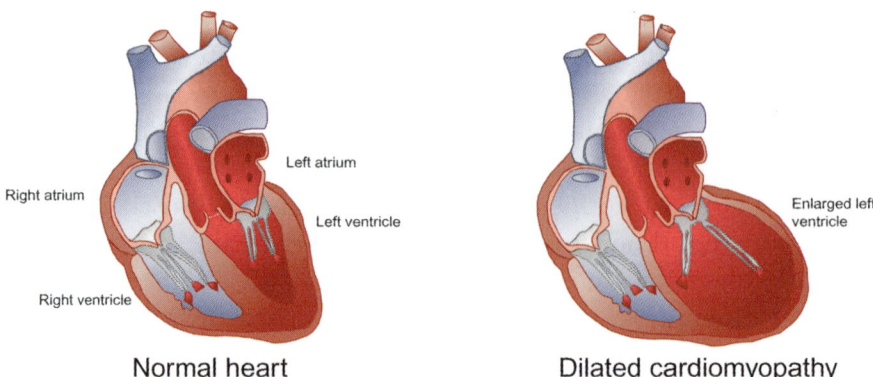

Normal heart   Dilated cardiomyopathy

Figure 14.   Dilated cardiomyopathy.

The normal heart consists of four chambers, the right atrium and ventricle and the left atrium and ventricle. Of these, the left ventricle is the pump that propels blood out of the heart to most parts of the body. In dilated cardiomyopathy, this chamber is enlarged and the contraction is weakened.

periods of rapid heartbeats,[428] hormonal disorders or autoimmue diseases.[84] However, the cause could not be identified in about half of the 1,280 patients with cardiomyopathy referred for further assessment at the Johns Hopkins Medical Center.[429]

It is estimated that there are 40 to 50 patients with dilated cardio-myopathy per 100,000 persons,[85] and occurs about twice more frequently among men. Again, the prevalence may vary with different geographical regions.[97] This condition may account for 2% to 4% of those with heart failure.[430] While the most common age of onset is in the third and fourth decade, it can also be found in children.[84] Although variable, the annual mortality rate was estimated to be as high as 20%.[431] Almost 30% to 50% of them died suddenly.[431]

About 30% to 48% of these patients may have associated with some form of genetic inheritance.[432] But the mode of inheritance is heterogenous, involving more than 40 genes.[84,93] While the predominant mode is autosomal dominant, less commonly, transmission is autosomal recessive or X-linked.[93] Importantly, the 2-year survival is less than 50%,[433,434] and 30% to 40% of them die suddenly.[433–435] Certain types of mutation are known to be associated with a poorer outcome.[436] Participation in competitive sports for these patients was associated with a greater risk for sudden death.[436]

Treatment for Dilated Cardiomyopathy

Management of patients with dilated cardiomyopathy is similar to treatment for heart failure. Beta-blockers have been shown to improve heart pumping function and reverse the morphological changes associated with dilated cardiomyopathy. This benefit may be mediated, at least in part, by modifying gene expression of the heart muscle cell.[437] When heart failure is severe, use of beta-blockers improved survival by more than a third.[438] Trimetazidine is a metabolic modulator which optimises the way the heart utilises energy. Indeed, not only heart function was improved but there were other metabolic effects in non-heart tissues.[439] Although statins, a group of potent cholesterol lowering medicines, have been shown to improve outcomes by preventing heart attack and stroke,[440] they also possess anti-inflammatory effects.[441] As such, there may be other effects of statins that may not be related to the cholesterol lowering effect. Indeed, the use of statins was associated with more than three-quarters reduction in the chance of dying among patients with dilated cardiomyopathy.[442] Co-enzyme Q10 supplementation may also be useful for this group of patients.[443] Since a significant proportion of patients with dilated cardiomyopathy died suddenly, implantation of an intra-cardiac defibrillator has been associated with a 31% reduction in mortality.[444]

Identifying Those at High Risk

Not every patient with this condition dies suddenly. In particular, the use of an intra-cardiac defibrillator did not show benefit to patients with dilated cardiomyopathy[445] but without potentially lethal rhythm disorder. This device is recommended for patients suffering from this condition with ejection fraction less than 30% to 35% and breathlessness on mild to moderate exertion despite being treated with adequate medicines.[374] However, only 30% of individuals who died suddenly in Oregon had severe left ventricular systolic dysfunction, with ejection fraction less than 35%.[446] On the other hand, left ejection fraction was greater than 30% in more than 56% of persons who died suddenly in Maastricht area in the Netherlands.[3] Moreover, about 20% of them had left ventricular ejection more than 50%. Using symptom and left ventricular ejection fraction as criteria for implantation of intra-cardiac defibrillator to prevent sudden death, the sensitivity and specificity is 71% and 51%, respectively.[447] As such, the left ventricular ejection is only moderately effective in identifying those who require the device. So using this measurement alone is inadequate to determine who needs and does not need the device. In fact, it is as good as tossing a coin. Hence, better techniques to determine who is at risk for sudden death are required.

Micro-volt T-wave Alternans

As such, other tests have been designed to identify those who are at greater risk for sudden death and who are more likely to benefit from device implantation. Indeed, novel techniques have been developed to better risk stratify this group of patients.[448] Presence of

T-wave alternans indicates that the heart muscle may be electrically unstable.[57] The T-wave represents repolarisation of the heart muscle cells, the period when the heart muscle recovers after stimulation. When the heart muscle is stimulated, there are alterations in the electrical activity caused by movement of various ions in and out of the cells. These changes result in the contraction of the heart muscle. After which, the movement of these particles reverses and the muscle relaxes. The electrical activity of these complex activities is reflected on the surface electrocardiogram as the T-wave. As such, T-wave alternans refers to the alternation in the shape, amplitude and timing of the T-wave, and has been found to be associated with electrical instability of the heart. This phenomenon may be induced[449] or it may occur spontaneously.[449] However, macroscopic T-wave alternans, when changes can be seen with the naked eye, is uncommon (Figure 15). In a review of 6,059 patients in 1948, there were only five cases (0.08%) with the alternating amplitude of the T-wave that was visible on routine ECG tracing.[450] This pattern may be a marker for potentially lethal heart rhythm.[451] One of them was a 70-year-old man from Belgium. Fortunately, he was in an Intensive Care Unit and the patient was successfully resuscitated by the hospital staff.

Using sensitive equipment, computerised processing techniques and mathematical algorithms, scientists were able to detect minute changes in electrical voltages of the T-wave in 1982[452] which is not seen with the naked eye. They occur especially when the heart rate is increased to a slightly higher rate. However, several technical

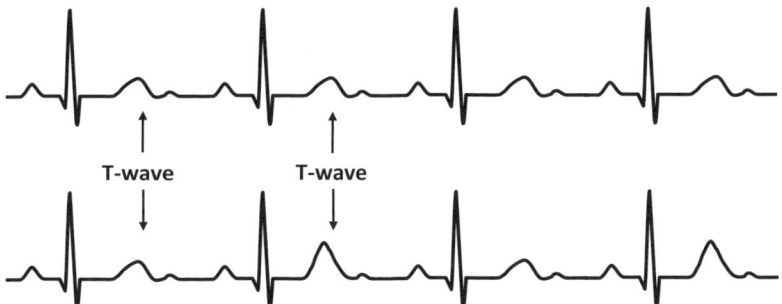

Figure 15.   Macroscopic T-wave alternans.

While the T-wave (arrowed) appears similar with every beat in the upper panel, the size of the T-wave (arrowed) changes with alternating beats in the lower panel.

requirements must be met before the findings can be interpreted accurately[453] and its presence has been associated with a greater likelihood of potentially lethal heart rhythm in a variety of heart conditions.[454] From a pooled analysis from two clinical trials consisting of 129 patients with previous heart attack and severe impairment of left ventricular pumping function (ejection fraction of 30% and less), the presence of T-wave alternans was evaluated.[455] They found that 27% were tested negative, 60% were positive and 13% were indeterminate. At 24 months, none of those tested negative died suddenly or suffered from cardiac arrest. On the other hand, 15.6% of patients who were tested positive or indeterminate had these events! The overall mortality was 12.5%, 21.4% and 21.3% in the T-wave alternans negative, indeterminate and positive groups, respectively. These results were corroborated by a single-centre report of 768 patients with poor heart function from narrowing of blood vessels.[456] Five hundred and fourteen (67%) of them did not have a negative T-wave alternans test, and their risk for death from any cause or rhythm abnormality was two times higher. In another study, the presence of T-wave alternans was associated with a higher likelihood of inducing a potentially fatal heart rhythm during an invasive electrophysiology study.[457] In addition, it also had predictive value for subsequent rhythm disorder comparable to systematic stimulation of the ventricle to induce abnormal heart rhythm. Indeed, a study comparing the predictive value for potentially fatal rhythm disorder showed that T-wave alternans was superior to invasive study.[458] For a positive result, the risk for abnormal rhythm was eight times higher for T-wave alternans but only three times higher for invasive assessment.

More recently, the value of T-wave alternans testing was also compared with invasive testing in a multi-centre study among 566 patients with narrowing of heart arteries, impaired heart function (ejection fraction less than 40%) and short runs of rapid heart beats.[459] The investigators found that the ability of the non-invasive technique to detect potentially lethal heart rhythm and sudden death was comparable to the invasive technique after 1.9-year follow-up. The risk for an abnormal result of either test was more than two times higher compared with a normal finding. In another single-centre study, 286 patients with impaired heart function (ejection fraction less than 0.35) with short runs of rapid heartbeats or fainting spells underwent T-wave alternans and invasive testing of electrical stability.[460] Similar to the earlier report, a positive T-wave alternans test was associated with a 2.4 times higher risk. Although T-wave alternans was a more effective predictor of occurrence of serious rhythm disorder at 2 years, the residual risk among those with a negative result remained relatively high. This finding was consistent regardless of the cause of abnormal heart function.

Among 446 patients with heart failure but without narrowing of coronary artery were followed up for 18 to 24 months.[448] The investigators reported that T-wave alternans was abnormal in 65% of the patients, and the rate of dying from heart disease or presence of life-threatening rhythms was 6.5%. Conversely, this rate was only 1.6% among those with normal T-wave alternans. Thus, an abnormal test result conferred a 4-fold higher risk. In a review of more than 2,600 patients from 19 studies, they found that the presence of T-wave alternans increased the risk of a potentially lethal abnormal rhythm disorder by four times.[58] Over a 21-month period, the rate of a serious rhythm event was 3% for those without T-wave alternans and 19% for individuals with T-wave alternans.

However, the usefulness of this technique has not been consistently demonstrated in patients with heart failure. In a multi-centre randomised trial of 490 patients with mild to moderate heart failure, T-wave alternans was assessed.[461] Only 37% of them were found to be positive and 22% were negative. The majority of them (41%) were indeterminate. While the proportion of patients with adverse rhythm events was higher among those with positive T-wave alternans, the difference was not statistically significant. In other words, the finding was likely due to chance. But a limitation may be related to a relatively small number of subjects in the study, the time to occurrence of sudden death in clinical trials and the ascertainment of endpoint.[462] Similarly in another multi-centre study in the United States, 575 patients with poor heart function (ejection fraction less than 30%) after a heart attack were studied.[463] They found that the result of T-wave alternans was not predictive of subsequent severe rhythm disorder. Total mortality was about two times higher among those who did not have a negative T-wave alternans test. A smaller multi-centre

European study corroborated with the finding that T-wave alternans testing was not useful in predicting abnormal rhythm disorder among patients that have recently recovered from a heart attack, even if the pump function has been affected (ejection fraction less than 40%).[464]

Despite these discrepancies, a recent study reported that the amplitude of T-wave alternans, recorded from intra-cardiac electrograms in intra-cardiac defibrillators, was greater immediately before spontaneous potentially lethal rhythms.[465] Indeed, in 2006, the American College of Cardiology, American Heart Association and European Society of Cardiology, in collaboration with the European Heart Rhythm Association and the Heart Rhythm Society[374] recommended the use of T-wave alternans when evaluating patients for palpitation, fainting or near-fainting spells. A later statement from the American Heart Association/American College of Cardiology Foundation/ Heart Rhythm Society concluded that the results of T-wave alternans were useful in identifying individuals at risk for sudden death.[466] While acknowledging the complexity in identifying subsets of patients who may or may not benefit from implantation of intra-cardiac defibrillator, the United States National Heart, Lung, and Blood Institute and Heart Rhythm Society recognised the potential value of T-wave alternans in assessment.[9] The International Society for Holter and Noninvasive Electrocardiology Consensus statement[467] recommended that T-wave alternans evaluation is a useful adjunct in assessing patients with or suspected to have a potentially lethal arrhythmia.

To extend the concept of T-wave alternans further, Finnish investigators evaluated its predictive value in individuals undergoing exercise testing.[468] Of the 1,037 patients, 24% suffered from a previous heart attack and 24% underwent exercise testing to determine adequacy of treatment. Heart pump function was not routinely assessed in this study. Out of the 529 (51%) evaluated, 1.5% of them had severely impaired pump function. Presence of T-wave alternans was detected in 8.4% of them. After a mean period of 44 months of follow-up, 59 (5.7%) of them died. Sudden death occurred in 20 subjects (1.9%). The occurrences of death and sudden death were 6.3 and 3.3 times higher for those with T-wave alternans. Thus, this technique may also be useful for patients without severe impairment of heart pumping function.

The Big White Killer Wolf

Bypass Tracts and Short-Circuits: the Pre-Excitation Syndrome

"A shortcut is the longest distance between two points."

The Path of Progress as part of the Issawi's Law of Progress
Charles Issawi
Ragnar Nurkse Professor of Economics, Columbia University

For several years in the 1920s, the folks in Montana have been terrorised by a huge white killer wolf. Its notorious reputation has extended beyond the confines of Jefferson forest to the neighbouring States. Cattle, deer and even elk were lost to its voracious appetite. Every night, as its haunting howls permeate through the hills, chills were sent down the spines of man and beasts — both farmed and wild. The 1.8 m long unbridled maverick, with a 50 cm bushy tail, declared itself as the outlawed monarch of the mountains and valleys and ruled on the east side of Rocky Mountains. Since a bounty of $1700 had been placed on its head by the authorities, this free-roaming slayer had been hunted from the ridges to the plains with ropes, guns, traps, dogs, horses and even with help from the air. However, its strength, speed, agility and cunningness had allowed it to evade capture. Once, even a car tried to run it over but failed. When its mate was killed in a trap a few years earlier, it became more daring, brutish and cruel. On April or May 1930,

A. E. Close and Earl Neill were chasing the white wolf with their two dogs. After several tiring hours of pursuit, the dogs managed to catch up and attack the 18-year-old creature. Being much larger and stronger, the elderly animal was still able to fight back ferociously and drove the dogs slowly back to their masters. Fully engaged in battle, it did not realise that Close was only 40 yards away, hiding behind a tree. As he raised a 0.30-inch rifle, Close hesitated and thought, "What a shame to kill such a smart fellow…" before firing. The fatal shot landed on the front left cheek, just below the eye of the animal and the sniper remarked unassumingly, "…and that's all there was to it." It marked the end of more than a decade of fear and uncertainty, silencing the last call of the wild. For its "misdeeds", the majestic 38 kg animal was preserved and displayed in the County Courthouse for several decades. Finally, it was moved to a glass case in its simulated habitat at the Basin Trading Post in Stanford, Montana, in the United States.

A Fruitful Trans-Atlantic Collaboration

Interestingly, in the same year in August, three doctors from both sides of the Atlantic Ocean described an electrocardiogram with unique features that was associated with abnormal heart rhythm, a condition which now bears their names, the Wolff-Parkinson-White syndrome.[469] In those days, interaction between colleagues across the vast body of waters was limited. This collaboration started with the consultation of a young otherwise healthy man who presented to Dr Paul Dudley White on 2 April 1928 at the Massachusetts General Hospital with intermittent episodes of palpitation. He was found to suffer from atrial fibrillation.[470] Atrial fibrillation is a condition when rhythm in the atrium becomes totally disorganized and is at a rate of 400 to 600 beats per minute.[471] Since not all of these impulses are conducted into the ventricle, the transmitted beats stimulate the main pumping chamber at varying intervals. Hence, the pulse rate is commonly described as irregularly irregular. But when the rhythm is normal in patients with Wolff-Parkinson-White syndrome, the electrocardiogram may be abnormal. During his sabbatical writing leave in Europe, Dr White discussed these

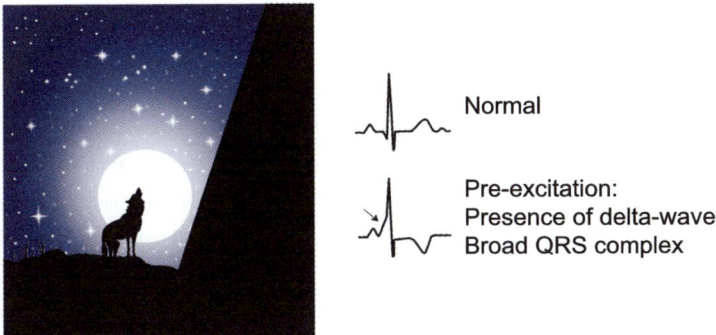

Figure 16. Pre-excitation wave.

A lone wolf howling in the Rockies. The delta-wave (arrowed) of the Wolff-Parkinson-White syndrome. Image of wolf modified from Shuttlestock image (Image ID: 67263736).

electrocardiograms with several cardiologists. Only Dr John Parkinson in London showed interest because he had seven patients with comparable electrocardiograms with similar pattern. These distinctive signs in the electrocardiogram include shortened duration of the conduction from the atrium to the ventricle but prolonged duration of the electrical impulse in the ventricle. The abbreviated electrical circuit from the atrium to the ventricle is manifested in the electrocardiogram as delta-wave (Figure 16). Together with another four patients from Boston, Massachusetts, Dr Louis Wolff, Sir John Parkinson and Dr Paul Dudley White published their seminal manuscript,[469] despite the fact that this electrocardiographic pattern has been unknowingly described 17 years earlier.[472] Other than annoying episodes of palpitations, patients with Wolff-Parkinson-White syndrome without atrial fibrillation were considered to be of low risk for sudden death. Thus, they were not routinely discouraged from participating in competitive sports.[473]

It Does Not Always Occur during Sports

Jörg was an active 18-year-old soccer player in Austria (*personal communication, Prof Christian, J Wiedermann*).[474] Despite having two to three brief episodes of palpitations yearly, he continued to play his soccer games with his friends. The young man was well-built and did not have chest discomfort, giddiness or fainting spells. Just like any ambitious teenager, Jörg brushed away his symptoms so that he could continue with soccer. Furthermore, none of his family members had heart disease or died suddenly. During his routine medical examination, the electrocardiogram showed features consistent with Wolff-Parkinson-White syndrome. He was considered to be asymptomatic and was not disallowed to participate in sports.

One day, his symptom recurred. This time, it was more severe and prolonged. He had giddiness and chest discomfort, and his lips turned blue. His heart rate was very fast, more than 300 beats per minute, and the rhythm was irregular. A drug to treat the potentially fatal rhythm disorder, ventricular tachycardia, was administered and fortunately (or rather unfortunately), his heart rhythm normalised. The resting electrocardiogram showed the abnormality diagnostic of Wolff-Parkinson-White syndrome. Instead of escalating his cardiac evaluation, an oral medicine used to prevent ventricular tachycardia was prescribed. While shopping 10 days later, he collapsed suddenly. Resuscitation attempts were unsuccessful and Jörg passed away when he was brought to the Emergency Room. Subsequent post-mortem examination did not show abnormalities of the heart structure, valves, muscle and coronary arteries. However, an extra electrical pathway connecting the atrium and ventricle was detected which was consistent with the diagnosis of Wolff-Parkinson-White syndrome.

Much earlier, in 1942, a 16-year-old boy died suddenly two hours after drinking cold water.[475] Like the previous patient, he had been complaining of palpitations for the previous three years and his electrocardiogram showed features consistent with the Wolff-Parkinson-White syndrome. Though autopsy showed normal heart structure, there were microscopic evidence for three muscular connections between the right atrium and right ventricle. For the first time, these anomalous pathways, electrocardiographic findings and sudden death were found together in the same patient.

Bypass Tracts and Circus Movement

The atriae and ventricles of the heart are pumps that drive blood to various parts of the body. Contraction of these chambers are coordinated and synchronised so that blood flows efficiently. Within the heart is a complex network of specialised muscle tissue that makes up the conduction system which controls these harmonised well-coordinated actions. Between the atriae and ventricles, there is an insulating ring and electrical signals can only cross to the ventricles through a unique connection, known as the atrio-ventricular node and the bundle of His. Not unlike an immigration checkpoint, these specialised tissues slow down the conduction of electrical impulses from 0.5 m/s to 0.05 m/s. Due to this delay, the maximal number of heart beats that can conduct through this channel is about 220 beats per minute. This limitation was "built-in" to prevent the ventricle from beating too fast, which can be potentially fatal (Figure 17).

However, the discovery of this intricate system and the abnormality associated with Wolff-Parkinson-White syndrome have been convoluted, and somewhat analogised to putting the cart before the horse. Unlike invertebrates, it was previously believed that the electrical activities of the atrium and ventricle were independent of each other because of the fibrous ring that separated the two chambers. In March 1892, Stanley Kent from the University of Oxford was the first to establish the connection between the atrium and ventricle when he studied the heart of various mammals,[476] although these muscular bridges were on the outer aspect of the heart. In 1913, Kent, who had moved to University of Bristol, described the connection between the right atrium and right ventricle at the back of the heart in a man and believed that it was one of the normal pathways to the ventricle.[477] Not surprisingly, he erroneously postulated that in the normal heart, there were multiple links between the atrium and the ventricle.

It was not until 1906, that the discovery of the atrio-ventricular node was reported.[478] Dr Sunao Tawara, a young Japanese medical graduate studying pathology under the supervision of Ludwig Aschoff at the Philipps University in Marburg, Germany, found a

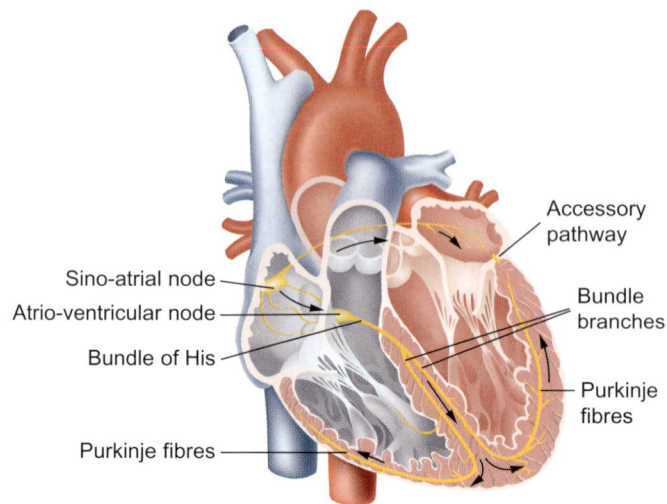

Figure 17.   Accessory pathway.
The electrical conduction system of the heart consists of specialised tissue (in yellow) that propagates electrical impulses within the muscle. A fibrous ring (which acts like an insulator) separates the atriae and ventricles. In a normal person, electrical impulse travels through the atrioventricular node from the atrium to the ventricle. An accessory pathway provides an alternate connection between the two chambers.

compact network of fibres at the base of the inter-atrial septum as he traced backwards from the ventricle. For his work, it is also named as the Node of Tawara. This is the principal pathway connecting the atrium and the ventricle. Subsequently, the muscular fibre bridges between the atrium and the ventricle described by Kent were termed para-specific conduction, and later known as accessory pathways or bypass tracts.[479] In patients with Wolff-Parkinson-White syndrome, these abnormal accessory tracts connect the atrium to the ventricle, bypassing the atrio-ventricular node.

The underlying mechanism for rapid heart rate was elucidated by a young promising physiologist at Cambridge University. Due to the unique electrical properties of the accessory pathway, George Ralph Mines described impulses from the ventricle back to the atrium in one direction.[480] When the circumstances were conducive, the electrical activities travel in a circular fashion, from the atrium to the ventricle via the atrio-ventricular node and back to the ventricle via the accessory pathway, resulting in rapid heartbeats.[481] As a result of his then cutting-edge research, it was not surprising that he assumed the Professorship and Chair of Physiology at McGill University in McGill University in Montreal, Canada, in August 1914 at a very young age.[482] On the Saturday evening of 7 November 1914, the 29-year-old was found unconscious in the laboratory by the janitor. Apparently, there was still equipment attached to him for the recording of his breathing. He was brought to the Royal Victoria Hospital and regained consciousness for a short period. Mines then developed seizures and passed away shortly before midnight. The autopsy did not show any abnormality, and his death was assumed to be the result of self-experimentation. However, this conclusion has been an issue of contention. As such, his paper on circus movement of electrical impulses was published posthumously in 1914.[481]

This concept was subsequently expanded two to three years following the description of the Wolff-Parkinson-White syndrome.[483,484] These researchers corrected the originators, Dr Wolff, Sir John and Dr White, because they attributed the abnormal electrocardiogram pattern to conduction abnormalities in the ventricles. Instead, they postulated that a bypass tract resulted in these changes.[484] This extra pathway allows electrical impulses to travel to and from the atrium and ventricle, moving round and round, causing the heart to beat rapidly. Eventually, it was recognised that circus movement is one of the principal mechanism for the generation of abnormally rapid rhythm, and has been termed the Rosetta stone of electrocardiography.[485]

From Wolff-Parkinson-White to the Pre-Excitation Syndrome

In 1942, Professor Richard F. Öhnrell from the Karolinska Hospital in Stockholm, Sweden, described the concertina effect among patients with Wolff-Parkinson-White syndrome. It referred to the electrocardiographic pattern between the activation of the atrium and ventricle. He attributed the characteristic electrocardiographic pattern to earlier stimulation of the ventricle by impulses from the atrium as it traversed via the bypass tract instead of travelling through the normal route via the atrio-ventricular node. Thus, the term "pre-excitation" was coined. By March 1944, after studying several cases of Wolff-Parkinson-White syndrome extensively, Öhnrell was confident of his findings and reported his observations as the sole author in an entire supplement issue of *Acta Medica Scandinavica* (currently known as *Journal of Internal Medicine*).[486] Around the same time, the unique electrocardiographic feature of pre-excitation was given the name, "delta" wave.[487] In 1942 or 1943, the three French investigators used the figure "Δ" rather than the fourth letter of the Greek alphabet "delta" to describe the shape of the electrocardiographic abnormality (Figure 16).[235]

Frequency of the Pre-excitation Syndrome

The Wolff-Parkinson-White syndrome is an uncommon condition. Electrocardiography was routinely performed among United States Air Force men since 1957.[488] Of 122,043 tracings studied over a 4- to 5-year period, 187 (1.5 per 1,000) electrocardiograms were consistent with the diagnosis of Wolff-Parkinson-White syndrome. Correspondingly, the Royal Canadian Air Force shared the same experience in their 67,375 subjects.[489] They found that occurrence rate for Wolff-Parkinson-White syndrome was 1.6 per 1,000. However, not every patient with this condition can be detected with one electrocardiographic recording because the tracing can be normal. Every year, the incidence rate of newly diagnosed Wolff-Parkinson-White syndrome was estimated to be four per 100,000 residents in the Olmsted County in Minnesota.[490] This figure corresponded to the findings in a Greek population where the rate of discovering new cases was 4.4 per 100,000 residents per year.[491] Of note, these patients did not have symptom and the abnormality was detected during this study. In a group of military aviators (more than 80% were without symptom), the occurrence of rapid heartbeats was estimated to be 1% annually.[492] Although most patients with Wolff-Parkinson-White syndrome have only one accessory pathway, some have reported that 20% of their patients may have two or more bypass tracts.[493]

It is believed that the accessory pathways were remnants of the connection between the atrium and ventricle during formation of the heart in the foetus. Hence, the condition may occur more frequently in families. Researchers at the Duke University Medical Center in Durham, North Carolina, found that 0.55% of first-degree relatives of patients with Wolff-Parkinson-White syndrome had pre-excitation.[494] This rate was three to four times higher than that reported in the general population (0.15%).

From Pre-Excitation to Premature Death

Despite reports of cases of sudden death associated with Wolff-Parkinson-White syndrome, the risk was unlikely to be high. Indeed, the occurrence of sudden death in the Olmsted County community was low, at 0.15% per year.[490] Subsequently, by grouping the findings of 20 studies enrolling only *asymptomatic* patients with Wolff-Parkinson-White syndrome, the occurrence of sudden death ranged from 0 to 4.5 events per 1,000 person-years of follow-up, with an annual average rate of 0.13%.[495] Even among patients with symptoms and Wolff-Parkinson-White syndrome, the risk of sudden death did not appear to be extraordinarily high. In Maria Cecilia Hospital in Cotignola, Italy, there were 8,575 patients with Wolff-Parkinson-White syndrome who had palpitation and were referred for electrophysiological testing.[496] However, 369 of them declined catheter ablation and were followed up for five years. Despite the fact that most of them were not treated with medicines on a regular basis, only about 8% experienced a serious rhythm disorder. Cardiac arrest occurred in four patients (1.4%) over this period, which translated to approximately 0.8% per year.

However, sudden death could be the initial presentation of a patient with pre-excitation.[493] Indeed, at the Academic Hospital in Maastricht, the Netherlands, more than 50% of victims of aborted sudden death from ventricular fibrillation were their first presentation of Wolff-Parkinson-White syndrome.[497] The underlying rhythm disorder associated with sudden death among patients with Wolff-Parkinson-White syndrome was believed to be ventricular fibrillation. This rhythm resulted in disorganised contraction of the ventricle so that blood could not be effectively pumped out.

Although this relationship was appreciated in as early as 1934,[498] documentation of the abnormalities was unclear. It was only in 1951 that a patient with pre-excitation developed ventricular fibrillation four hours following administration of a medicine to control abnormal heart rhythm.[499] However, the initiation of ventricular fibrillation remained unclear.

In November 1969, a 63-year-old woman with Wolff-Parkinson-White syndrome was admitted to a hospital for persistent palpitation.[500] As she remained unwell, the patient was transferred to Hahnemann Hospital in Philadelphia, Pennsylvania, for further management. Since she was ill and in atrial fibrillation, various medicines were administered in an attempt to control the heart rate and rhythm. But a few hours later, the patient collapsed in ventricular fibrillation. Although she was successfully resuscitated with electrical cardioversion, her cardiac rhythm degenerated into ventricular fibrillation again about six hours later. Electrical cardioversion normalised the rhythm once more. Several medicines were then used to maintain her heart in normal rhythm. In the analysis of this case, the attending doctors postulated that during atrial fibrillation, electrical impulses were conducted from the atrium to the ventricle via the accessory pathway. Due to the rapid atrial rate, the rhythm in the ventricle quickly deteriorates into fibrillation. This complication arises because the accessory pathway is able to recover faster than the atrio-ventricular node to allow impulses to be conducted at a much faster rate. The association of atrial and ventricular fibrillation was subsequently corroborated by a larger series.[493]

In another study of 273 individuals (35 years or younger) who died suddenly in Padua, Italy, a prior electrocardiogram was available in 93 of them.[501] Ten of the deceased (3.6%) had documented pre-excitation in the tracing prior to death. Of the six who had palpitation, three fainted before. In other words, 40% of them did not have any warning symptom. In another multi-centre European review of 23 patients with Wolff-Parkinson-White syndrome, ventricular fibrillation was the first presentation in six patients (26%).[502] Thus, when determining the proportion of patients who had died suddenly, previously asymptomatic patients were unlikely to be included in the analysis. As such, the risk of sudden death could have been under-estimated in post-mortem analysis. Nonetheless, it is important to identify who is at risk because transecting or ablating the accessory pathways can prevent sudden death.[501]

Who is at Risk?

Based on earlier experience, patients with Wolff-Parkinson-White syndrome who have experienced previous episodes of atrial fibrillation, especially when impulses are conducted from the atrium to the ventricle via the accessory pathway, are at increased risk for sudden death. Those with rapid heartbeats during episodes of palpitation are also likely to be of greater risk.[493,497,502,503] The risk of ventricular fibrillation is higher when the ventricles contract at more than 270 beats per minute. In addition, males are also more likely to suffer from sudden death.[497,502] While fainting spells may be a predictor for subsequent sudden death in other rhythm disorders, this symptom lack prognostic value among patients with Wolff-Parkinson-White syndrome.[504,505]

There are several other indicators that have been associated with lower risk of sudden death among patients with Wolff-Parkinson-White syndrome. Most of these characteristics are related to electrocardiographic features, which indicate that the accessory pathway takes a longer time to recover after electrical stimulation. So, the intermittent appearance of the delta-wave in the electrocardiogram suggests that the recovery period of accessory pathway is long.[502] In other words, when the delta-wave is present, the electrical impulse travels via the bypass tract from the atrium to the ventricle.[506] When it has not recovered from the next signal, the impulse travels through the normal passage, and hence the delta-wave is lost. So the electrocardiogram appears normal. Therefore, when the accessory pathway is not able to conduct electrical impulses from the atrium to the ventricle at a rapid rate, the ventricle is less likely to end up with fibrillation.

Exercise may be used to increase the heart rate to assess the electrical property of the bypass tract at different beat intervals. Although physical activity may shorten the recovery period of the accessory pathway,[507] it may not conduct electrical impulses when the heart rate becomes too fast. Under this circumstance, the delta-wave is lost and the electrocardiogram normalises.[507,508] However, it may re-appear in the tracing when the heart rate slows down after exercise. Ambulatory electrocardiography can also sometimes detect abnormal cardiac rhythm.[509]

The doctors at the San Raffaele University Hospital in Milan, Italy, evaluated whether invasive electrophysiologic testing was able to predict the occurrence of abnormally fast heartbeats.[509] This procedure involves positioning electrodes to various cardiac chambers so as to record and stimulate the heart. By analysing the information, the electrical properties and the manner in which impulses are conducted can be characterised. From 1993 to 1996, a total of 162 asymptomatic patients with Wolff-Parkinson-White syndrome were studied and were followed up till end of December 2001. About 20% of them developed symptoms and they found that abnormal cardiac rhythm events occurred more frequently among younger patients, and those with multiple accessory pathways or when the pathways recovered more rapidly after stimulation. Other researchers have also corroborated the fact that patients with multiple accessory pathways are more likely to have a potentially lethal rhythm disorder.[493,496,497] Children also share these adverse determinants.[510] Conversely, those with longer recovery period after a laboratory-induced stimulus during electrophysiological studies were also less likely to experience a potentially lethal rhythm disorder.[496,503] In the Italian study,[509] they also found that individuals who developed atrial fibrillation, spontaneous or induced during electrophysiological testing, were more likely to die suddenly. Although there were eight patients who developed spontaneous atrial fibrillation, only four of them were symptomatic. Three patients had dizziness and one had palpitation. These four patients underwent successful ablation of the accessory pathways and no further rhythm disorder was recorded. For the remaining four patients, three had ventricular fibrillation.

Unfortunately, the individual that had this lethal rhythm died suddenly while playing soccer. Conversely, the other two patients were successfully resuscitated.

To further test their strategy of using an invasive approach to risk stratify patients with Wolff-Parkinson-White syndrome and who had fast heart rate induced by electrophysiological study, the researchers randomly assigned them to be treated with or without ablation.[511] Of 37 patients treated with ablation, two (5%) had an episode of rapid heart rate. However, rapid heart rate events occurred in 21 (60%) of the 35 patients who did not undergo ablation. One of these patients suffered from ventricular fibrillation. The researchers estimated that the procedure reduced the occurrence of rapid heartbeats by 92%. As such, they concluded that prophylactic ablation markedly reduced the frequency of rapid heartbeats in asymptomatic high-risk patients with Wolff-Parkinson-White syndrome. Based on their results, this group of Italian doctors[512] and others[513] advocated the use of electrophysiological studies to ascertain the risk of these patients, particularly for those with high-risk occupations or lifestyles. Some physicians also believed that short recovery period the bypass tracts, multiple pathways and atrial fibrillation together make up the electrical milieu for the development of ventricular fibrillation and subsequent sudden death.[512]

Other doctors have extended this concept by using various drugs[514–516] to determine the recovery period of the accessory pathways is short. These patients would then be considered at increased risk. However, this approach has been questioned due to the lack of correlation with adverse events.[517,518] The reason may be related to the low rate of sudden death for asymptomatic patients, making such correlation statistically challenging.[490–492,503,519,520]

Destroying the Tracks

In 1968, physicians at the Duke University Medical Center reported a 32-year-old fisherman who had recurrent episodes of fast heartbeats since the age of 4.[521] Although most of them occurred spontaneously, it was brought on by exercise or emotional stimuli. However, in 1965, he developed heart failure and was unable to continue with his work. After extensive evaluation with various medicines, the physicians were able to locate the accessory pathway. When the incision was made at the right atrium and ventricle, the delta-wave disappeared. The patient recovered well from the procedure and his medicines were discontinued. His heart size also normalised and he was able to return to his normal activities. By the 1980s, surgical interruption of the accessory pathway has been recommended as a clinical service for patients who did not respond well to medicines or if they have atrial fibrillation and, as such are at higher risk of sudden death.[522] During this procedure, the chest is surgically cut opened, and after the accessory pathway has been identified by a comprehensive mapping exercise, it is truncated. Since there are significant risks and complications associated with relatively high costs, arrhythmia surgery is performed as a last resort for patients who are not well-controlled with medicines or if the rhythm disorder is potentially life-threatening.[522]

Subsequent technological innovations have led to the development of steerable pacing electrodes and advanced mapping techniques. Although various methods of energy delivery have been employed for ablation, such as cold (cyroablation) and micro-wave, the most common source used today is radiofrequency waves. In 1983, the procedure was able to be performed by merely inserting the equipment into the heart, without the need of opening up the chest.[523] By 1991, the success rates were reported to be high when employing these minimally invasive techniques.[524,525] However, there is no procedure that is totally risk-free. Since multiple electrodes are inserted through blood vessels, both veins and arteries, complications include bleeding, clotting, perforating the heart, damaging the valves, heart attack, stroke, puncturing the lung and radiation. During the ablative process, adjacent tissues, such as normal conduction tissue, nerves, coronary artery and the oesophagus (gullet), may be injured. Although the incidence of significant complications has been estimated to be 1% to 2%,[513] in experienced centres, it may be less than 1%.[512] While opinion is varied on whom to perform this procedure on, 70% of cardiologists who specialises in rhythm disorder supported its use in asymptomatic patients with Wolff-Parkinson-White syndrome.[526]

For young athletes, the Wolff-Parkinson-White syndrome accounted for about 1% of sudden death.[60] Training does not alter the electrical properties of the heart, in particular the accessory pathway.[527] The 36th Bethesda Conference recommended that asymptomatic patients with Wolff-Parkinson-White syndrome without other heart abnormalities may be allowed to participate in sports.[528] However, for those taking part in moderate or high level activities or who are symptomatic, invasive electrophysiological study is recommended to determine the electrical properties of the accessory pathway. Ablation of the bypass tract may be needed for the athlete to continue with sports. On the other hand, the European Society of Cardiology recommended all athletes to undergo a comprehensive risk assessment including an electrophysiological study.[529] For a young patient, the Pediatric and Congenital Electrophysiology Society (PACES) and the Heart Rhythm Society (HRS) recommended a more pro-active approach.[530] Those with electrocardiograms showing pre-excitation should be referred to a paediatric cardiologist who specialises in rhythm disorder. A low risk profile has to be clearly demonstrated in these sportsperson before they are allowed to participate. Otherwise, they would be subjected to invasive testing and possibly ablation.

But Sometimes, It just Vanishes!

Interestingly, about 13% of asymptomatic patients with Wolff-Parkinson-White syndrome lose the delta-wave after five years, indicating that the bypass tract did not allow electrical activity to pass from the atrium to the ventricle. However, it continued to conduct impulses from the ventricle to the atrium.[509] In another study, 29 asymptomatic patients with Wolff-Parkinson-White syndrome underwent electrophysiological testing twice over a period of more than 36 months.[519] Of note, nine (31%) lost the capacity for pre-excitation and were unable to conduct impulses from the atrium to the ventricle via the accessory tract. These patients tended to be older and the bypass tract takes longer to recover after an electrical stimulus. Nonetheless, it remains unclear if getting older increases the risk of scarring and damages the accessory pathways.

This phenomenon was also observed in other spectrums of life. In a study of 90 infants who presented with fast heartbeats in their first four months of life and found to have Wolff-Parkinson-White syndrome, after 6.5 years, the abnormal electrocardiographic pattern disappeared in 36%.[531] Maturation of heart tissue could have led to the removal of remnant muscular connections, and hence the disappearance of pre-excitation.

After more than 80 years, Wolff-Parkinson-White syndrome is a well-characterised uncommon condition with a relatively low risk of sudden death. Diagnosis is usually made by an electrocardiogram and there are validated approaches to risk stratification. Definitive treatment is also available for this condition.

It's not Only the Heart

Time Bombs Ticking in the Head

A Messy Brainy Entanglement: Arterio-Venous Malformation

*"He had passed the preceding day in the bosom of his family, and,
excepting a bilious attack under which he had laboured for some days,
there was nothing in his appearance to create the least apprehension that
the fatal hour was so near."*

Obituary of Sir Thomas Stamford Raffles
The Gentleman's Magazine, July 1826

The death of the founder of modern Singapore, Sir Thomas Stamford Raffles, on Wednesday, 5 July 1826, a day short of his 45th birthday, was considered as sudden and unexpected. In fact, his household was in the midst of preparing the birthday celebration of what was supposed to be a joyous occasion. As with his usual habit, Raffles slept at about 10 to 11 pm. Although his usual waking hour was 6 am, Raffles was not found in his room at 5 am. Lady Sophie Raffles rose and found him lifeless at the foot of the spiral staircase in his country home at Highwood in Hendon, Middlesex, England. They promptly summoned whatever emergency medical services available at that time. The attendants made a courageous and comprehensive attempt to revive him but were sadly unsuccessful.

Some have thought that a heart attack could be the cause. However, Sir Everard Home, who performed the autopsy that evening, did not confirm the suspicion since the heart appeared normal. Instead, the "right frontal bone was twice the thickness of the left; this must be imputed to the effects of the sun in India, since it is a common occurrence in those who have resided long in hot climates... thickness of coats of the vessel... vasculosity exceeded anything I had ever seen." He added that in the cavity of the right brain, "there was a coagulum of the size of a pullet's egg, and a quantity of bloody serum escaped, which measured six ounces." Although Sir Everard was uncertain regarding the cause of the bleeding, he believed it resulted in immediate death. A fall could have caused bleeding in the head. However, there was no other injury to suggest that Raffles tripped and fell down the stairs. On review of the post-mortem report, Dr James Khoo, a well-known Singapore neurosurgeon, inferred that the cause of death was likely due to bleeding in the right frontal lobe of the brain from an arterio-venous malformation.[532] His episodes of vomiting could also have been a symptom attributed to bleeding in the brain. The skull is a non-expandable structure that holds the brain. So when there is bleeding, as the blood volume increases, other parts of the brain may be compressed. As a response to increase pressure within the skull, the patient vomits.

From his many letters in his memoir, Raffles complained of severe headache and had an irritable disposition, which kept him from his duties. These symptoms could have been a harbinger of an arterio-venous malformation in his head. It was also one of the reasons for him to give up his position at Fort Marlborough in early 1824 and returned to England under semi-retirement. In 1825, Raffles bought Highwood House, a fine classical building and the largest house in Mill Hill, which is a suburb 7 miles (11.2 kilometres) northwest of London. He was a keen botanist and naturalist. Although enriched by his experience in South-east Asia, Raffles often lamented about missing England in his correspondences. Unfortunately, he was unable to enjoy the rest of his life in this undulating area with abundance of pleasant greenery. Although Raffles lived there for barely a year, his wife, Lady Sophia, stayed there until 1858, when she died. In 1954, the estate has been restored to a nursing home. Subsequently, it became a hostel for the owner's employees and was vacated in January 2008 and is being rented out.

Arterio-venous malformation in the head

Normally, the blood in the arteries flows into a network of capillaries before entering into the veins. Capillaries are lined by a single layer of cells to allow oxygen and nutrients to flow from the blood to the tissue and waste products from the tissue to the blood stream. Arterio-venous malformation is an uncommon congenital condition in which the capillary system and the tissue are bypassed. Its cause is unknown and the person is likely to be born with the condition. Normally, the capillaries also act like a sponge and dampen the pressure in the venous system. With lower pressure in the system, the walls of veins are much thinner than arteries. Arterio-venous malformations look like a messy tangle of blood vessels and have relatively fragile walls. Without passing blood through the capillaries, these abnormal vessels are subjected to higher pressure. Hence, they are prone to rupture and bleeding. Although they do not grow in numbers, the channels of the abnormal vessels may widen as the weakened wall stretches. As such, the size of the group of vessels may enlarge. Sometimes, clots may form in these vessels, obstructing blood flow. In these situations, they may become smaller.

Population-based detection rates of arterio-venous malformation in the head were 1.1, 1.2, 1.3 and 1.4 per 100,000 in Scotland,[533] Sweden,[534] New York[535] and California,[536] respectively. On the other hand, using a mathematical model to compute the prevalence of arterio-venous malformation in the brain in the Lothian area of Scotland, it was estimated to be 15 to 18 per 100,000 adults.[537] With increasing utilisation of imaging for a variety of reasons, the frequency of this condition may be higher. In a review of 16 published studies on magnetic resonance examination of the head, arterio-venous malformation was discovered incidentally in 0.05% of them, which translates to 50 per 100,000.[538]

Likely, most arterio-venous malformations in the brain are unde-tected. Occasionally, there may be abnormal blood vessels on the face, such as a nexus or "pot-wine" stain, which could suggest the presence in the head. The types of symptoms that are produced by the condition have been documented by various studies. In a cohort of 1,289 consecutive patients with arterio-venous malformation from three independent databases in Europe, Asia and North America, the characteristics of patients were described.[539] The mean age was 31 years and 45% were female. The most frequent presentation was, unfortunately, bleeding in the brain (53%). Generalised and focal seizure accounted for about 30% and 10%, respectively. Chronic headache occurred in 14% of the patients and persistent weakness or numbness was found in 7%. The weakness and numbness became progressively worse in 5% of the patients.

A Striking Berry Burst: Intracranial Aneurysms

"Rebooting my brain: how a freak aneurysm reformed my life"

Maria Ross

She was cycling along Riverside Drive in New York as part of her 8-month programme to prepare herself for her first Ironman com-petition at Lake Placid in July 2007. Cynthia Lynn Sherwin was an experienced athlete, creative dietician and energetic elite fitness instructress. By the age of 33, she completed the New York Marathon five times and competed in several triathlons. Committed to her beliefs, she appeared frequently on radio and television to promote healthy living. In her drive to influence her ideals of proper exercise and sound nutrition to a new generation, Cynthia had just started giving talks to elementary and middle-school students. On that early Monday morning of 23 April 2007, Cindy left her Lower East Side apartment in Manhattan to train for her arduous 112-mile (180 kilo-metres) ride. She was to meet her clients that afternoon followed by a run through Central Park in the evening. But Cynthia never made it. Halfway through the journey, she collapsed and died suddenly from a ruptured intracranial aneurysm. By the following year,

TeamCindy was established to encourage athletes to participate in triathlon events under her banner to raise awareness regarding this condition. Her supporters expanded her vision and founded the Cindy Lynn Sherwin Memorial Foundation. Their objective is to continue her passion into inspiring individuals to achieve personal wellness through keeping fit physically and eating healthily.

An aneurysm is an out-pouching of a weakened blood vessel wall. Aneurysms can occur in any blood vessel in the body and come in various shapes and sizes. They may protrude from one side of the blood vessel wall or an entire section may be enlarged circumferentially (which may look like a miniature version of a python after it has swallowed a rat). When the aneurysm occurs in the head, where the blood vessels are relatively small, the "ballooned" section from one side of the wall looks like a berry, and hence the term, "berry" (saccular) aneurysm is coined (Figure 18). Persons are not usually born with an

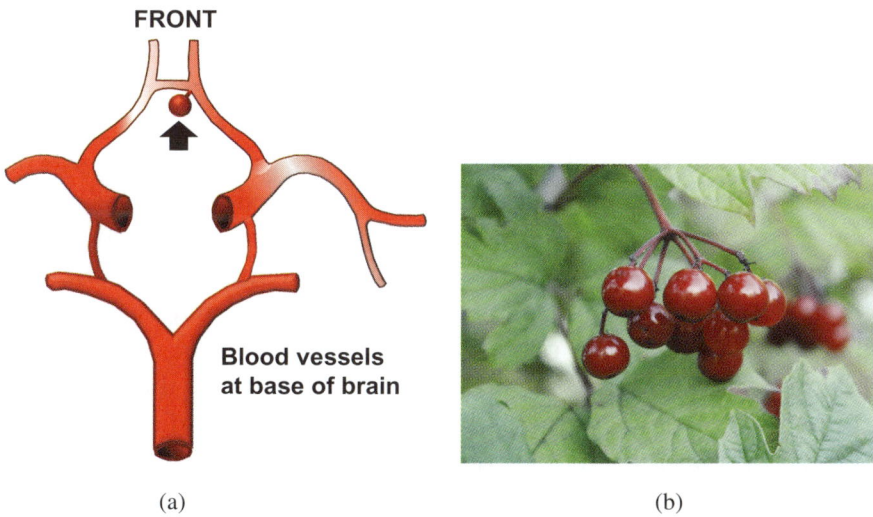

(a) (b)

Figure 18. Intracranial aneurysm.

A small aneurysm is present in the front arteries of the brain (arrowed) (panel A). The out-pouching of the blood vessel, may look like a berry (Panel B), and usually arises from the branch points. (B) Viburnum berries hanging from a green shrub. Although it is red, the fruits may be purple, blue or black. Some of them are edible but several others may be toxic. They may have a peculiar after-taste (Image obtained from Shuttlestock; ID: 150504095).

aneurysm. They develop after the age of 40 years and usually at the branching of vessels. As they are under constant pressure, the sac enlarges gradually and the wall becomes progressively thinner and weaker.

Several conditions have been associated with intracranial aneurysms. Most of them are related to atherosclerosis (or thickening of the blood vessels), such as hypertension and cigarette smoking, or weakening of the blood vessel wall as a result of congenital abnormalities, inflammation, infection or injury to the head. Not uncommonly, about 15% to 20% of patients have more than one intracranial aneurysm.

When the aneurysm ruptures, blood usually leaks into the space between the linings within the head, between the skull and the brain, known as subarachnoid haemorrhage. Less commonly, blood may accumulate in the brain tissue or flow into the brain cavities. Similar to arterio-venous malformation, no one knows when the aneurysm will rupture. They occur frequently between the ages of 35 and 60 years, and occur 2.5 times more commonly among women.[540] In a Finnish study of 142 patients with 181 unruptured intracranial aneurysms followed up for about 20 years, there were 33 episodes of bleeding. The annual rate of rupture was 1.3%.[541] In a review of several studies, the overall risk of bleeding was estimated to be 1.9% annually.[542] As expected, the larger the aneurysm, the greater the likelihood for rupture.[541,542] For every 1 mm increase in size, the risk increased by 11%.[541] When the diameter of the aneurysm was less than 10 mm, the annual risk for bleeding was only 0.7% compared to 4% for those 10 mm or larger.[542] On the other hand, the chance of rupture decreased with increasing age at the time of diagnosis. The risk fell by 3% for each older year. The risk for rupture was 7.5 times higher when an intracranial aneurysm was diagnosed at an age younger than 50 years.[540] There are also several other factors[540] that have been associated with greater odds for rupture including those who are suffering from hypertension, smoke cigarettes and have a family member with subarachnoid haemorrhage. Aneurysms located in the brain-stem are also more likely to rupture.[542] Any condition that suddenly increases blood pressure may increase the risk of rupture.

Once bleeding has occurred, the consequences are devastating. In a large cohort of more than 64,000 Finnish residents,[543] there were 437 patients who suffered from subarachnoid haemorrhage. Of these, 79 (18.1%) died outside the hospital or at the emergency room. In other words, as many as 1 in 6 patients with such type of bleeding in the head would have died before receiving optimal medical attention. For those who have survived the initial episode, the blood vessel may go into spasm to stop further bleeding. In doing so, blood supply to the brain is cut-off resulting in further damage to the brain. The brain may become swollen and may lead to even more injury. Normal automatic function, such as breathing, may be affected. Within the next 30 days, 95 (21.7%) of 437 patients died.[543] Even for those who have survived for a year, the risk of dying for patients with subarachnoid haemorrhage continued to be approximately two times higher than the general population. The heightened risk was attributed to the effects of the subarachnoid haemorrhage, subsequent damage to the brain or bleeding in the head. Sadly, less than a third of those who survive retain adequate neurological function.

How Common is Intracranial Aneurysm?

In a population-based cohort of 2,000 persons in Rotterdam, with a mean age of 63 years, using high-resolution structural brain magnetic resonance imaging, the aneurysms were present in 35 (1.8%).[544] For this group of individuals between the ages of 45 and 97 years, the prevalence of aneurysms did not increase with age. In a post-mortem study in Japan, there were 84 deceased with 102 unruptured intracranial aneurysms from 10,259 autopsies,[545] with a prevalence of 0.8%. The detection rates of intracranial aneurysms varied substantially because of different study designs and populations. Based on review of autopsy reports, it was estimated to be only 0.4%.[542] But when the information was collected prospectively; that is data were obtained when the post-mortem was conducted, the prevalence was estimated to be 3.6%. Correspondingly, in a review of angiographic studies, intracranial aneurysms were reported in 3.7%. However, they were detected in 6.0% of patients undergoing angiography. In the review of 23 studies, the prevalence was estimated to be 2.3%.[542] When the review was expanded to 68 studies with 1,450 intracranial aneurysms detected in 94,912 patients from 21 countries, the prevalence was estimated to be 3.2%.[546] The latter review included higher quality studies and imaging techniques were superior in detecting aneurysms.

Unlike, the Rotterdam experience, aneurysms in the Japanese study were found more frequently among older individuals. This trend of increasing prevalence of intracranial aneurysm with older persons was also observed in a review of 23 clinical studies.[542] However, most of these aneurysms in the Japanese study were small.[545] About 54 % of them were 4 mm or less in diameter and 35% were between 5 mm to 9 mm in diameter. There are other co-existing conditions that increase the likelihood for intracranial aneurysm. This abnormal protruberance of blood vessels occurred almost seven times more frequently among those with adult form of autosomal dominant polycystic disease of the kidney[546] and 3.5 times more likely when there were family members with intracranial aneurysm or subarachnoid haemorrhage.[546] Patients with atherosclerosis were 1.7 times more likely to have intracranial aneurysms.[546] The occurrence of intracranial aneurysms was 3.6 times higher for those with brain tumours.[546] Overall, intracranial aneurysms occurred more than 60% more frequently among women.[546]

What are the Symptoms?

Most individuals with aneurysms do not have any symptom. In the United States, 3 to 5 million Americans have been estimated to have intracranial aneurysms. The individual may complain of pulsating headache or localised pain. When an aneurysm compresses on a nerve or brain structure, it may produce symptoms corresponding to the site. For example, when the nerve to the eye-lid is affected, the person may blink frequently and the face may twitch. Hence, it may be summarily dismissed as a tic.

Sometimes, there may be an acceleration of the frequency and severity of headache before the aneurysm rupturing. Once the wall of the vessel is breeched and starts to bleed, the patient would have felt the most severe headache. When the pressure within the skull increases, the afflicted would start vomiting and become drowsy. Eventually, the person would fall into a coma. At other times, the patient would die suddenly. In a review of 113 patients with this form of bleeding in Rochester, Minnesota, 12 (13%) died outside the hospital.[547] If the bleeding occurs within the brain tissue, there may be weakness of one side of the body, the upper or lower limb, difficulty with speech and language, visual disturbance and seizure, depending on the territory of the brain that is affected.

When the Bleeding Starts

Once bleeding has occurred, treatment should be initiated as soon as possible. While treating the aneurysm does not reverse the brain damage, it will prevent further bleeding and damage. On stabilising the patient, physical rehabilitation may be beneficial.

The challenge is to manage a patient with an unruptured intracranial aneurysm. A team of specialists — consisting of neurologist, neurosurgeon and interventional neuro-radiologist — may have to be assembled for the task. Every patient should be considered individually based on symptoms, location, size and shape of the aneurysm. For small aneurysms in asymptomatic individuals, patients are followed up regularly for new signs and symptoms, optimising blood pressure and lipid control, treated for other medical conditions and advised to quit smoking. Repeated imaging examination may be useful to determine if the size of the aneurysm increases. Other treatment modalities include use of surgical clips or coils to occlude the aneurysm. As with any form of intervention, the accompanying risks include damage to normal blood vessels and brain tissue, bleeding and infection.

Detecting Abnormal Blood Vessels in the Head

While these two conditions are different, both arterio-venous malformation and intracranial aneurysm are abnormalities of the blood vessels in the head. Thus, some form of imaging of the blood vasculature is used for diagnosis. There are two types of non-invasive procedure that can be used to see the blood vessels. The first is computed tomographic cerebral angiography. This is a sophisticated X-ray machine in which contrast is injected into a vein so as to visualise the blood vessels in the head. Another test is magnetic resonance angiography in which strong magnetic fields are applied to the head to generate images. In both types of procedures, the patient is placed on a table and slid into a "tunnel" to obtain the images. The time taken to acquire the images for computed tomography is considerably shorter than magnetic resonance angiography. However, there is X-ray radiation in computed tomography and contrast material, which may be toxic to the kidney or the patient may develop an allergic reaction. These techniques have evolved and dynamic images may be obtained to provide higher quality pictures to make more precise diagnosis, in particular for arterio-venous malformation, the type of vascular network and drainage.

Diagnostic cerebral angiography is an invasive procedure in which a small tube is inserted and guided to each of the blood vessels that go to the brain. Similar to coronary angiography, contrast material is injected into each of the blood vessels and X-ray is performed so that all cerebral arteries are seen. This is the most reliable test to detect abnormalities in the blood vessels of the head.

Can We Stop the "Time Bomb" from Ticking?

An arterio-venous malformation is meshwork of blood vessel pulsating with every heart beat. It may appear similar to a biological improvised explosive device. On the other hand, the intracranial aneurysm may look like a balloon, being inflated with every heart beat, and may burst at any time. Indeed, no one knows when it will happen.

A brain arterio-venous malformation and its association with bleeding have been described for more than 120 years, with the risk being initially quantified two to three decades ago. However, it is an uncommon cause for sudden death, accounting for about 1%.[548] Early estimate for the annual rate for haemorrhage for untreated brain arterio-venous malformation is about 2% to 4%.[549,550] But this is not a uniform condition and the risk of bleeding depends on the size of the anomalous vessel, the location on the brain and the vein which the anomalous vessel is draining into.[551] In one study, the yearly risk for bleeding is 0.9% for arterio-venous malformation that is located superficially on the brain and draining to superficial veins compared with 34% for one that is sited deep in the brain and draining to deep veins.[552] A total of 678 patients with arterio-venous malformation in the brain were identified at the Toronto Western Hospital in Canada.[553] After a mean follow-up period of 2.9 years (or 1,932 patient-years), the rate of bleeding was 4.6% per year. Of the 89 who bled, 5 died (6%) and 31 (35%) suffered from significant functional impairment. The risk of bleeding was higher in the first year of diagnosis. Presence of an intra-cranial aneurysm increased the risk for bleeding by about 60%. The risk of bleeding was about 14 times higher among those who had bled in the brain within the first year.[554] It was also nine-fold higher for men. Although it is challenging to estimate, the risk of dying after bleeding in the brain is 10% to 15%. Significant brain damage, leading to paralysis or weakness of limbs, may be as high as 20% to 30% after bleeding in the brain.

An international multi-centre clinical trial was conducted from 2007 to determine if some form of intervention could prevent death or stroke in patients with unruptured arterio-venous malformation.[555] Interventional therapies are procedures used to remove or destroy the arterio-venous malformation and include surgery to remove the abnormal blood vessels (neurosurgery), using X-ray to guide doctors to use material to occlude the abnormal blood vessels (embolism using interventional neuro-radiological technique) or using high energy radiofrequency waves that are focussed on the abnormal blood vessels and annihilate them (stereotatic radiotherapy). However, the study was prematurely terminated on 5 April 2013 because patients who did not receive intervention were

3.7 times less likely to die or suffer from a stroke. Of the 114 patients who were randomly assigned to intervention, the rate of stroke or death after 33 months of follow-up was 31%. However, these adverse outcomes occurred in only 10% for the 109 patients who did not undergo any form of intervention. But some doctors were critical of their findings. Early risk increased with intervention treatment and the 3-year duration of the study might not be sufficiently long to provide information on long-term outcome. The investigators were also admonished for not stratifying the risk of the patient and the arterio-venous malformation. Patient's age, size, location (which part of the brain is involved), how the veins flow and presence of other abnormality in the blood vessels could have influenced the risk and danger of rupture. Since the mode of intervention was not specified in the study, success and complication rates differed leading to varying results.[556] Despite these criticisms, a long-term observational study of up to 24 years among 204 patients with arterio-venous malformation in Scotland showed comparable findings.[557] After about 7 years of follow-up, the likelihood for death or disability due to bleeding in the head for those treated without intervention was lower, at about 0.6 the rate of those who received intervention. Treatment techniques and operator skills improve with time.[556] Published and follow-up studies have almost been limited by evolving technologies in a rapidly changing environment. As such, the use of intervention therapies should be carefully considered individually.

In most instances, the approach to a patient who was discovered an arterio-venous malformation, especially when it cannot be removed, is conservative management. Patients with intracranial aneurysms should also be cautious about their daily activities. Smokers are strongly encouraged to quit smoking. The patient is to avoid activities that increase the risk of head injury or blood pressure. Hence, activities such as contact sports — rugby or soccer, high-demand physical activity — marathon running and long distance cycling, leisure activities that increase the risk of fall or head injury — skiing or bungee jumping, and extreme sports — iron-man competition and rock climbing, should be avoided. Lifting heavy objects or straining may increase blood pressure and the risk of rupture. As such, these activities should not be performed. Violent and explosive emotions such as rage or grave sadness have also been associated with bleeding. Blood thinners — aspirin or warfarin, stimulants — pseudoephrine and amphetamines and recreational drugs — cocaine, increase the risk of rupture. They should be followed up regularly by a neurologist or neurosurgeon and control blood pressure adequately.

The Sporadic Killers
Less Common Causes of Sudden Death

Flight to Eternity: Pulmonary Embolism

"The sensation I had was fantastic. I was flying as free as a bird. It was so peaceful up there. It was the first time in my life I thought I was going to burst with excitement. It is not every day you can see your own shadow on top of a cloud."

Diary of Emma Christoffersen
September 2000

She loved travelling and the trip to Australia was an opportunity that could not be missed. Although it was not her first long haul flight, sadly, it was certainly the last. Emma Christoffersen was a 28-year-old fit healthy woman from Newport, South Wales, and was planning to get married after returning from Australia. Despite working as a sales assistant in the confines of a Marks and Spencer outlet, she loved the outdoors, especially the outback. It was indeed a trip of her life-time to spend three weeks of vacation with her best friend, Rhian Bevan. They went parachuting and scuba diving. On return to London from Sydney, via Singapore, Rhian recalled that half-way through the 12,000-mile journey over 20-odd hours, Emma complained of an irritating rash at the bottom of her leg. However, Emma did not make a fuss out of it. To avoid disturbing her sleeping neighbouring passengers, she slept most of the time. On disembarking the flight, Emma complained of breathlessness and was unable to catch up with Rhian in Heathrow Airport. Suddenly, she stopped, slumped against the window and collapsed slowly on to the floor. The paramedics arrived within minutes and administered oxygen. Emma woke up struggling and complained of pain, and said that she was scared and cold. Using a tunnel beneath the runways, Emma was quickly brought to Ashford Hospital. Even though she was rushed immediately to the resuscitation room, it was too late. Emma had already died. Her premature death made headline news worldwide. Post-mortem examination identified the cause to be deep vein thrombosis and massive pulmonary embolism. These two conditions are related, and collectively known as venous thrombo-embolism (VTE).

Having lost their child, Ruth and John Christoffersen campaigned fervently to bring others to attention this potentially fatal condition and the perils of long distance travel. Her parents were perplexed as to how Emma could have died when she did not smoke and had lived an active life. Ruth's message was simple and straightforward. Deep vein thrombosis and pulmonary embolism "... can hit young people. It seems to strike at random and in a way is just like Russian roulette." About eight months later, they were able to tell the story of their beloved daughter to a global audience. The programme "Economy Class Syndrome" was telecasted on 10 June 2001 in the British Broadcasting Corporation (BBC) television current affairs documentary series, Panorama. With such extensive publicity on this condition, the international media frenzy made the medical, aviation and regulatory communities raise the issue to a higher priority.

When Symington and Stack identified eight patients suffering from pulmonary embolism shortly after air travel, they have earlier coined the term "Economy Class Syndrome" in 1977.[558] But others felt that the term "economy class" was misleading because the condition can occur at any class or mode of travel. So in 2000, the United Kingdom House of Lords Select Committee on Science and Technology preferred to use "Traveller's Thrombosis" instead.[559] However, this fanciful name did not catch on with the popular media.

Lack of mobility was likely to be the contributory factor for deep vein thrombosis. Indeed, the association between immobilisation was also observed during the Second World War of London in 1939.[560] During a simulated bombing exercise, there were 23 persons who slept on deckchairs underground who died mysteriously. Dr Keith Simpson found that those deaths were due to clots in the lungs. The authorities acted on this information promptly by replacing deckchairs with bunk beds. Then the deaths stopped. Subsequent analysis quantified the risk associated with travelling. Travellers were more than two times more likely to suffer from deep vein thrombosis or pulmonary embolism compared with non-travellers.[561] Air travel poses a unique environment for clotting, such as cramped seating with a compressed thigh and limited room for leg movement, lower oxygen, humidity and pressure in the air. For every 2-hour increase in the duration of travel by any mode, the risk for VTE was raised by 18%. However, the risk was increased by 26% for air travel.

Deep vein thrombosis occurs when clots develop in the deep veins of the legs. The word thrombosis refers to formation of clots. There are two sets of venous systems in our legs: the superficial and deep veins. Those vessels that can be seen on the surface of the leg, beneath the skin, belong to the superficial system. On the other hand, the deep veins run through the calf and thigh muscles. Since we have adopted an upright posture, after blood has flowed to the legs, the return of blood to the heart may be slow and requires assistance. So when the leg muscles contract, they act as an accessory pump to drive the blood back to the heart. Although a person may not be aware when there are small clots that are formed in the veins. The patient may complain of pain, swelling, redness and warm at the site of the thrombosis. Though the clots by themselves are not dangerous, it may result in long-term swelling of the feet and damage to the skin if the veins remain blocked. Based on studies of patients who had developed deep vein thrombosis in the calf following surgery, about half of them resolve spontaneously within 72 hours, and in a sixth of the patients propagate towards the veins in the thigh.[562,563] However, if the patient

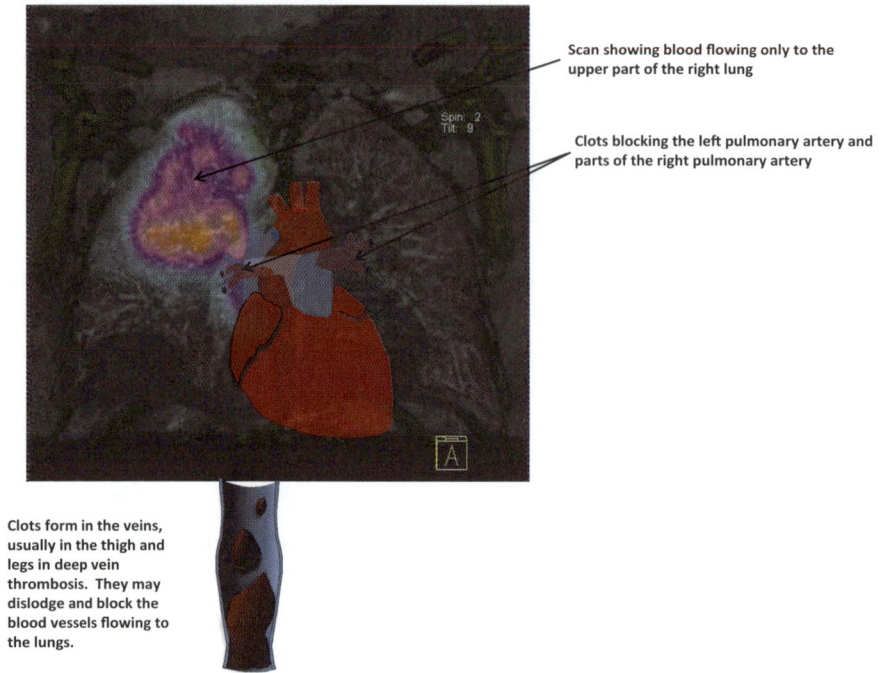

Scan showing blood flowing only to the upper part of the right lung

Clots blocking the left pulmonary artery and parts of the right pulmonary artery

Clots form in the veins, usually in the thigh and legs in deep vein thrombosis. They may dislodge and block the blood vessels flowing to the lungs.

Figure 19.   Deep Vein Thrombosis and Pulmonary Embolism.

develops pain or swelling, the rate of progression increases to one in four.[564] It is believed that when the clot extends above the knees, the condition can become life-threatening. At this site, the clot is more likely to break off and then lodge at a vessel whose size is smaller than that of the clot. After returning to the heart, blood continues to flow in the artery to the lung (Figure 19). When the flow is obstructed, it gives rise to a condition known as pulmonary embolism. Depending on the location of interruption of blood flow, the patient may have chest pain, shortness of breath and in the worst case scenario, sudden death. In hospitalised patients, about 11% to 12% succumb during the early phase of the ill-ness.[565,566] For the next two years, the annual recurrence rate for VTE was 4.4%.[566]

This less well-known condition has been estimated to account for 100,000 deaths in the United States yearly.[567] The annual incidence of VTE was 1 per 1,000 Americans.[565,568] However, there were ethnic differences in the occurrence of VTE.[569] In California, the rate was highest for African-Americans (141 per 100,000) followed by Caucasians (104 per 100,000) and Hispanics (55 per 100,000). Asians and Pacific-Islanders had the lowest incidence (21 per 100,000). Approximately 25% of patients had acute pulmonary embolism, and the first manifestation is sudden unexpected death.[570] Correspondingly, 10% of patients with symptomatic acute pulmonary embolism following surgery died within an hour.[564] Over a 32-month period in Seville, Spain, 2,447 autopsies were conducted in the Institute of Legal Medicine. There were 29 individuals who died from pulmonary embolism.[571] This number constituted 4.3% of all sudden deaths. In New York City, the overall annual incidence for out-of-hospital fatal pulmonary embolism was 1.6 per 100,000 residents.[572] When the diagnosis of pulmonary embolism is made, mortality rate ranged from 3% to 8%. Conversely, when the diagnosis is missed, mortality is 4 to 6 times higher.

Patients with VTE are treated with blood thinners. Initially, the medicine may be administered by injecting heparin followed by oral anticoagulants. Heparin may be infused intravenously or injected under the skin, a technique similar to injecting insulin. Alternatively, oral anticoagulation alone may be used. The traditional medicine used orally is warfarin. This medicine prevents the formation of certain clotting factors by blocking the action of Vitamin K. However, the therapeutic range of thinning of blood to prevent clotting is narrow. If the blood is not sufficiently thin, it may not be efficacious. Conversely, if the blood is too thin, the risk of bleeding is high. Importantly, certain foods and other medicines can affect the efficacy of warfarin. Thus, the thinness of the blood needs to be assessed regularly. To reduce the inconvenience of clinic visits, home monitoring is available. A new anticoagulation, known as rivaroxaban (Xarelto), has been approved for treatment of patients with VTE. Compared with warfarin, the number of food and medicines interaction is considerably less than warfarin. Blood testing is not routinely needed and the test for the degree of blood thinning for rivaroxaban is currently not freely available. Antidote for rivaroxaban is also not easily available. Not unexpectedly, the new medicine is more expensive than warfarin. However, the overall cost may be comparable because patients treated with rivaroxaban do not require frequent clinic visits and blood testing. The duration of treatment depends on the extent of deep vein thrombosis, presence of pulmonary embolism, provocation and predisposing factors for VTE. For those who are unable to use blood thinners for whatever reason, filters may be inserted in the large vein in the abdomen to prevent clots from reaching the lungs. These filters may be removed subsequently.

When there is a large amount of clots in the arteries in the lungs, especially when the blood pressure is low and there is not enough blood flowing to the body, more potent medicines may be used. These medicines may dissolve clots but is accompanied by a higher risk of bleeding. One of the most feared complications using this group of medicine is bleeding in the brain. Although uncommon (1%), the risk of dying is very high when it occurs. Alternatively, surgery may be performed to remove the clots from the pulmonary arteries. Catheters have also been developed to remove the clots without opening the chest.

To prevent deep vein thrombosis is to prevent pulmonary embolism. General measures include adequate hydration, exercise or leg massage, avoid crossing legs, use of compression stockings or foot pumps, avoid alcohol or caffeinated beverages and walk about when possible. However, there are several characteristics that increase the risk for the conditions and specific precautionary steps may have to be undertaken before long distance travel. Individuals older than 40 years, who are very short or very tall, pregnant or suffer from cancer, heart failure or metabolic disorders such as diabetes mellitus and obesity, have a greater tendency to develop clots. Risk is also higher for smokers, oral contraceptive users, those with previous deep vein thrombosis, who have undergone recent surgery to the abdomen, pelvis or legs and individuals with family members with clotting disorders. There are certain medical conditions such as cancers, antiphospholipid syndrome and genetic disorders that increase the risk of clotting and VTE.

Mayhem in the Highway: Acute Aortic Syndromes

"Was there anything in the health care system could have done to save my brother?"

Vivian Ho
James A. Baker III Institute Chair in Health Economics
Rice University
Houston, Texas

As Hurricane Katrina was battering through the streets of New Orleans, destroying properties and lives, Michael Ho was suffering quietly in his home when his principal artery in his chest tore apart on 13 August 2005. Several days earlier, while on vacation golfing in Ireland, the body of the 42-year-old bank executive began to swell. By the time he returned home to Beverly Hills in California, Michael felt extremely ill and complained of swelling and severe chest pain that radiated to the back. His family physician was unable to determine the cause of his pain but noticed that the heart was not in the normal position in the chest X-ray. The doctor attributed the swelling to an allergic reaction from the food he ate earlier on that day and treated him with anti-histamines. Nonetheless, Michael was referred to a cardiologist on a non-urgent basis. His somewhat sudden death was attributed to an aortic dissection. When recounting the symptoms to her friend and medical colleagues, it was clear that her brother was suffering from a medical emergency. What his sister, who is also an Associate Professor in the Department of Medicine at Baylor College of Medicine, was upset about was whether her brother could have been saved. Aortic dissection is part of the group of potentially life-threatening disorders known as acute aortic syndrome, which includes intramural haematoma, penetrating atheromatous ulcer, aortic aneurysm leak and rupture. Some doctors felt that aortic dissection, intramural haematoma and penetrating atheromatous ulcer belong to the spectrum of aortic dissection.[573] Nonetheless, these patients complained of severe pain in the chest or the abdomen, and the blood pressure is low due to loss of blood volume. Since the aorta is a long conduit, other symptoms may arise depending on the site. It includes heart failure (7%) with presenting symptoms of shortness of breath and swelling, loss of consciousness (9%), stroke (6%), heart attack, weakness of one limb or both legs and sudden death.[574]

The aorta is the main conduit and the largest blood vessel that carries blood to all parts of the body. When blood is pumped out of the heart, it enters the aorta. It starts in the chest and moves towards the neck before doing a U-turn at the back of the chest and descends into the abdomen. Eventually, the aorta terminates in the lower abdomen by branching to the right and left side of the pelvis so that the arteries continue into the legs. As with any blood vessel, the wall is made up of three layers. The inner layer, known as intima, separates blood and its components from the rest of the blood vessel wall. Unlike a pipe, the intima is biologically active and controls substances entering and exiting the arterial wall. The outer layer is the adventitia which holds the vessel in its position and interacts with surrounding tissues. In between the layers, is a muscular layer which controls the tone of the aorta.

For reasons unclear, a tear may occur in the inner lining of the aortic wall extends to the middle layer (Figure 20). However, it usually occurs in an area of the aorta that has been damaged or degenerated. Blood rushes in and forms a double-lumen aorta, consisting of the original channel, which is known as the "true" lumen, and the new channel, which is known as the "false" lumen. Generally, the "false" lumen is larger than the "true" lumen. The torn vessel wall is known as the intimo-medial flap or the entry point. Blood in the false lumen may then break through at another site and re-enter the true lumen. There may be more than one exit points. Besides being thinner, the wall of the "false" lumen may also be weaker. Due to the pressure in the vessel, it may rupture and the consequence may be catastrophic. Alternatively, the enlarged portion may compress other tissues giving rise to symptoms such as pain. In other situations, the torn vessel wall may obstruct blood flowing into vital organs. If the blood vessel to the head is affected, the patient may suffer from a stroke. The blood column in the "false" lumen is not always static. As such, it may propagate forward or backward to extend the degree of damage.

Slanted side view of the chest cavity

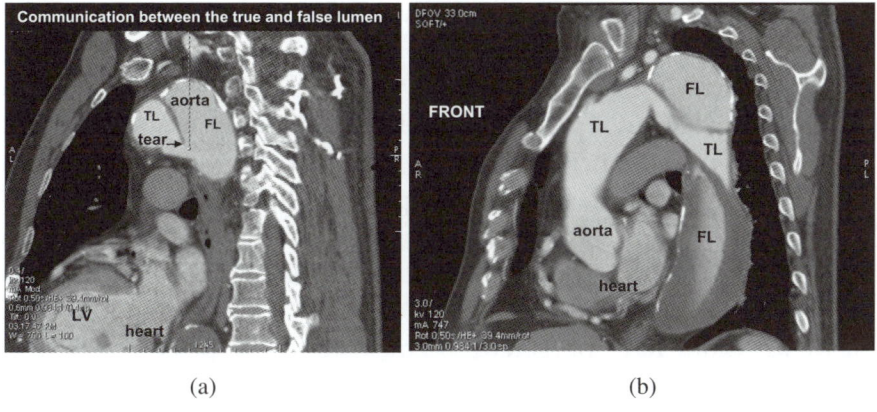

(a)   (b)

Slanted side view of the chest cavity

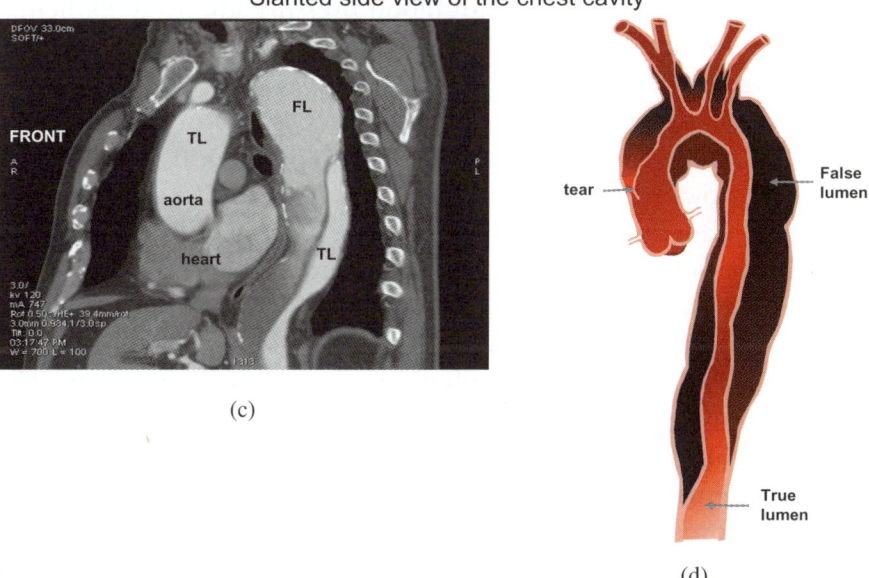

(c)   (d)

Figure 20. Aortic dissection.

The aorta arises from the left ventricle (LV) of the heart. Panel A shows the tear (dissection) of the main blood vessel (aorta) and the entrance from the true lumen (TL) to the false lumen (FL). The false lumen (FL) compresses on the true lumen (TL) near the arch of the aorta because of the accumulation of the blood (Panel B). As the aorta continues in its course, the true lumen is the smaller and brighter channel (Panel C). Panel D shows aortic dissection diagrammatically.

The most common predisposing factor for aortic dissection is hypertension (72%) followed by atherosclerosis (31%).[575] Those with previous cardiac surgery (18%) and connective tissue disorder, such as Marfan or Ehlers Danlos syndrome (5%) accounted for a smaller proportion of patients. The key to management of a patient with aortic dissection is to control blood pressure. Unfortunately, dissection involves the proximal aspect of the aorta in about two-thirds of the cases.[576] When it occurs, the chance of dying is 1% to 2% per hour for the first 24 to 48 hours. By 48 hours, about 30% of these patients would have died, by a week, 40% and by a month, half of them would have perished.[575] Thus, when the proximal part of the aorta is affected, surgery or some form of intervention is required. If the dissection occurs at the descending or abdominal aorta, the patient is treated with blood pressure lowering medicines unless the risk of rupture is high or when blood flow to a vital organ is compromised.

Another uncommon aortic emergency is rupture of an aneurysm. An aneurysm is an enlarged portion of a blood vessel. As the segment grows bigger, the wall becomes thinner. Most of the time, the person does not know if an aneurysm is present unless it presses on some structure that cause symptoms such as pain. When the wall is breeched, blood may leak out slowly or rupture, which is similar to a balloon. The patient may experience severe pain and low blood pressure. There may be a pulsating mass in the abdomen. The chance of dying is 80% to 90% for those who are admitted to hospital. With surgery, it is lowered to about 50%. Approximately, about 5% of patients are symptomatic before an aortic emergency occurs. In other words, for the remaining 95%, the first symptom is death. The risk of rupture was four times higher in women and two times higher in smokers.[577]

Since patients with aortic aneurysms do not usually have symptoms, ultrasonic examination of the abdomen may be a suitable technique to identify and follow-up this group of patients. In a review of 127,891 men and 9,342 women between the ages of 65 to 79 years, the chance of dying from rupture of the aneurysm or from emergency or elective surgery for repair of the aneurysm was 40%

lower for men after 3 to 5 years of screening.[578] Correspondingly, the rate of aneurysmal rupture was lowered by 55%. Due to a smaller number of women in the study, these benefits were not observed for female. However, screening increased the likelihood for men undergoing aortic surgery by two-fold. In a smaller subgroup of 67,770 men in the United Kingdom, when the follow-up period was extended to 7 years, the risk of dying was reduced by almost 50%.[579] Notably, when the ultrasonic examination was normal, the risk of rupture was low at 0.54 per 10,000 person-years. In other words, one of these subjects with normal scan was expected to have a rupture of the abdominal aorta after 20,000 years. Thus, it appears that screening is useful for men in this age group, especially for smokers and those at risk for aneurysm. Indeed, in January 2014, the United States Preventive Services Task Force reaffirms its 2005 recommendation of one-time ultrasonography screening for abdominal aneurysm for men aged 65 to 75 years who have ever smoked.[580]

Several studies have been conducted to determine if medicines can prevent the enlargement of an aortic aneurysm. Importantly, blood pressure must be adequately controlled. Aneurysm growth is generally slow, estimated to be 2.21 mm annually.[577] While growth rate was increased in smokers (by 0.35 mm yearly), it was decreased in patients with diabetes (by 0.51 mm every year). Traditionally, beta-blockers — anti-hypertensive agents — have been used. This group of medicines blocks the effect of adrenaline, and hence prevent the effect of pressure on the wall of the aorta. Long term administration of propranolol, a beta-blocker, was shown to slow down the rate of aortic enlargement in a study of 70 patients with Marfan's syndrome and mild to moderate dilated aorta.[581] Of the 38 patients who did not receive propranolol, four patients suffered from aortic dissection after 9 years. After 11 years, only 2 of the 32 patients who were treated with propranolol had aortic dissection. One of these two patients did not receive beta-blocker. However, others found that beta-blockers may increase the mortality of patients treated with beta-blockers.[582]

Molecular biological techniques have not only identified the defect that cause Marfan's syndrome but have created mice with the condition by inducing changes in their genetic make-up. Based on their experiments, therapeutic approaches were developed to strengthen the connective tissue. In addition to the usual treatment with beta-blockers, an angiotensin converting enzyme inhibitor, perindopril (Coverysl), was shown to lower the stiffness of the large arteries and aortic diameter in a small study of 17 patients.[583] Angiotensin receptor blockers, another type of blood pressure lowering medicine, were also found to be useful in preventing the enlargement of the aorta in 18 patients with Marfan's syndrome and were younger than 16 years.[584] Statin therapy also showed potential in preventing the aorta from growing larger.[585]

Doxycycline, a commonly used antibiotic, has also been shown to inhibit an enzyme which can weaken the aortic wall. A multi-centre Dutch clinical trial evaluated the efficacy of this drug in preventing progression of abdominal aortic aneurysm in 286 patients.[586] After 18 months, doxycycline did not slow down the enlargement of the aneurysm, lower the need for elective surgical repair and reduce the time to repair. In fact, the diameter of the aneurysm for those receiving doxycycline grew 0.8 mm more than patients receiving placebo, especially during the first six months of the study.

Damaged Gates and Leaking Valves

"Runner down, runner down!"

A spotter yelling in his bullhorn
30th Chicago Marathon Event

The date, 7 October 2007, was not a day that marathoners can easily forget. Although 45,000 participants were to be flagged off at 8 am on that morning of the 30th Annual Chicago Marathon, about 10,000 of them did not turn up. It was a relatively warm and humid autumn day and temperature reached higher than 31°C (88°F) in the late morning. For the first time in 30 years, the run was stopped prematurely at about 11:30 am. Almost 11,000 participants did not complete the run, more than 300 requiring medical attention, 49 were hospitalised, with at least three in critical condition and one man dead. The 15 first-aid stations and ambulances were over-whelmed and there was chaos and confusion in the course. It was like a war zone with runners carried away in stretchers, people yell-ing for medics, screaming sirens from emergency vehicles and deaf-ening noises from helicopters hovering overhead.

As with several of them, it was his first marathon. Chad Schieber, a 35-year-old physically fit police officer from Midland, in Lower Michigan, had been training hard for the previous six months. At about noon, he collapsed at the 18th mile mark at the South Side. Chad was evacuated to a hospital and pronounced dead at 12:50 pm. Sadly, his wife and brother, who also participated in the race, only knew about his death after they returned to their hotels. Initially thought to have succumbed to heat injury, Dr Nancy Jones, Chief Medical Examiner of the Cook County announced that he had sig-nificant mitral valve prolapse after an autopsy.

Mitral valve prolapse is a common medical condition found in 2.4% of the population.[587] Previous estimate was higher, at about 5%, and the likely reason was that less stringent criteria were used for diagnosis.[588] The mitral valve is a complex two-leaflet structure that separates the left atrium and left ventricle. When the left ventri-cle contracts, blood is pumped out into the aorta, which is the main conduit. At the same time, the mitral valve closes to prevent blood from flowing back to the left atrium. In mitral valve prolapse, the leaflets, which are like two panels of a door, are thickened and redundant, and bulge into the left atrium, otherwise known as pro-lapse. Sometimes, the leaflets do not close completely and it may leak. The rate of sudden death in patients with mitral valve prolapse was estimated to be 16 to 41 per 10,000 per year, or approximately 0.2% to 0.4% annually.[589,590] Although the figure was low, it was still about twice the expected rate in the general population. For several years, abnormal heart rhythm has been postulated to be the underly-ing mechanism of sudden death among patients with mitral valve prolapse.[591] The risk was greater for those with severe back-flow or leakage, reduced heart function, prolapse of both leaflets, frequent missed beats and women.[592,593] When the apparatus to hold the mitral valve breaks, the leakage is severe and the rate of sudden death increases to about 1.8% yearly.[594]

Patients with mitral valve prolapse do not have specific symptoms. However, they may complain of chest pain, palpitation, shortness of breath or giddiness. On listening to the chest, there is a clicking sound which may be followed by a murmur. In most cases, echocardiogram will show the diagnostic features of mitral valve prolapse. The majority of patients with this condition can live a normal life and enjoy most physical activities.[592] However, they should avoid extreme sports.

Another more commonly recognised valve disorder known to cause sudden death is aortic valve disease. Instead of two leaflets, this valve has three cusps which separate the aorta from the left ventricle. After blood is pumped out from the heart, the valve prevents it from flowing backwards. Bicuspid aortic valve is one of the most common congenital malformation of the heart affecting 0.4% to 2.3% in the general population.[595] Since there are only two cusps, the valve does not function normally and it becomes narrowed or leak. Among older individuals, the aortic valve may be thickened and calcified. The cusps may then be fused together, making the opening smaller, a condition known as aortic stenosis. In those cases, the narrowing becomes more severe and the heart needs to pump harder. When the valve opening is small and the output is limited, the heart may fail. At other times, there may be abnormal heart rhythms which could be fatal. For those without symptoms, such as breathlessness, chest pain, palpitations, giddiness or fainting spells, the risk of sudden death is estimated to be about 1% annually.[596,597]

Although these individuals may not have symptoms, auscultation of the chest would reveal a heart murmur. Echocardiography generally confirms the diagnosis.[598] Among those without symptoms and with mild aortic stenosis may participate in low impact sports.[132] However, competitive sports should be avoided for individuals with moderate to severe aortic stenosis. Aortic valve surgery may be performed for some cases.

Fit to Death: Sudden Unexpected Death in Epilepsy

"[Patsy Custis] *rose from dinner about four o'clock in better health and spirits than she had appeared to have been in for some time; soon after which she was seized with one of her usual fits and expired in it in less than two minutes without uttering a word, a groan, or scarce a sigh. This sudden and unexpected blow ... has almost reduced my poor wife to the lowest ebb of misery.*"

Writing to his brother regarding the death
of his 12-year-old step-daughter
George Washington

In the community-wide Oregon Sudden Unexpected Death Study[445] over a 2-year period from 2002 to 2004, there were 121 individuals who died suddenly and had left ventricular function assessed prior to death. Among these, 58 (48%) had normal heart function, and a seizure disorder was present in 8 of them (14%). These individuals did not die from an accident, prolonged life-threatening seizure, known as status epilepticus, or any other cause of death. Prior to their death, they were in fairly good health and were performing their usual activities. In some cases, there may be abnormalities after careful examination of the brain stem.[599]

A group of three British investigators described the accounts of 15 deaths which were attributed to sudden unexpected death in epilepsy (SUDEP).[600] This number constituted 11% of all the patients who died from this condition. There were 9 men and 6 women with ages ranging from 17 to 47 years. The most frequent location was in the bed and all seven of them who died there (47%) had generalised seizure. In fact, 12 (80%) had the typical generalised tonic-clonic seizure. There was a 47-year-old man with generalised tonic-clonic seizures after sustaining injury to his head and subsequent infection of the brain. Since there was no recurrence of the fits for eight years, he did not receive anti-convulsant therapy. One day, he returned home early from work because of a headache and went to bed. His wife heard strange noises in the bedroom. She found him lying on his side and jerking. After about a minute, he flipped on his back suddenly and the fit stopped. As he was blue and not breathing, his wife performed mouth-to-mouth resuscitation. When he was able to breathe again, she left the room to telephone for assistance without putting him in the recovery position. When she returned a few minutes later, breathing had stopped again and there was no pulse. Cardiopulmonary resuscitation recommenced until the arrival of the paramedics. One of the other three deceased who did not suffer from a convulsion shouted, "I'm going to have a convulsive seizure" before collapsing and died without have a fit. Another regained consciousness following a seizure but collapsed 5 minutes later. A 17-year-old girl was found lying in the street with a pool of urine and was incoherent. She then stopped breathing, but a pulse was felt initially. Cardiopulmonary resuscitation was initiated as the pulse faded. But it was unsuccessful.

Of 1,000 persons with epilepsy, about one of them died of sudden unexpected death in epilepsy. However, the incidence ranges from 1 in 370 to 1 in 1,110 of patients with epilepsy per year.[601] Among those with poorly controlled seizures, this condition occurred more commonly, approximately 1 in 150 to 1 in 200.[601] The risk of sudden unexpected death in epilepsy may be higher among those in the 20- to 40-year-old age group, of African American descent, with structural abnormality in the brain, who abuse alcohol and have poor compliance with anti-epileptic medicine.[601] Although the use of two or more anti-epileptic agents was associated with a higher risk of sudden death, no specific medicine was identified to have a higher risk.[602] Thus, rather than the drug, the frequency of seizure was more likely to be associated with SUDEP.[603] For patients with more than 50 seizures a year, the risk of SUDEP was more than 10 times higher than those with not more than two attacks annually.[604] In addition, epileptic patients with longer duration of disease (more than 10 years), mental retardation and psychiatric disease were more likely to die suddenly.[605] Another report stated that if there were three or more tonic-clonic seizures in the preceding year, the risk of sudden, unexpected death is increased by more than eight times.[602,604] However, absence or myoclonic seizures were not known to increase the risk of sudden death.

There may be several underlying mechanisms for SUDEP. During a seizure attack, breathing may be interrupted and airway may be obstructed. After a seizure, the upper airways may collapse and block the passage of airflow. Another probable reason may be the brain signals for spontaneous breathing were lost, resulting in death. There may be changes in the pressure of the blood vessels in the lungs leading to water leaking into the lungs.[606] The patient then drowns. Due to disorganised electrical activities, the heart may also be affected and the patient can also suffer from a cardiac arrest. Indeed, there were structural abnormalities in the hearts of patients with epilepsy who died suddenly.[607] In particular, there were scars detected in the heart muscle and could be the source of lethal heart rhythms. The scars may be the result of lack of oxygen delivery to the heart muscle during seizures because the patient stopped breathing, spasm of the coronary artery or sudden rise in acute stress hormones.[607] Increase in the autonomic stimulation has also been found in patients with SUDEP.[608] Conversely, the seizure may be the result of an abnormal heart rhythm. Among 19 patients with refractory focal seizures from the Institute of Neurology at the University College London, an implantable electrocardiographic recorder was implanted.[609] The investigators found that during a seizure, 4 patients (21%) had slow heart rate, requiring implantation of a permanent pacemaker. Importantly, 3 (16%) of them had potentially fatal episodes when the heart stopped beating.

Since the cause for sudden death is unknown, there is no specific measure that could be undertaken. About two-thirds of patients with SUDEP died in their bed.[600] Monitoring them during sleep, by physically checking or using devices, may reduce the risk of sudden death by 2.5- to 10-fold.[610] Importantly, persons living with patients with epilepsy should be instructed on first-aid responses during a convulsion, in particular, the positioning of the individual and keeping the airway patent. Optimisation of seizure control may prevent convulsion, and hence SUDEP. For patients, comply with anti-epileptic medicines to reduce the frequency of seizures and subsequent risk for SUDEP, especially during periods of stress.[606] However, control of fits can be challenging in up to 30% of patients, and these individuals have the highest risk of sudden death. Among those whose seizures were controlled with surgery, the occurrence of SUDEP was lower.[611,612]

PART III

Can Sudden Death be Prevented?

History ... Checked ... Examination... Checked ... Investigations ... Checked ...

The Role of Routine Medical Examination

"Every time you get a movie, you get a medical. So you know, you know you're alright for a couple of weeks."

Sir Michael Caine
British Actor and Academy Award Winner

Or is it?

Most of us would be aware of a routine car maintenance programme. This is a regular activity when the owner brings the vehicle to a mechanic to inspect and test the car, service or replace certain parts, lubricants or other fluids. As a result, the automobile is deemed safe, functional and reliable, and that its expected life-span may be ensured. Not surprisingly, this concept of preventive maintenance is also being extended to our bodies. Routine medical examination is expected to identify problems early and manage them appropriately to optimise health outcomes. Thus, can routine medical examination prevent sudden death? How much does it cost? Is it affordable?

While the occurrence of sudden death was highest among individuals from the general population, the incidence is the lowest.[30,36]

This paradox, which was somewhat explained earlier, remains to be one of the greatest public health challenge (Figure 3). As such, many of them, even those with conditions associated with sudden death syndromes, do not have any symptoms and may not be detected. Since coronary artery disease, in particular heart attack, narrowing of the coronary artery and heart failure, account for the majority of sudden death, identifying these groups of patients would help to ascertain who is at greater risk. Therein lies the difficulty in identifying individuals, in general, who are at high risk of sudden death.

For those who are symptomatic from coronary artery narrowing, heart failure or rhythm disorder, they may complain of chest pain, breathlessness or palpitation. The symptoms are particularly of significance when they occur with physical exertion which last for a few minutes and relieve following rest. Other symptoms such as explained tiredness, deterioration of physical performance, fainting or near-fainting episodes also require evaluation. There are also those without symptoms but at increased risk for sudden death. These are individuals with family history of unexpected death, particularly for first-degree relative (siblings or parents) who are younger than 50 years of age, or specific inherited sudden death syndromes. Recently, a biomarker obtained from blood testing, *high sensitivity* troponin-T assay, has been found to be associated with increased risk for sudden death.[613] Elevated level of this substance indicates injury to the heart muscle and has been used for diagnosis of heart attack.

Currently, the most common cause for unexpected sudden death is coronary artery disease and almost half of patients who suffered from a heart attack did not have previous symptoms. Hence, to reduce the risk of sudden death, effort is focussed on detecting risk factors, such as high blood pressure, high cholesterol level and diabetes, and effects of coronary artery narrowing. Since this proposition appears reasonable, it is widely adopted.

The role of routine medical examination in an otherwise healthy person to promote health, screen risk factors and subclinical illnesses has been an issue of contention for several decades. First advocated in the United States by the American Medical Association in 1923,[614] routine annual physical examination for healthy individuals was gradually abandoned by the American College of Physicians, the Canadian Task Force on the Periodic Health Examination and the United States Preventive Services Task Force in 1991 in favour of a more targeted approach.[615] Indeed, the British National Screening Committee has recommended an informed choice for participants in all screening programmes and the risks plus the uncertainties for cardiovascular diseases including treatment modalities have to be clearly explained.[616] More recently, the findings of a group of Danish investigators showed that although routine medical examination was able to detect new medical conditions, it failed to improve death rates in a systematic review of the literature.[617] In their study, routine medical examination also did not alter the individuals dying from cardiovascular disease or cancer.

Screening Young Athletes

Sudden death in a young healthy competitive athlete is always a tragedy. In the United States, the prevalence of unsuspected cardiovascular disease is estimated to be 0.3% of the general athlete population. The incidence of sudden death in high-school and college sportsperson (12 to 24 years old) was estimated to be 1 in 100,000 or lower.[618,619] Unexpectedly, the overall chance for dying was more than two times higher for young competitive athletes than non-athletes.[283] Likely, several of the diseases associated with sudden cardiac death are related to physical exertion. Furthermore, 60% to 80% of athletes who suffered from a sudden cardiac arrest did not have prior symptoms.[99] Therefore, recognising these symptoms prior to participation in sporting activities may prevent premature death. However, the impact of routine medical screening on a high-risk group of individuals may be different.

One of the first countries to promote routine medical examination for young competitive athletes was Italy. Over a 26-year period, a systematic screening programme in Northeast Italy, including resting electrocardiogram, was able to reduce the incidence of sudden death from 3.6 to 0.4 per 100,000 yearly.[33] The improvement was substantial as it amounted to almost 90% relative reduction in the occurrence of sudden death. The overall disqualification rate was 2%. Most of the benefits were attributed to exclusion of a sportsperson with various forms of cardiomyopathy. The proportion that died from cardiomyopathy fell from 36% to 17%. Correspondingly, the percentage of athletes who were disqualified because of cardiomyopathy increased from 4.4% to 9.4%. Importantly, there was no change in the death rate among those who did not participate in competitive sports and were not screened. However, the false positive rate was 7% in this study. In other words, out of 14 individuals with an abnormal test, one of them was falsely abnormal. These persons would require further investigations to determine the significance of the abnormal result.

The procedures include taking the individual and family history and physical examination. A standardised pre-participation questionnaire is used to assess young athletes at risk for sudden death.[132,620] The evaluation consisted of eliciting symptoms of heart disease such as chest pain on exertion, fainting or near-fainting spells, a sensation of rapid heartbeats, undue shortness of breath or deterioration of effort tolerance and unexplained seizures. Family history of sudden death or unexplained fainting spells, particularly when the affected individual was younger than 50 years old, was also sought for. The clinical examination was directed to detect abnormal signs in the cardiovascular system. Since they are highly motivated, minor symptoms may be ignored. These highly competitive individuals may be willing to risk their health for glory and money. Thus, the examiner should be sufficiently skilled to elicit relevant history from the participants. The challenge during screening is to minimise missing potentially life-threatening conditions in well and physically fit individuals without increasing the number requiring further investigations. Referring them for evaluation can affect training schedules adversely. It can also have a negative psychological influence on young minds. Emotional and adjustment disorders can also affect these young active individuals emotionally and spiritually. As they are asymptomatic, they and their parents or guardians do not understand the gravity of the situation. For those who are allowed to participate in competitive sport in the United States, they are to be reviewed every two years.[621] On the other hand, in Italy, the athletes are examined annually.[622]

Resting Electrocardiogram

A standard resting 12-lead electrocardiogram is useful in determining abnormalities that is associated with increased risk of sudden death.[374] There are various patterns in the tracing that can identify conditions such as previous heart attack, Brugada syndrome, arrhythmogenic right ventricular dysplasia and cardiomyopathy, in particular hypertrophic cardiomyopathy. Of the various measurements ascertained from the electrocardiogram, the QT-interval — a measurement of repolarisation — is critical (Figure 13). Sudden death is associated with those with prolonged or shortened QT-interval. However, as the duration of the QT-interval is dependent on heart rate, interpretation can be a challenge. When the heart rate decreases, the absolute period increases. Correspondingly, when the heart rate increases, the QT-interval decreases. Other conduction abnormalities may also be recognised.

However, the yield is generally low. Due to this limitation, the routine use of the resting electrocardiogram as part of pre-participation medical examination is a matter of debate. Identification of certain conditions may prevent sudden death by not allowing these individuals to take part in the sports temporarily or permanently, or by administering appropriate treatment.[33,233,623] While the European Society of Cardiology[529] and the International Olympic Council[624] adopted the routine use of resting electrocardiogram in addition to history taking and physical examination as part of the evaluation for young athletes. However, the American Heart Association did not make this recommendation in 2007.[620] In the recent Minnesota State High School League games and practices for athletes between the ages of 12 to 19 years, the incidence of sudden death was 0.24 per 100,000 athlete-years over 19 academic years.[625] These high school students underwent the routine 3-yearly health screening examination. Due to the low occurrence of event, the investigators recommended that the decision to perform an electrocardiogram should consider age, training intensity and genetic predisposition of the individual. Among the general athlete population, college students was higher, with an annual rate for sudden cardiac death of 2.3 per 100,000 athlete-years.[626]

One of the key reasons for performing a routine electrocardiogram is to detect hypertrophic cardiomyopathy. This condition is the most common cause of sudden death among young competitive athletes, accounting for more than a third of cardiovascular causes of sudden death.[620] Although some of these patients may have symptoms or abnormal physical findings, many of them are asymptomatic and the electrocardiogram is abnormal in more than 90% of the cases.[133,627] Hence, individuals found to have this condition would be disqualified from active competition. Indeed, this strategy has been shown to be life-saving in Italy, with almost 90% decline in sudden death from sporting events over a 23-year period.[33] On the other hand, there was little change among non-athletes who were not screened. However, the electrocardiogram may not be normal in many competitive athletes due to physiological changes of training, a condition otherwise known as the athlete's heart.[628] The likelihood for a false positive examination is not insignificant and ranges from 10% to 25%.[233,629] Furthermore, an abnormal finding would require further evaluation, including echocardiogram, and may create unnecessary anxiety to the young person and the family. Therefore, the American Heart Association estimated the increased cost associated with the routine use of electrocardiogram for screening of young athletes to be US$2 billion in 2007.[620] Based on their assumptions, the estimated cost to prevent a sudden death was US$3.4 million. As such, routine electrocardiography was not routinely recommended by the American Heart Association because of the excessive recurrent annual cost of US$2 billion. But in their computation, this estimated cost should be only applicable to the first year of implementation. Subsequent analysis depends on the number of new athletes each year and the frequency of repeat examination for the incumbents.

Medical history, physical examination and electrocardiogram have been routinely performed on school children in grades 1, 7 and

10 in Japan since 1973.[630] Resting electrocardiogram was more sensitive in identifying high-risk heart conditions that are associated with sudden death.[631] The usefulness of the resting electrocardiogram was ascertained at the Center for Sports Medicine in Padua, Italy.[233] Among 33,735 young men and women, 3,016 (8.9%) of them were referred for additional testing. Subsequently, 621 (1.8%) were not allowed to participate because of cardiovascular reasons. Of the 22 athletes with asymptomatic hypertrophic cardiomyopathy, 18 (82%) had abnormalities in the electrocardiogram and 5 of them (23%) had a family history or heart murmur. This finding suggested that the electrocardiogram alone was able to detect asymptomatic individuals with hypertrophic cardiomyopathy. In fact, in another study on young athletes, electrocardiogram can identify 99% of the abnormalities found on echocardiogram.[632] When the Italian experience was updated with 42,386 participants, the findings persisted.[33]

This experience was also shared across the Atlantic Ocean. In the United States, 5,615 high school athletes were screened over a three-year period in northern Nevada.[633] History was obtained and they were examined. An electrocardiogram was also performed. On completion of the assessment, 22 of them (0.4%) were disqualified. History alone did not identify any of these individuals. Abnormal heart sound could be only heard in one of them. However, the electrocardiogram detected 16 athletes. The authors concluded that these procedures could be performed efficiently on large groups of high school athletes and that the electrocardiogram alone was superior to history and auscultation in detecting serious or potentially serious cardiovascular abnormalities. Approximately 10% of these participants required echocardiography. More recently, but with a smaller number of athletes, investigators from Massachusetts showed that electrocardiogram improved the identification of individuals with cardiovascular disease.[634] However, the electrocardiogram may falsely categorise 1 in 6 athletes to have cardiovascular disease. But, the abnormalities differed from the earlier studies with valvular disorders accounting for the majority of the heart conditions. Only one of the eleven athletes who were found to have an abnormality was due to hypertrophic cardiomyopathy. Therefore, the value of including the electrocardiogram as part of routine screening for athletes could depend on the causes and incidences of sudden death.[635]

Despite all these controversies, this test has been introduced into the International Olympic Council, European countries,[529] Japan and Israel. On the other hand, it is used at the discretion of the examiner in the United States.[620] While the United Kingdom does not support a national cardiac screening programme for athletes, pre-participation screening, especially for those who self-fund, is recommended.[636] However, the charitable organisation, Cardiac Risk in the Young (CRY) in the United Kingdom, provides subsidy for individuals between the ages of 14 to 35 years who desired to be examined for conditions predisposing to sudden cardiac death regardless of symptoms, family history of sudden cardiac death or athletic status.

Specific changes in the electrocardiogram can be seen in certain sudden death conditions. It is believed to be abnormal in more than 90% of individuals with hypertrophic cardiomyopathy and greater than 75% of those with arrhythmogenic right ventricular cardiomyopathy.[637] On the other hand, intensive exercises, particularly among endurance athletes, can result in abnormalities in the electrocardiogram, a condition known as the athlete's heart. These high performance athletes may produce changes in the electrocardiogram which may mimic those who are at increased likelihood of sudden death.[638] The pattern, known as early repolarisation, may be misinterpreted as Brugada syndrome. Using software to magnify the tracings, 139 of 155 (89%) top-ranking male Italian athletes were found to have this abnormal pattern. On the other hand, only 18 of 50 (36%) male students were found to have this pattern. Notably, the changes were more marked among the athletes. Furthermore, the site of these changes also differed between athletes and normal. So, readers of the electrocardiograms have to be highly skilled and experienced in interpreting the tracing.[134] Nonetheless, the falsely, equivocal or borderline abnormal finding may account for 4% to 7% of positive cases[622] and could generate more investigative tests, thereby escalating cost.

From 2008 to 2012, the value of the electrocardiogram was evaluated in 11,845 consecutive young subjects between the ages of

14 to 35 years in the United Kingdom.[636] About two-thirds of them were non-athletes. Abnormal patterns in the electrocardiogram, classified as Group 1 or 2,[134] were prevalent. Changes in Group 1 were considered common and minor and were present in 49% of non-athletes and 87% of athletes. But the alterations in Group 2 are less common and may be associated with cardiomyopathy. As such, echocardiogram is recommended for those with Group 2 abnormalities. Although these changes were present in 22% of non-athletes and 33% of athletes, electrocardiographic changes suggestive of an abnormal heart was found in 10% and 21%, respectively. After performing echocardiography on 784 non-athletes with Group 2 electrocardiographic changes, 16 (2%) of them had features consistent with mild cardiomyopathy. As such, the investigators concluded that significant abnormalities occurred commonly in more than a fifth of young persons. After further evaluation, structural heart abnormality was found in only 2%. Hence, they recommended that electrocardiogram should not be routinely performed because of the small number of cardiac conditions that were detected. Furthermore, the definition of Group 2 electrocardiogram patterns should be refined.

Likely, cost-effectiveness may partly account for the differences in recommendations across the Atlantic Ocean. The American Heart Association estimated that the routine use of electrocardiogram would cost $330,000 to completely screen each athlete for suspected relevant heart disease in 2007.[620] The annual budget for mass screening would be a staggering $2 billion for the United States. In a different economic-decision model on the addition of electrocardiogram to cardiovascular history and physical examination for competitive high school and college participants, the investigators found that the incremental cost was $89 per athlete.[639] For each life-year saved, the additional cost-effectiveness ratio was $42,900 when electrocardiogram was added to history and physical examination. Compared to no screening at all, the cost-effectiveness ratio was $76,000 per life-year saved. More recently, another group of investigators, using a cost-projection model, estimated that it cost more than $10 million to save a life if electrocardiography was routinely performed as part of the screening programme for competitive athletes in the United States.[640] But professional sports have grown into a multi-billion dollar business. An avid jogger may know that an echocardiogram could cost less than the latest performance running shoes. Should a sudden death event occur and the athlete is resuscitated but survived in a vegetative state, there is also the additional expenditure to take care of the unfortunate victim. Therefore, as the debate on cost-effectiveness continues, it has to extend beyond the traditional statistical modelling techniques and healthcare financing. Another consideration was the potential delay caused by additional testing and sometimes leading to unnecessary disqualification. During the period of evaluation, training schedules would be interfered. The potential participant may feel left-out and have an adverse impact on the emotional well-being.

Unlike high school or college athletes, the rate for sudden death among professional sportsperson is estimated to be 1 in 3,500 yearly in the United States. A survey was conducted to determine screening practices on 122 major professional sports team in North America.[641] While information on personal and family history was obtained and physical examination was performed on every member of all the teams, electrocardiogram was conducted in 92% and lipid profile was assayed in 89%. The National Basketball Association required electrocardiography to be performed routinely. However, the test was performed only when it was clinically indicated for participants of the National Football League. Stress electrocardiography and echocardiogram were performed less frequently. Since the risk was higher and the number was considerably smaller for this group of individuals, the authors recommended that electrocardiogram should be part of pre-participation examination to enhance the safety of professional athletes.

Exercise Electrocardiography

Overall, coronary artery disease is the most common cause of sudden death.[13] Since the exercise electrocardiography is able to detect coronary artery narrowing and other anomalies associated with insufficient blood supply, it may be a useful test to determine those at higher risk for coronary death.

To further refine the screening process for athletes, the value of stress electrocardiography performed during a pre-participation examination for competitive sports was ascertained.[642] Among 30,065 persons who were examined at the Institute of Sports Medicine in Florence, Italy, 1,812 (6.0%) had abnormal resting electrocardiograms. The majority (>80%) were insignificant changes. Exercise electrocardiography was abnormal in 1,459 (4.9%) of the potential participants. Of these, resting electrocardiogram was normal in 1,227 (67.7%). Of 196 (0.6%) who were considered ineligible for competitive sports, 159 athletes (81.1%) were disqualified due to a cardiac reason. The authors highlighted that although 126 (79.2%) of them did not show significant abnormality in the resting electrocardiogram, the exercise electrocardiography was abnormal. Therefore, the investigators concluded that exercise electrocardiography was able to detect abnormalities of the heart better than resting electrocardiogram. Whether this approach further improved the outcome was unclear. Nonetheless, this test is mandated by law in Israel since 1999.

In Italy, those younger than 40 years of age, electrocardiograms were performed before and after a 3-minute step test.[622] But for competitive athletes older than 40 years, a formal stress electrocardiography is conducted.[643] Indeed, the risk of sudden death is greater among athletes older than 35 years of age, and highest for those in their forties.[644] At this age group, coronary artery disease was the most likely cause of sudden death. Among asymptomatic individuals, the rate of detection of severe coronary artery disease by exercise treadmill testing was 0.44%.[645] To further enhance the diagnostic ability, various forms of cardiac imaging and stress testing were recommended to identify asymptomatic athletes who are at risk of sudden cardiac death.[646]

Although the echocardiogram is a useful tool to differentiate between patients with hypertrophic cardiomyopathy and thickening of the heart muscle wall as a result of high level competitive sports, an indeterminate zone still exists.[647] As such, a more sophisticated form of exercise testing has been proposed to further distinguish these two conditions.[648] Between 1995 and 1999, eight active asymptomatic sportsmen were found to have mutations of genes which were observed in patients with hypertrophic cardiomyopathy. Other than thickening of the heart muscle on echocardiogram, there were no other indices that support the diagnosis of hypertrophic cardiomyopathy. This first group of eight individuals constituted those whose diagnosis of hypertrophic cardiomyopathy was uncertain. The investigators also enrolled another eight highly trained asymptomatic athletes with thickening of heart muscle wall but without family history of sudden death. There were 12 other elite athletes without left ventricular hypertrophy and another 12 other recreational athletes who participated in this study conducted at the St George's Hospital Medical School at the United Kingdom. In addition to exercising on a stationary bicycle and the usual parameters, such as heart rate and blood pressure, instruments were used to measure oxygen consumption, carbon dioxide output and work rate. Of these four groups of athletes, those with hypertrophic cardiomyopathy had the lowest peak oxygen consumption, albeit the value was substantially better than what was predicted for his age. Subsequently, the investigators were able to determine values of peak oxygen consumption, oxygen uptake per beat and the time when the oxygen in the body is unable to meet the increased demands of exercise. However, this test can only be performed in a specialised test centre and is not routinely available in clinics and hospitals.

Even prior to the start of exercise, the amount of heart rate increase was able to determine the risk for sudden cardiac death. The Paris Prospective Study I enrolled 7,749 French civil servants in Paris from 1967 and 1972. They were followed up for 23 years. The heart rate change from rest and just prior to an exercise test was ascertained.[649] On the average, the mild mental stress increased heart rate by about 9 beats per minute. Compared with those whose heart rate increased by less than 4 beats per minute, the risk of sudden death was more than two times higher for participants whose heart rate was increased by more than 12 beats per minute. Although the precise mechanism for this association is not certain, it is believed to be attributed to dysfunction of the autonomic nervous system. Indeed, a study on 1,284 patients with recent heart attack showed that the likelihood of dying for those with impaired heart rate variability and baroreflex sensitivity were three times higher.[650]

Echocardiography

While echocardiography is useful for assessing patients who have survived from a cardiac arrest, it is useful to determine the structure and function of the heart. The size of the heart and the thickness of the wall chambers can also be determined. In particular, hypertrophic cardiomyopathy, which is the most common cause of sudden death among young competitive athletes, can be readily detected with echocardiogram.[104] However, the left ventricle is generally better visualised than the right ventricle.

Cardiac Magnetic Resonance

Magnetic resonance imaging generates strong magnetic waves to obtain images of the body. Unlike echocardiography, it is less dependent on the operator and subject. As such, certain conditions such as arrhythmogenic right ventricular cardiomyopathy and sarcoidosis may be better visualised with cardiac magnetic resonance.

Traditionally, the echocardiogram and radionuclide scan have been used to determine left ventricular systolic function. When the left ventricular ejection fraction is less than 35% for patients with heart failure, implantation of an intra-cardiac defibrillator is recommended.[651] However, less than a third of them receive an appropriate shock.[53] Furthermore, those with low ejection fraction alone may not be a strong predictor for subsequent risk of sudden death.[55] Similar to echocardiography, the structure and function of the heart can be determined by cardiac magnetic resonance. In addition to determining left ventricular systolic function, this technique is able to detect scars in the heart. Gadolinium can be administered during cardiac magnetic resonance imaging and is able to localise at damaged heart muscle cells. Due to its para-magnetic properties, these areas appear bright and the size, location and the pattern of a scar can be ascertained in the heart. The area of scarring has been shown to correlate with gross and microscopic examination of the heart.[124,652] Indeed, the presence of fibrous tissue in the heart provides the substrate for the association with potentially fatal heart rhythm disorder regardless of left ventricular ejection fraction.[653] A report from the Duke University on 137 patients undergoing evaluation for possible placement of intra-cardiac defibrillator helps clarify the relationship between heart function and scarring.[654] They found that the risk for abnormal heart rhythm increases with decreasing left ventricular ejection. When the size of the scar tissue was more than 5% of the mass of the left ventricle, the rhythm disorder risk increased by more than 5-fold. Indeed, risk was greatest among those with left ventricular ejection fraction less than 30% and with scar tissue greater than 5%.

While scars in the heart may be present in up to 71% of patients with dilated cardiomyopathy,[655] its significance in prediction of sudden death is less certain.[656]

Keep on Movin'
Physical Activity and Exercise

"If we could give every individual the right amount of nourishment and exercise, not too little and not too much, we would have found the safest way to health."

Hippocrates c. 460 BC to c. 370 BC

As the Greeks flourished militarily, politically and economically, the fields of arts, literature and sports grew correspondingly. From their various statues that we can still see in several museums around the world, the human body form has been sculptured to perfection. According to tradition, only upper-class men had the time, resources and opportunities to train and compete in various athletic events. The Olympic Games was believed to be inaugurated in 776 BC at Olympia in the Peloponnese peninsula of Greece. By the sixth century BC, the Games had expanded to include Greek-speaking city-states. Winners were honoured publicly in the form of palm branch, red ribbons, olive tree wreath or kotinos, statues and poems. But there were no huge monetary awards or lucrative advertising contracts.

With the decline of the Greek civilisation, physical activity has been relegated to tasks for servants and manual labourers. Despite the revival of the modern Olympic Games in 1896 in Athens, medical practitioners did not sanction the relationship between physical activity and health. Even in the 1950s, running was believed to be harmful because it stressed the heart. People older than 40 years were recommended to move from a two-storey to a single-storey house to reduce physical exertion. After the Second World War, Dr Jeremiah Morris attempted to determine the relationship between occupation and a rising potentially killer condition, coronary artery disease. As he was in London, he decided to study conductors and drivers operating the double-decker buses. The conductors climbed an average of 500 to 750 steps daily while drivers sat almost all the time during their job. These two groups of workers were followed up and conductors were less likely to develop coronary artery disease. If the conductor had the disease, it occurred later and less likely to be fatal.[657] Sudden death was a frequent first presentation. Initially, his findings were largely ignored by the medical community. His persistence in proving his hypothesis that physically active work protected the individual from coronary heart disease was eventually vindicated. Dr Morris was able to demonstrate similar findings among different jobs and social classes, and vigorous activity at leisure time.[658]

Health Paradox in Exercising

However, exercise is a double-edged sword. While physical activity promotes health, strenuous activity can be transiently associated with sudden death.[659] The risk of cardiac arrest was highest among those with the lowest levels of regular exercise. Overall, the risk of dying for asymptomatic male during exercise was 25-fold higher. Among healthy men, the risk of sudden death was 56 times higher during vigorous exercise compared with low level of habitual activity. On the other hand, for those who exercised frequently, the corresponding risk was increased by only 5 times. For habitually vigorous men, the risk of sudden death was only 40% of those who had a sedentary life.[659] Overall, the risk of sudden death during vigorous activity is low, at 1 per 1.51 million episodes for men.[660] Among women, the risk of sudden death during exercise was estimated to be considerably lower, at 1 in 36.5 million hours of exertion.[661] The risk of dying suddenly for a female exercising with moderate to vigorous intensity was only 2.4 times higher compared to lesser or no exertion. Similar to men, the likelihood for dying suddenly was lower for women who exercised regularly.

Exertion may increase the likelihood of acute plaque rupture resulting in occlusion of a coronary artery. This phenomenon is one of the underlying mechanisms for sudden death.[662] However, endurance sports are also known to impair the contractility and relaxation of the heart. While the reduction in the force of contraction is transient occurring shortly after running a marathon, the disturbance with relaxation of the heart persists for at least a month.[663] After running a marathon, there was also release of cardiac biomarkers, suggestive of damage to heart muscle. This deleterious event occurred particularly among non-elite marathoners.[664] However, the long-term significance of these changes has not been established. In a group of 114 world-class *young* (average age of 22 years) Italian Olympian endurance athletes who had undergone uninterrupted intensive training and competition for at least eight years, their doctors did not find any adverse impact on heart structure or function.[665] All of them have participated in at least two consecutive Olympic Games and some have taken part in as many as five events. On the other hand, among 286 participants of the Tour de France, the left ventricle size was larger[666] than normal. In addition, the pump function of the heart was reduced in more than 10% of them. These findings suggested that endurance sports have been associated with deterioration of heart function. But others were critical about their findings and attributed the detrimental impact on the heart to probable doping.[665]

Cardiorespiratory Fitness

Cardiorespiratory fitness has been found to be associated with sudden death.[667] In other words, the longer a person can run or cycle, the greater the likelihood that he or she would live longer. Among 2,368 Finnish middle-aged men, there were 146 sudden cardiac deaths after 17 years. In this study, cardiorespiratory fitness was assessed by using a cycle ergometer. The investigators found that for every increase of a metabolic equivalent, the risk for sudden death was reduced by 22%. Furthermore, earlier studies have reported that by improving physical fitness by 1 metabolic equivalent, overall mortality was lowered by 10% to 24%.[668–670] Better physical fitness may improve parasympathetic modulation and possibly reduce the occurrence of potentially lethal rhythm disorders.[671] Cardiorespiratory fitness may be determined, at least in part, by genetic factors.[672] As such, physical fitness may not be able to be improved in some individuals.

Since narrowing of heart vessels is an important cause for sudden death especially among the middle-age, interventions that reduce the risk for heart attacks are likely to be beneficial. Of these, physical activity and exercise have been consistently shown to prevent death from heart and vessel (cardiovascular) diseases. It is estimated that a 55-year-old man who is able to walk 1.6 km in 15 minutes has a low level of fitness and the lifetime risk of dying from heart and vascular disease is 30%. Conversely, this risk for another 55-year-old man who completed the same distance in 10 minutes or less is only 10%.[673] Even for an individual with traditional risk factors for heart disease, exercise has been shown to mitigate the likelihood of succumbing to heart disease. Thus, a person with conditions such as hypertension, diabetes mellitus or high blood cholesterol level but has high level of fitness has a lifetime risk for cardiovascular death comparable to a person with low risk burden.[673]

Get Off the Couch

Physical activity is defined as "any bodily movement produced by skeletal muscles that results in energy expenditure."[674] It may be structured or incidental. A structured physical activity, otherwise known as exercise, is planned purposeful activity that is performed with the aim of promoting health and fitness. On the other hand, incidental physical activity is unplanned and is generally part of activities of daily living or leisure undertaken at home, work, elsewhere or when running errands. In 2008, the United States Federal Government issued guidelines on physical activity for adults[675] and proposed that all adults should avoid inactivity. For substantial health benefits, physical activity of moderate-intensity should be performed for at least 150 minutes weekly, and each session should be more than 10 minutes. The duration should be at least 75 minutes weekly for vigorous-intensity aerobic physical activity. For additional and more extensive health benefits, the duration of exercise should be at least 300 hours a week for moderate-intensity or 150 minutes a week for vigorous-intensity. These recommendations have led to the axiom, "Some physical activity is better than none and more is better than some." By grouping various clinical studies on the intensity of coronary artery disease, a group of investigators provided quantitative information to support the recommended.[676] By engaging 150 minutes of moderate-intensity leisure-time physical activity, the risk of coronary heart disease was reduced by 14% compared with those without leisure-time physical activity. When the duration was doubled to 300 minutes weekly, the risk was lowered by 20%. In addition to aerobic exercises, muscle-strengthening activities involving all muscle groups are also recommended on two or more days a week. For older persons or those with conditions that limit physical activity, exercises should be performed to a level that is permitted.

Increasingly, our lives have been more and more sedentary with the changing work environment. Over a 50-year period in the United States, the number working in the service sectors was increasing and the number in manufacturing and agricultural jobs were decreasing. Dr Timothy Church and his colleagues found that there was a reduction of more than 100 calories in daily occupation-related energy expenditure, which accounted for the significant increase in mean body weight among men and women.[677] It is unlikely that this trend will reverse. To the disciplined, setting a schedule for specific periods to perform physical activity may be achievable for some. However, we know that only the minority exercise regularly. In the United States, this proportion was 31%[678] and for Singapore residents between the ages of 18 to 69 years, it was 24%.[679] Instead of setting aside time, integrating physical activity in our daily activities may improve our health. Nowadays, instead of using lifts or elevators, we are encouraged to use the stairs. Since most of us move from one place to another several times daily, walking is increasingly promoted as a form of exercise.

Exercise and Health Benefits

Several clinical studies have shown numerous health benefits of exercise. Of these, the risk of dying from a heart attack was reduced by 23%.[680] High and moderate intensity exercise reduced the occurrence of stroke by 25% and 21%, respectively.[681] The risk of sudden death may be lowered by 60% for healthy men who habitually took part in vigorous exercise.[659] Correspondingly, the risk for sudden death for women who exercises regularly (at least 4 hours weekly) is reduced by almost 70%.[661] Exercising more than 150 minutes weekly for overweight individuals reduces the chance of sustaining diabetes by 58%. Using a medicine that treats diabetes, the condition was only prevented in 31% of them.[682] Several of the risk factors related to cardiovascular diseases also improved with exercise.[683]

One of the key mechanisms of benefit of exercise is restoration of endothelial function, allowing the blood vessel to relax and improve blood flow. An important mediator is nitric oxide. Subsequent biochemical pathways help reduce stiffness of blood vessel, mobilise cells for regeneration of tissue, form new blood vessels and neutralise damaging reactive chemicals.[684] Inflammatory and haemostatic biomarkers, blood pressure and lipid level were lowered with exercise.[685] There are also changes in the nervous system which improve cellular function and enhance hormonal responses.

Not uncommonly, weight loss is one of the goals for exercise. But most daily energy expenditure is consumed for vital activities (Figure 21). The proportion of energy spent by a person with sedentary lifestyle to an exercise enthusiast ranged from 5% to 35%. For a 2000-calorie daily intake, this amounted to 100 to 700 calories. The euphoria following physical exertion may be rewarded by various treats. To lose weight, exercises must be accompanied by a healthy diet; as the saying goes, "Diet is about pounds, exercise is about inches. Diet is about weight, exercise is about health."[686]

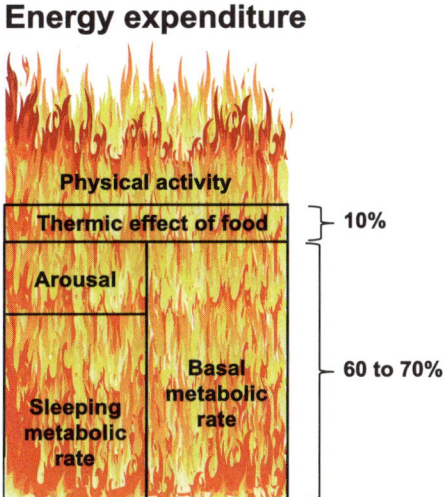

Figure 21. Estimated Proportion of our Daily Energy Expenditure.

In the normal individual, physical activity accounts only for the minority of energy expenditure. Most of the energy is consumed by basal metabolism, activities that keep one alive. The thermic effect of food is the energy required for digestion, absorption, and disposal of ingested nutrients. For carbohydrates, it is 5% to 15% of the energy consumed. It is 20% to 35% for proteins and 5% to 15% for fats.

While fat is lost with exercise, muscle and bone mass are built up. Furthermore, muscle and bone are denser than fat. Hence, exercising can certainly make one look trimmer but not necessarily lighter.

The 10,000 Steps

Runners count rounds, swimmers count laps, cyclists count clicks. Well, walkers count steps. To incorporate physical activity in our daily activity, one method is to determine the number of steps we walk during the usual activities that we do. As such, the use of pedometers and accelerators are gaining popularity.

Counting steps is certainly not novel. The ancient Chinese philosopher, Lao Tzu (c.604 BCE to c.551 BCE), once said, "A journey of a thousand miles begins with a single step." In different words regarding life, Peter A. Cohen said, "There is no one giant step … it's a lot of little steps." In the 15th century, Leonardo Da Vinci was credited for the design of such an instrument which was subsequently used by Roman soldiers to estimate the distance they walked. As a result of his invention on self-winding mechanism of pocket watches in the 1770s, Abraham-Louis Perrelet developed the mechanical pedometer. An average individual takes 3,500 to 5,000 steps daily. Normally, a mile (or 1.6 km) can be covered by 2,000 to 2,500 steps. For a 70-kilogramme person, approximately 80 calories are consumed. By increasing to 10,000 steps a day, Dr Yoshiro Hatano estimated that it would use up 20% of our total caloric intake, balancing the daily energy intake for healthy living. So the manpo-kei ("万步计"or 10,000 step meter) was developed in 1965 in Japan, and marketed. Subsequently, walking clubs flourished as an easy achievable way of promoting health.

Using such a device can also serve as an incentive to enhance the quality of physical activity. Indeed, the pedometer has been shown to increase by more than 2,000 steps a day based on a review of several small clinical trials.[687] This number translates to the distance of a mile (1.6 km) and is associated with reduction in body weight and blood pressure. The body mass index is also lowered by 0.4 kg/m^2 and systolic blood pressure by 4 mmHg. A 2 mmHg fall in systolic blood pressure is associated with a 10% reduction in chance of dying from a stroke and 7% reduction in death from diseases of blood vessels in a middle-age population.[688]

For a sedentary person to embark on a walking programme, start off with 2,000 steps daily. The number of steps may be increased gradually and comfortably. Avoid over-exertion and straining. Listen to your body. Although the goal is 10,000 steps a day, the number of steps may be raised by 2,000 to heighten physical challenge. Furthermore, younger persons should aim to achieve 12,000 steps a day.

However, walking may not be suitable for everyone. For the elderly and those with illness or joint problems, they may not be able to walk this distance. Hence, there are other forms of exercises, such as cycling (preferably on an ergometer or stationary bicycle) or walking along the edge of the children's swimming pool. Water provides buoyancy and reduces weight-bearing. There is also resistance when walking in the pool.

Another criticism of this technique of merely counting steps is the lack of assessment of intensity of exercise. Walking 1,000 steps in 10 minutes was found to be of moderate intensity for men and women.[689] The recommendations on amount and intensity of physical activity[675] may be met by walking 3,000 steps in 30 minutes five times a week.[689] However, the duration may be divided into three 10-minute of 1,000-step intervals daily.

Today, there are even more sophisticated devices that not only monitor the number of steps. It can record heart rate, rhythm, blood pressure, oximetry, amount of energy consumed and other parameters as well. There are numerous apps available for the smartphones or tablets that are related to health. To the more technologically adapted, they have found these apps useful.

Gamercising or Exergaming: Exercising in the Virtual World

The rise of computers more than seven decades ago has changed our lives drastically. We have moved considerably faster than ever before. With the integration of graphics and subsequently three-dimensional visualisation technology, the virtual world was born. By the late 1980s, complex machines with primitive pictorial displays were developed as the first generation of active gaming by allowing the play to respond to the events in the game. When motion sensors are available together with greater computing power, sophisticated devices were designed to further enhance the participation experience of the gamer. The attractiveness of these novel activities is that they are designed to please ... the player, of course. First, they provided a route to vicarious escape from mundane real life. In this virtual world, we can become super-heroes and sports champions. Although the games can be challenging, its level of difficulty can be modified to suit the beginner and the expert. Thus, these games are self-paced. To continue to keep them playing, gamers are given the opportunity to achieve small wins. There is always a high score to beat. When a game is lost or when the mission is unsuccessful, the player can try and try again, often in secret. Just press the reset button and there is no one to jeer.

Today, gamercising, exergaming or active gaming has evolved into a giant industry using technology to drive physical activity to become a fun and enjoyable experience. It ranged from simple finger and wrist movement to total body motion with sensor monitors and pads while performing various types of virtual sports. As our lifestyle becomes increasingly sedentary, the ability to exercise without leaving the house is an attractive alternative. Instead, one can go for a jog in the park, cycle in the hills or ski in the mountains. Using other technologies such as Global Positioning System (GPS), players can move from place to place as they progress in the game. Accelerators, heart rate and blood pressure monitors can also be incorporated into the hardware to determine the posture and physiological parameters of the players. Likely, there is an exergame for everyone.

But can these activities replace the outdoors? Among children and youth, active video games have been shown to provide light to moderate physical workload.[690,691] In a review of clinical studies published on active video gaming, heart rate, oxygen consumption and energy expenditure were increased with the use of exergaming.[692] However, the amount consumed may not be comparable to the corresponding sporting activities.[693] These devices can be designed to suit individuals with various physical limitations. Nonetheless, the American Heart Association mooted the Power of Play Initiative to explore "the potential opportunities and benefits of the use of active-play video games to help child and adults avoid sedentary behaviour and find enjoyable, accessible ways to be more physically active."[694]

Other Peril of Endurance Activity

Although the more common conditions that may cause cardiac arrest in a sportsperson have been discussed, there are also several other causes. In a 27-year United States registry of 1,866 athletes who had died suddenly or successfully resuscitated from cardiac arrest, about 20% of the events were not related to exercise.[60] There were 416 (22%) who died from blunt trauma, 65 (4%) from commotion cordis and 46 (2%) from heat stroke. The significance of heat injury was highlighted by the Israeli marathon experience. From 2007 to 2013, there were 14 long distance running events in Tel Aviv.[695] Over the 7-year period, 2 of 137,580 participants died, and so the mortality rate for these events was 1.45 per 100,000. Unlike what was expected, both of them suffered from heat stroke, one in 2011 and 2013. There were 12 additional patients with near-fatal heat injury. The number of participants with heat-related injuries may be as high as 1 to 2 per 1,000 runners. Hence adequate rest, hydration and training are required for those intending to take part in endurance events. On the other hand, only one 38-year-old man suffered from a heart attack when he was at the 20-km mark in 2011. This patient was successfully treated by coronary angioplasty. The lack of sudden cardiac death events may be attributed partly to mandatory pre-participation examination. In Israel, an electrocardiogram is required by law for participants who are organised in teams or associations. However, other runners needed to submit a declaration of good health.

Longevity Potions and Elixir of Health

Omega-3 Fatty Acid Supplementation

Donovan: *"Which one is it?"*
Knight: *"You must choose. But choose wisely…"*

From the movie, Indiana Jones
and the Last Crusade on the pursuit of the Holy Grail:
Screenplay by Jeff Boam
Story by George Lucas and Menno Meyjes

Indeed, coronary heart disease is the major cause of sudden death. Approximately 50% of cases, sudden death is the first manifestation of coronary artery disease.[696] One of the principal strategies to prevent sudden death is to maintain a healthy lifestyle by eating wisely and exercising regularly. Have adequate rest, manage stress well and keep your ideal weight. Look out for the risk factors, such as hypertension, diabetes mellitus or dyslipidaemia. These conditions increase the likelihood for coronary heart disease.[697,698] If they are present, treating them to achieve therapeutic goals would lower this risk and the corresponding likelihood of sudden death.[699] Meanwhile, it is not unexpected that a common question asked in a clinic is; "Is there anything I can eat to prevent sudden death or a heart attack?" Although severely criticised by recent commentators regarding the cholesterol hypothesis of coronary heart disease,[700,701] Ancel Keys[702,703] raised the interest of the Mediterranean diet in lowering death rates related to narrowing of coronary arteries. Fatty acids became the subject of interest.

Biochemically, fatty acids are carbon atoms linked together as a chain, with branches of hydrogen atoms, and an acid group at one end. In our body, they are used to form membranes of cells and stored or used as fuel for energy, an alternate source from glucose. They are also messengers found in hormones or within cells to transmit information. In 1929, Herbert McLean Evans and George O. Burr in the United States discovered essential fatty acids. Humans do not have enzymes to generate double bonds at the third (omega-3 or ω-3) and sixth (ω-6) positions of the carbon chain. In order words, our body is unable to manufacture them and needs to be ingested (or injected). Plants provide linoleic acid (ω-6 fatty acid) and alpha-linolenic acid (ω-3 fatty acid). When the length of the carbon chain is increased, they found eicosapentaenoic acid (EPA) and docosahexaenoic acid (DHA). Both EPA and DHA are ω-3 fatty acids and found in fish oils. Since EPA is involved in the production of substances that prevent the clumping of platelets together, it makes the blood thinner. On the other hand, DHA is found in abundance in the brain, retina and testicles. About 50% of the weight of the membrane of brain cells is made up of DHA.

After visiting Evans in 1937, Hugh Sinclair, a British physiologist, thought that deficiency in some fatty acids might account for the rise of heart attacks in the Western world.[704] When he visited the Greenland in 1944, Sinclair found that the Eskimos did not have grey rings around their eyes, which is a sign suggestive of high cholesterol levels, and tended to suffer from nose bleeding. Subsequently, two Danish investigators found that the rate of cardiovascular disease was low and the absence of diabetes among the Eskimos who consumed large amounts of fatty fish.[705] The Eskimos consumed about 400 g of seafood daily and their average intake of ω-3 fatty acids was 14 g each day compared with 3 g for the Danes. When they examined the lipid profile of 130 Eskimos and their wives in the northern part of the west coast of Greenland, they found that most types of lipids, including total cholesterol, triglyceride, low-density and very low-density lipoproteins, were lower than Danish or Eskimos living in Denmark.[706] They also found that ω-6 fatty acids were replaced by ω-3 fatty acids, especially when the concentration of arachidonic acid was compared with EPA. Correspondingly, due to the action of EPA on anti-platelet function, bleeding time was increased among Eskimos compared with Danish subjects.[707] Conversely, high-density lipoprotein was higher among men.

During the Second World War, after Germany had invaded Norway in 1940, the diet of Norwegians changed to lower fat intake and higher fish consumption.[708] During this period, there was a fall in deaths from heart attacks. The ω-3 fatty acids, particularly EPA, present in these marine mammals were believed to have contributed to the low occurrence of heart attacks.[709] Likely, other socio-economic factors could have also played a role. Sinclair conducted an experiment by putting himself on an Inuit diet, eating food obtained from marine animals, especially seal, for 100 days.[710] His bleeding time rose from 3–5 minutes to 50 minutes with a fall in platelet and red blood cell counts. The concentration of very low-density lipoprotein fell and the high-density lipoprotein increased. Based on these and other findings of numerous investigators, the properties of anti-clotting, anti-inflammatory, anti-atherogenic and anti-arrhythmic effects are the likely mechanisms for its benefits.

Wonders of Oily Fish

One of the earliest studies to document the benefits of eating fish was conducted in the town of Zutphen, in the Netherlands.[711] In 1960, dietary information was collected from 852 middle-age men. After 20 years, the researchers found that the rate of dying from heart disease was 50% lower for those who consumed at least 30 g of fish daily compared with participants who did not eat fish. As such, the investigators concluded that eating as little as one or two fish dishes per week may prevent heart disease. Among 84,688 nurses in the United States, there was an inverse relationship between fish consumption and risk of dying from heart attack or coronary heart disease.[712] The risk was lowered by more than a third among those who eat fish at least twice weekly compared with nurses who eat fist less than once monthly. The eating oily fish hypothesis was further strengthened by an evaluation of 334 cases, aged 25 to 74 years, who were free of heart and other major diseases and suffered from a cardiac arrest in Seattle-King County of Washington State from 1988 to 1994.[713] Their fish eating habits were evaluated from their spouses and were compared with 493 healthy individuals with comparable age and sex (control) in the population. Blood specimens were obtained to determine the fatty acid composition in the red blood cell, which is a biomarker of dietary ω-3 polyunsaturated fatty acid intake. Compared with those who did not take fatty fish, the risk of cardiac arrest was significantly reduced by 50% for individuals who consumed at least one fatty fish meal weekly. This result was corroborated by the fatty acid composition analysis in the red blood cells.

But not all observational studies have been associated with improved outcomes. In the Chicago Western Electric Study, among 1,822 healthy men who were 44 to 55 years of age, those who consumed at least 35 g of fish daily, the risk of dying from heart disease was almost 40% lower than individuals who did not eat fish.[714] However, sudden death was not prevented. The effect of fish consumption studied in 57,053 Danish men and women were followed up for a mean period of 7.6 years.[715] Among men, intake of fatty fish was associated with a lower occurrence of heart attack. But this benefit was not observed among women or men eating lean fish. The authors attributed the lack of benefit for women to the small number of heart attack cases.

Therefore, the question of the benefit of eating oily fish needed to be addressed and the study, Diet and Reinfarction Trial (DART) was reported in 1989.[716] In this trial, three dietary strategies among 2033 men with heart attack were studied; (1) low-fat intake with an increase in the ratio between polyunsaturated to saturated fatty acid; (2) increase in fatty fish intake; and (3) increase in cereal fibre intake, was reported. At the end of two years, there was a 29% reduction in all-cause mortality, particularly death from heart attacks, among those who were advised to eat 200 g to 400 g of fatty fish twice weekly. Of note, and rather surprisingly, there was no significant difference in recurrent non-fatal heart attacks. Correspondingly, serum cholesterol level did not differ significantly among the three groups of patients. Sudden death was believed to be the basis of the benefit of consuming fatty fish because as many as half of the patients with heart attack die abruptly. Indeed, in the United States, approximately 70% of coronary deaths occur out of the hospital in 2008.[5] The findings from these studies formed the basis of the recommendation of eating fatty fish to prevent death after a heart attack. Generally, cardioprotection may be achieved by eating at least one fish meal weekly, with greater benefit up to five servings weekly. However, the heart protection afforded by eating fish was somewhat attenuated in a land such as Japan where marine animals were widely consumed.[717]

The benefits of eating fish were also shown in individuals without pre-existing heart attack or stroke. Among 20,551 United States physicians, fish consumption habit was evaluated at baseline and followed up for 11 years.[718] The risk for sudden cardiac death for men eating fish at least once weekly as about half of those who ate fish less than once a month. Interestingly, this benefit was obtained by those taking shellfish, such as shrimps, lobsters and scallops, as well. On the contrary, when the amount of fish oil was measured in the blood among the 254 United States male physicians with heart attack, the investigators found that higher concentration was not associated with a lower occurrence of this adverse event.[719] The researchers attributed the lack of association to the greater awareness of eating fish among doctors.

As with any dietary study, while the amount consumed may be measurable, how much ω-3 fatty acid consumed is less certain. The amounts of EPA and DHA provided vary with season, location where the fish is caught and the species. White fish, such as cod, coley, plaice and haddock, contains only about 1% of fat. On the other hand, oil fish, like trout, salmon, mackerel, herring, pilchard and sardine, may contain 5% to 25% of fat. The effect on blood lipid profile may also differ with various marine animals. While consuming an Eskimo diet,[710] mackerel (200 g/d),[720] cod liver oil supplement[721] or fish oil concentrate[722] may raise high-density lipoprotein levels, eating salmon or vegetable oil[723] did not.

Probable Protective Mechanisms

As such, lowering the risk of sudden death by eating fish may be related to consumption of ω-3 fatty acids by providing electrical stability of the heart which prevents abnormal heart rhythm[724] and fatal disorganised rhythm disorder.[725] This benefit may be mediated by several complex pathways, including various ion channels present on the surface of the heart muscle cells and several enzymes mediating responses to hormones, stimuli and inflammation.[726,727] Various inflammatory markers are reduced with regular fish consumption.[728] Fish eating also lowers heart rate.[729] Another possible mechanism for the benefit of ω-3 unsaturated fatty acid was the enhancement heart rate variability.[730,731] Heart rate variability is a measure of the autonomic nervous system which has been shown to be an independent predictor for death from abnormal heart rhythm after a heart attack.[732] Fish oil also lowers serum triglyceride[733] and "stickiness" of platelets.[734] Platelets are found in the blood and are the first to respond when the vessel wall is breeched. Subsequently, blood clots are formed to prevent further blood loss. Although the heart attack rate was not lowered in some studies, the severity of the damage to the heart muscle may be reduced by eating fish.[735] Another mechanism that fish oil may confer is the stabilisation of lipid deposited in the blood vessel wall.[736,737] Currently, it is believed that a break in the weakened blood vessel introduces the contents to the blood. This interaction leads to clot formation as discussed earlier. Fish oil may stabilise the wall and prevents it from breaking by lowering the number of cells and substances associated with inflammation.[738–742] By doing so, a heart attack may be avoided.

More Studies Greater Challenges

To further explore the dietary pattern, the Mediterranean diet was evaluated in another clinical trial.[743] Again, patients with a previous heart attack were chosen for the study, 302 were randomly assigned to Mediterranean alpha-linolenic acid diet and another 303 to prudent diet. Alpha-linolenic acid is an 18-carbon ω-3 polyunsaturated fatty acid. Although the trial was discontinued prematurely at

27 months because of the significant benefit in the treatment arm, the risk of adverse events remained lower at 4 years.[744] At 46 months, the risk of dying was 70% lower among those in the Mediterranean diet group suggesting the durability of this dietary strategy.

However, the definition of a Mediterranean diet can be challenging because the region encompasses a wide geographical area with dissimilar culture, practice and beliefs. In general, the diet is high in fruits, root (legumes) and green vegetables, bread and grains. Olive oil is the principal fat source but dairy products, fish and poultry are to be consumed in low to moderate amount. Saturated fats and red meat should be eaten sparingly. Wine may be drunk in low to moderate amounts.[745] Indeed, plasma levels of alpha linolenic acid were higher among those randomly assigned to the Mediterranean diet compared with patients receiving usual care.[744]

However, marine animals may contain several environmental contaminants, including methylmercury, polychlorinated biphenyls and dioxins.[746] These undesirable chemicals tend to concentrate in older, larger predatory fish. Thus, the concentrations of mercury in big marine animals such as swordfish and sharks are the highest, at about 1 μg/g. Tuna, trout, pike and bass have intermediate concentrations (0.1 μg/g to 0.5 μg/g). Although removing the skin and fats may reduce the amount of polychlorinated diphenyls, methylmercury is found in the muscle and not removed by skinning and trimming. Mercury consumption may attenuate the beneficial effects of ω-3 fatty acid,[747] and mercury accumulation has been shown to accelerate the progression of atherosclerosis in the neck arteries.[748] Earlier studies showed that increased levels of mercury in the hair or toenail were associated with a higher likelihood of heart attacks and dying from it.[749,750] In a European study of 684 men with a first heart attack, the amount of mercury in toenail was compared with 724 otherwise normal men.[750] Among those without heart attack, the mean mercury level was 0.25 μg/g of nail, and it was 25% higher for patients with heart attack. Indeed, higher mercury concentration was associated with increased risk of suffering from a heart attack. Although high level of DHA in the fat tissue was associated with lower risk of heart attack, high mercury content diminished the cardioprotective effect of fish intake. Despite eating a large amount of fish in Eastern Finland (almost 50 g daily), high level of mercury in hair and toenail were associated with increased risk of heart disease.[751] Mercury content in Finnish lakes was particularly high because of industrialisation, shallow waters and acidic soil. On the other hand, a recent study in two large United States populations did not show that increased exposure to mercury was associated with a higher risk for heart disease or stroke.[752] Although the researchers were unable to explain why their result was different from previous investigations, it may be attributed partly to variation in selenium levels. However, there are other risks associated with seafood intake as well. While the inhabitants of Greenland have lower rates of heart attack, the likelihood of bleeding in the brain is increased.[753] Another potential hazard of consuming fish oil is fibrosis of the heart and may be caused by rancid oils. Vitamin E may prevent this potential limitation of storing fish oil.

From Oily Fish to Fishy Oil

Having identified the likely substance that provided the health benefit, it was not surprising that ω-3 fatty acids supplementation were subsequently evaluated in clinical studies. In a large cohort of 45,722 male healthcare professionals, followed up for 14 years, those who consumed ≥250 mg of long-chain ω-3 polyunsaturated fatty acid were found to lower the risk of sudden death by 40% to 50%.[754] Dietary linolenic acid has also been shown to be inversely associated with calcified atherosclerotic plaque in the coronary arteries.[755] An early small clinical trial suggested the beneficial effects. Among 360 patients who were admitted to hospital for suspected heart attack, they were randomly assigned to one of three groups: fish oil (containing 1.08 g of EPA daily), mustard oil (containing 2.9 g of alpha-linolenic acid daily) and placebo (individuals in this group did not receive fish or mustard oil).[756] At the end of one year, nonfatal myocardial infarction occurred less frequently with fish oil (13%) and mustard oil (15%) compared with those taking neither of the two supplements (25.4%). However, the risk of dying from heart disease was lower only for those receiving fish oil (11.4% vs. 22.0%). The lack of benefit of consumption of alpha-linolenic acid has been observed in a Dutch 10-year follow-up study[757] and may be attributed to the reduced ability to convert it to EPA and DHA among young men.[758] In an experiment on rats, they were fed with standard diet, or diet supplemented with ascending doses of EPA plus DHA or ascending doses of alpha-linolenic acid.[759] After a week of their assigned diets, the rats were then randomly assigned to sham surgery or abdominal aorta banding. Sham surgery was an operation when an incision was made but the actual procedure was not performed. On the other hand, abdominal aorta banding was to create a narrowing in the main blood vessel thereby increasing the pressure that the heart needed to pump. Consequently, the heart muscle wall would thicken and the rat might end up with heart failure. After 12 weeks, the researchers found that supplementation with EPA plus DHA increased the secretion of an anti-inflammatory hormone, adiponectin, suppressed inflammation and prevented changes of the heart structure and abnormal function following pressure overload conditions. Although EPA, DHA and alpha-linolenic acid are ω-3 fatty acids, EPA and DHA are from fish oils and alpha-linolenic acid is from vegetable sources such as flaxseed. As such, their findings suggested that the effects provided by various ω-3 fatty acids may differ, and those from marine sources were likely to provide the benefits.[760]

Subsequent large clinical trials provided further support regarding the favourable effects of ω-3 fatty acids supplementation using fish oils. Among 18,645 Japanese patients with high cholesterol level, 14,981 without pre-existing coronary heart disease, were randomly assigned to receive statin alone or statin plus EPA 1,800 mg daily.[761] Since their cholesterol level was raised, all patients received a potent lipid lowering agent, statin. Statins have been previously shown to be effective in lowering death and adverse events such as heart attacks, especially for those with pre-existing vascular diseases and diabetes. After a mean follow-up of 4.6 years, the complications relating to coronary heart disease, such as dying from heart disease, heart attack, coronary angioplasty or bypass surgery, occurred 19% less frequently among those who were treated with statin and EPA. However, when important endpoints were studied, the risk of dying from heart attack and sudden death was not lowered by the addition of EPA. Yet the number of individuals who died suddenly was very small in this clinical trial and could have accounted for the lack of benefit. Of note was the proportion of women in the clinical trial. Unlike most other studies, 69% of the study population was female. Another interesting point was that the dose of statin administered to the patients in this study was relatively low, approximately 10 mg of pravastatin or 5 mg of simvastatin daily. These unique features could have accounted for the apparent discrepancies observed in this clinical trial.

In another clinical trial, 11,324 patients with a recent heart attack (less than three months) were randomly assigned to one of four groups in the GISSI (Gruppo Italiano per lo Studio della Sopravivivenza nell'Infarto miocardico)-Prevenzione trial.[762] The first group received a 1 g capsule of ω-3 fatty acids, containing 850 mg of EPA and docosahexaneoic acid (DHA) in a 1:2 ratio, once daily, the second group received 300 mg of vitamin E (synthetic α-tocopherol), the third group received both polyunsaturated fatty acid and vitamin E, and the last group, which served as the control, received neither fatty acids nor vitamin E. In this study, more than 70% of the patients were eating at least one serving of fish weekly and more than 80% of them were eating at least one serving of fruits daily. Only treatment with ω-3 fatty acid and not vitamin E improved outcome. After 3.5 years, the occurrence of death, heart attack and stroke was lowered by 15%; in particular, the risk of death was reduced by 20%. Of note, the risk of sudden death was significantly lowered by 45%. These benefits were obtained within 3 to 4 months following consumption of ω-3 fatty acids.[763] However, the rates of heart attack and stroke were not lowered. But others have suggested that the size of the heart attack may be smaller among those who were taking fish oils.[764] Notably, in the GISSI-Prevenzione trial,[762] combination of ω-3 fatty acids and vitamin E did not provide additional benefit. Although life-saving medicines were administered to the participants, statins (potent cholesterol-lowering medicine) were not used because the study was started before their efficacy has been proven.

Indeed, there were other clinical studies that did not demonstrate the beneficial effects of ω-3 fatty acid supplementation. Of 300 Norwegian patients with heart attack, they were randomly assigned to receive 4 g of ω-3 fatty acid or corn oil.[765] After 1.5 years, there was no difference in the occurrence of heart attacks or dying from one. But the authors explained the lack of benefit by the fact that their patients were enrolled from a region of relatively higher intake of fish and greater proportion of them using aspirin compared with previous studies. But the dose of ω-3 fatty acid was higher than the previous trials. Some others have even shown the detrimental effects of ω-3 fatty acid supplementation. In the Finnish Alpha-Tocopherel, Beta-Carotene Cancer Prevention Study, the dietary intake of specific types of fatty acids was recorded in 21,030 middle-age smoking men.[766] A subsequent systematic review of published clinical trials showed that ω-3 fatty acid supplementation reduced death from heart diseases but not sudden death.[767] However in another meta-analysis (a mathematical systematic review of studies relating to the subject),[768] death rates from any cause and heart attack were reduced by 20% and 30%, respectively. Importantly, sudden death was also lowered by 30% with dietary and non-dietary intervention of ω-3 polyunsaturated fatty acid. The benefit provided by ω-3 fatty acids appeared to be obtained from both seafood and plant sources.[754]

Modern large clinical trials have been conducted to address the potential for benefit for other patient groups. Among 12,536 patients who were at high risk for cardiovascular events, including heart attack and stroke, and had impaired glucose tolerance or diabetes, they were randomly assigned to receiving 1g of ω-3 fatty acids or placebo.[769] As expected, the level of serum triglyceride was significantly lowered compared with placebo. But after 6.2 years, the risk for death from cardiovascular causes did not differ between the two groups. There was also no difference in the rates of major vascular events, death from any cause or death from arrhythmia.

When the use of ω-3 fatty acid was studied to include individuals with multiple risk factors for heart attack or had vascular disease, its benefit was also not shown. Importantly, patients with heart attack were excluded from the study.[770] Of 12,513 individuals enrolled, 6,244 of them were randomly assigned to receiving 1 g of ω-3 fatty acid daily, consisting of EPA and DHA in a ratio of 0.9:1 to 1.5:1. Another 6,269 participants received placebo capsules, consisting of olive oil. After five years, there was no difference in the occurrence of death, heart attack or stroke between the two groups of patients (overall rate was 11.8%). Nonetheless, as expected, the fall in serum triglyceride was greater among those who received ω-3 fatty acids. One of the criticisms for the lack of benefit for use of ω-3 fatty acid in these two clinical trials was the relatively low doses used in the study.

Refining the Oil in the Fish

Nonetheless, with the results of these clinical trials and other epidemiological studies, the American Heart Association recommended that adults should eat fish, particularly fatty fish, at least twice weekly. Consumption of 1 g capsule of ω-3 fatty acids, containing 850 mg of EPA and DHA, for patients with heart attack was also recommended.[771] Similar to any substance that we consume, adverse or side effects can be expected. With intake of less than a gramme of ω-3 fatty acids, the likelihood of fishy aftertaste was low and a very low risk in developing gastrointestinal upset, bleeding or rise in low-density lipoprotein (LDL) cholesterol level. But when the dose increases to more than 3 g daily, the likelihood of fishy aftertaste is likely with a moderate risk of gastrointestinal upset. The LDL-cholesterol level is likely to be increased and there is moderate risk of worsening the control of blood glucose level among those with diabetes or pre-diabetes. However, the risk of bleeding remains low. Heavy metal, particularly mercury,[772] dioxins and organochloride pesticide contaminants,[773,774] are generally very low but may be present in poorly-controlled preparations.[775–777]

When the DART investigators attempted to extend the benefit of fish consumption among 3,114 men with angina instead of heart attack in a clinical trial, the findings were not what they had expected.[778] Among those who were randomly assigned to the fish advice group, the risk of dying from heart disease was 26% higher. More surprisingly, the risk of sudden death was 54% higher! But this study was terminated after a year because of inadequate funding. Hence, the interpretation of the findings was less certain.

Recently, the role of ω-3 fatty acid supplementation was evaluated again in contemporary clinical trials. A total of 4,837 patients with recent heart attack, and who were receiving evidence-based life-saving medicines, were enrolled in the Netherlands.[779] Patients were randomly assigned to four groups; and the first three groups received margarines which were enriched with certain types of ω-3 fatty acids. The margarine in the first group was supplemented with EPA and DHA, with a target intake of 400 mg daily. Alpha-linolenic acid, with a target daily consumption of 2 g, was added to the second group. The margarine in the third group was supplemented with EPA, DHA and alpha-linolenic acid and the last group received placebo margarine. After a median period of 41 months, there was no difference in the clinical outcomes among the four groups of patients. The authors attributed the lack of benefit to contemporary efficacious treatment of patients with heart attack. A major criticism of this study was the dose of ω-3 fatty acids. It was lower than the earlier studies and could have explained why the supplement was not efficacious.

In another study conducted in Germany, 3,851 patients with heart attack were recruited. More than three-quarters of them underwent primary angioplasty, a life-saving procedure to re-establish blood flow in the blocked artery causing the heart attack and more than 80% were treated with cholesterol lowering medicines. Conversely, in the GISSI-Prevenzione trial,[762] only 5% of their patients had either coronary angioplasty or bypass surgery and 4.7% received cholesterol lowering medicine. Furthermore, the design of the study was also different. In the GISSI-Prevenzione trial,[762] patients and investigators were aware which group participants were randomised to. However, in the recent study, neither of them knew which group they were in. This study design is generally accepted as being more scientific because the potential for bias is lower. Moreover, highly purified ω-3 acid ethyl esters-90 capsules, containing 460 mg of EPA and 380 mg of DHA, was used in this study. For those who were assigned not to receive ω-3 fatty acids, similar looking capsules were administered. After one year, the rate of sudden death was similarly low for both groups, at 1.5%. Although total mortality was higher for patients receiving ω-3 acid ethyl esters-90 capsules (4.6% versus 3.7%), it was not statistically significant. This means that a play of chance was likely to have accounted for the difference and there was no real difference. But the frequency of fish consumption after the heart attack increased substantially in both groups. However, the estimated rise in ω-3 fatty acid consumption was relatively low, at only about 1 g weekly. Some have suggested that the benefits may be shown with a longer duration of follow-up. On the other hand, the favourable mortality effects of ω-3 fatty acid supplementation was obtained in as early as 3 months following treatment in the GISSI-Prevenzione trial.[763] It would appear that when currently evidence-based medicines are appropriately administered to a patient after a heart attack, together with a healthy diet, ω-3 fatty acid supplementation may not be routinely needed.[780]

What about Omega-6 Fatty acids?

Moving away from fish, ω-6 fatty acids enter into the realm of plants, partly based on the success of cultivation and mechanisation. Over the past 100 to 150 years, the consumption of ω-6 fatty acids has increased substantially[781] due to an enormous increase in the intake of vegetable oil from corn, sunflower seeds, safflower seeds, cotton-seed, rape seed (canola) and soybeans. For a probable traditional ratio of ω-6 to ω-3 from 1 to 2:1, it rose to 16 to 30:1.[782] While the precise reasons for this shift were unclear, they may be related to the strong marketing techniques employed by the agricultural industry to boost sales.

It is believed that ω-3 fatty acids are anti-inflammatory and ω-6 fatty acids are pro-inflammatory. Thus, their effects on atherosclerotic plaque may be different. Among 188 patients who were to undergo a surgery to remove plaque from a major neck artery, they were randomly assigned to control, fish oil capsules (ω-3 fatty acid) and sunflower oil capsules (ω-6 fatty acid).[736] After the plaques were removed, they were analysed for stability of the blood vessel. Only those who had received ω-3 fatty acids showed that the lining on the blood vessel wall was thicker with less inflammation. These findings suggested that only ω-3 and not ω-6 fatty acid is potentially beneficial to patients with vascular disease. Furthermore, higher intake of ω-6 fatty acid may be pro-inflammatory and pro-thrombotic by increasing the production of substances such as thromboxane A2, which raises the tone of blood vessels making them narrower and promotes "stickiness" of platelets.[783] The relationship between ω-6 fatty acids intake and atherogenic lipid and haemostatic (clotting) profiles was shown in a small clinical trial.[784] It showed that as the consumption of ω-6 fatty acids increased, the level of LDL-cholesterol, platelet count and components also rose. However, in a large cohort of 45,722 men without heart disease, the protective effect of consumption of ω-3 fatty acids was independent of the amount of intake of ω-6 fatty acids.[754] Those who received ≥250 mg of long-chain ω-3 polyunsaturated fatty acids lowered the risk of sudden death by 40% to 50%. The lack of influence of ω-6 fatty acids on the benefits of ω-3 fatty acids was also shown in the Nurses' Health Study.[785] The American Heart Association recommends the consumption of 5% to 10% of the energy from ω-6 polyunsaturated fatty acids, compared with lower intake, decreases the risk of coronary heart disease.[786] Furthermore, the panel suggested that lowering this amount may increase coronary risk.

Recently, the findings of the Sydney Diet Heart Study provided greater insight into the role of consumption of ω-6 fatty acids.[787] This study was re-analysed to evaluate the effectiveness of replacing dietary saturated fat with ω-6 linoleic acid for the secondary prevention of coronary heart disease and death. It consisted of 458 men with a recent heart attack. Participants were randomly assigned to either replace dietary saturated fats (from animal fats, common margarines and shortenings) with ω-6 linoleic acid (from safflower oil or marga-rine) or no specific dietary instruction. At 12 months, serum total cholesterol was significantly lower among those taking ω-6 linoleic acid (13% vs. 6% reduction). However, their absolute levels would still be considered high under today's standards because the study was conducted about 40 years ago. Contrary to what was expected, they found that the death rate of those consuming ω-6 linoleic acid were 62% higher (17.6% vs. 11.8%) after a follow-up period of 39 months. The rates for cardiovascular and coronary heart disease were also increased by 70%. After combining their findings with other studies, the investigators did not find evidence that substituting ω-6 linoleic acid provided protection from death or heart disease. Instead, there was a trend towards increasing the risk of heart disease.

Better understanding of biochemical pathways has provided fur-ther insight into the adverse effects of ω-6 linoleic acid. Its breakdown products are incorporated into the oxidised low-density lipoprotein cholesterol and may form part of the atherosclerotic process.[788,789] Intake of ω-6 fatty acid was associated with increased concentrations of fasting triglycerides and remnant-like particles, and the size of very low-density lipoprotein size. The size of low-density lipoprotein was reduced. As such, these changes were associated with a more adverse lipid profile.[790] Conversely, by lowering dietary linoleic acid, the amount of the bioactive oxidised linoleic acid metabolites decreases correspondingly.[791] In fact, the Sydney Diet Heart Study investiga-tors[787] suggested that the previous recommendation on the consump-tion of ω-6 polyunsaturated fatty acids may need to be revised.[786]

Moving Forward

Based on current knowledge, routine supplementation with ω-3 fatty acids is probably not required to prevent sudden death. However, for patients with previous heart attack or heart failure, especially among women, this may be beneficial. Its usefulness in today's context of use of several life-saving medicines remains unknown. On the other hand, ω-6 fatty acid supplementation is probably not routinely needed and may be harmful for those consuming the modern diet.

Poisons and Medicines

Drugs that Prevent Sudden Death

"Poison is in everything, and nothing is without poison. The dosage makes it either a poison or a remedy."

Paracelsus (1493–1541)
Swiss German Physician and Founder of Toxicology

The next time an ambulance passes by, look for the Star of Life. Initially, the United States Highway Traffic Safety Administration drew an orange Omaha cross on a white reflective background to identify emergency medical services vehicles in 1972. But the American Red Cross complained it looked similar to their Red Cross symbol. So the next year, Leo R. Schwartz, the Chief of the Emergency Medical Services Branch of the United States National Highway Traffic Safety Administration, modified the Universal Medical Identification Symbol launched by the American Medical Association in June 1963.[792] In this design, a serpent curling on a rod was drawn in the centre of a six-point blue star with a white border. Subsequently, the Star of Life has been registered as a certification mark on 1 February 1977 with the Commissioner of Patents and Trademarks. Currently the symbol is used internationally to identify emergency medical services and unit.

Several sources have proposed the origin of this rod. Traditionally, it belongs to Aesclepius (or Asklepios), the god of healing and medicine in Ancient Greek mythology.[793] Not unexpectedly, many early Greek physicians claimed to be his direct descendents, and even Hippocrates was proud to be from the lineage of Poldaleiros, the son of Aesclepius. Plato also addressed the "Father of Medicine" as "the Aesclepiade." While being epitomised as the ideal blameless physician in Homer's Iliad, Aesclepius' role was expanded in the Roman Empire by building the temple known as Aesclepieia. Non-poisonous Aesculapian snakes crawled freely in these complexes where the sick slept. In ancient Greece, the snake represented wisdom, health and immortality. Every year, it gets a new skin, after shedding its old one. However, numerous other cultures perceive the serpent as a representation of evil. In the Bible, Satan has been portrayed as a snake and was the tempter of Adam and Eve in Genesis "the serpent was more crafty than any other beast"[1] (Genesis 3:1). When the Israelites were attacked by fiery serpents, "Moses made a bronze serpent and set it on a pole. And if a serpent bit anyone, he would look at the bronze serpent and live"[1] (Numbers 21:9). The Chinese has a saying "以毒攻毒" which translates to "using poison to overcome the effects of toxin." Similarly, for the ancient Greeks, products from snakes and even the venom have been used for treatment.

A substantial number of sudden cardiac deaths are due to coronary artery disease and heart failure. The changing pattern of causes of sudden death in the modern world has clearly shown the pre-eminence of coronary artery disease. From January 2002 to December 2006, there were 243 individuals, 40 years old or younger, who died suddenly and underwent post-mortem examination in two hospitals in Montreal, Canada.[794] Coronary artery disease accounted for 37% of the deaths between the ages of 21 to 30 years. It accounted for up to 80% of those in the next decade. More surprisingly was that almost 40% of those who died from coronary heart disease had severe and extensive (triple-vessel) disease. Regardless of the cause of death, about 40% had significant narrowing in one major heart artery. The principal approach for prevention is to optimise the management of these conditions and encourage the public to live healthily. Throughout history, the line between poison and potion is fine. Some of us may have heard of the conspiracy of pharmaceutical companies to mislead doctors and make big bucks. Fewer still appreciate heart aches associated with discovery of new molecules and the prohibitive cost of drug development. Evaluating a novel pharmacological agent is complex and several key issues have to be considered. In particular, design of a clinical trial has to be meticulous and takes into account several intricacies of each condition studied. After the initial cardiovascular event, the risk for another is highest in the first 6 to 18 subsequent months.[36] Therefore, in consideration of the safety and efficacy of any intervention, not only is the type of patients important, the timing of the treatment is also critical. There are several other modulating factors that could influence the results of a clinical study.

Beta-Blockers

This is a group of agents that inhibits the effect of adrenaline on the heart and blood vessels. Adrenaline is secreted in times of stress, anger, fear or physical activity. The hormone triggers the "fight or flight" mechanism to heighten the body's response to increase the chance of surviving a treacherous situation. It acts on specific proteins on the surface of the heart to increase the rate and strength of contraction and on certain blood vessels to cause them to narrow so that the blood is diverted to vital organs. In addition, the hormone also induces the release of glucose from its stores to provide energy to effect the responses. As such, heart rate and blood pressure rise, and the workload of the heart increase correspondingly. The beta-adrenergic receptor is one of these mediators. By blocking its actions, the deleterious effects on a diseased heart are prevented.

In 1958, dichloroisoproterenol was made in the Eli Lilly Laboratories as the first beta-blocker. Due to its low potency and that it also stimulates instead of merely blocking the receptor, it was considered to be not of clinical value. Pronethalol was then developed but withdrawn due to its potential to cause cancer in mice. Eventually, Sir James Black, a Scottish physician and pharmacologist working in the Imperial Chemical Industries in Great Britain, designed a non-specific beta-blockers, propranolol, in 1962 and was introduced into clinics and hospitals as an anti-anginal agent two years later. Indeed, the success of beta-blockers has been touted to be one of the most important contributions in the field of pharmacology. For this achievement, he was awarded the Nobel Prize for Medicine and Physiology in 1988. Subsequently, this group of medicine was found to be useful in treating high blood pressure, rhythm disorders, hypertrophic cardiomyopathy and heart failure.

Subsequently, beta-blockers were also found to reduce the tendency of the heart muscle to develop ventricular fibrillation.[795] In 1982, a randomised double-blind and placebo-controlled clinical trial sponsored by the United States National Heart, Lung, and Blood Institute evaluated the efficacy of propranolol in reducing mortality in more than 3,800 patients after a heart attack.[796] After 27 months, the proportions that died were 7.2% and 9.8% for patients randomly assigned to receiving propranolol and placebo, respectively. Correspondingly, the chance of dying suddenly was also lower for those treated with propranolol (3.3% vs. 4.6%). This finding was corroborated by an independent Norwegian study.[797] Following a heart attack, 560 high-risk patients suffered from potentially lethal or severe rhythm disorder, or mild to moderate heart failure. At 12 months, the rate of sudden death was 4.0% for those receiving propranolol, which was 52% lower than patients receiving placebo (8.2%). There were another four patients in the placebo group who were successfully resuscitated from ventricular fibrillation. On the other hand, there was only one such patient in the propranolol group.[798] Similar result was obtained in another earlier Norwegian study with almost 1,900 patients using a different beta-blocker, timolol.[799] After 33 months, the rate of sudden death was lowered by 45% for those treated with timolol (7.7% vs. 13.9%). In particular, the benefit was more striking for patients with heart failure.[800]

Previously, it was believed that patients with heart failure should not be treated with beta-blockers. The basis was that beta-blockers could depress heart function so its administration could worsen the condition. But the favourable results obtained from heart attack patients with heart failure led to several clinical trials evaluating the efficacy of beta-blocker in improving outcome. Indeed, the risk of dying and deterioration of heart failure were reduced. In particular, the incidence of sudden cardiac death in this high risk group of patients was reduced by 47% (5.5% vs. 10.4%) compared with 13% for those without heart failure (2.9% vs. 3.3%). When the results of 30 clinical trials were combined together with a total of almost 25,000 patients with heart failure, beta-blockers reduced the risk of sudden death by more than 30%.[801]

Beta-blockers have been shown to prevent sudden death among patients with previous heart attack and heart failure.

Angiotensin Converting Enzyme (ACE) Inhibitors

Besides adrenaline, the elucidation of another key hormonal control network of blood pressure began more than a century ago. Its progress was hampered because catecholamines, the group of adrenaline and related compounds, took centre stage for several decades. Nonetheless, one step at a time, building on the knowledge derived by preceding scientists, the renin angiotensin system was gradually characterised through analysis of urine, blood and various bodily organs with laborious experiments on Petri dishes over a period of more than 70 years. Indeed, through a series of chemical reactions, a potent hormone that constricts blood vessels, angiotensin II, was discovered. The bio-catalyst that is paramount in the production of this substance is angiotensin converting enzyme (ACE). From 1965, inhibitors to this enzyme was beginning to be uncovered. Sergio Ferreira, a Brazilian physician and pharmacologist, worked on bradykinin, a substance present in the venom of the Brazilian pit viper, *Bothrops jararaca*, which lowers blood pressure.[802] He found that the snake venom contained a mixture of enzymes and short-chain amino acids (peptide). Together, these substances lower blood pressure markedly and that is the mechanism in which the venom causes death. Although it is able to lower blood pressure, the substance was not useful because of the lack of activity when administered orally. Since the number of amino acids is small, the substance is easily broken down in the digestive system. Patients are unlikely to agree to long-term treatment with injections for the treatment of hypertension. Due to political instability in his home country, Ferreira brought his work to England in 1964 to begin his postdoctoral fellowship with Sir John Vane at the Institute of Basic Medical Sciences at the Royal College of Surgeons of England. Realising the potential of the peptide, Vane tried to convince E. R. Squibb and Sons, a pharmaceutical company in New Brunswick, New Jersey, to develop an ACE inhibitor for the management of high blood pressure. But at that time, ACE was believed to only play a part in a life-threatening condition known as "malignant hypertension" (which accounted for less than 5% of patients with hypertension) and thus, it was not considered to be commercially viable.[803] Furthermore, renin was not always elevated among patients with hypertension. In addition, antibodies against renin failed to lower blood pressure consistently in animal models. The peptides were expensive to manufacture and have to be administered by injecting a few times a day into patients.

One of the peptide that was shown to inhibit the action of ACE and found to be stable was Teprotide, a nonapeptide (9-amino acid peptide). In 1974, a group of investigators from the Columbia-Presbyterian Medical Center in New York, injected this compound into 12 patients with hypertension.[804] The mean diastolic blood pressure fell from 126 mmHg to 101 mmHg immediately, and lasted for up to 16 hours. The challenge was to design such a comparable agent that could be administered orally and able to lower blood pressure for a reasonable period of time. His former mentor, Dr Arnold D. Welch, who was the president of the Squibb Institute of Medical Research, supported his work, recognised the potential and was unafraid to make changes. Eventually, Vane managed to change the company's perception and expanded the role of the renin angiotensin system to include a far more common condition, "essential" hypertension. Filling the void of cardiovascular pipeline, a team was assembled. After testing approximately 2,000 chemical structures for ACE inhibition, a new oral drug, captopril, was finally developed in 1975.[805] When other researchers modified the structure and composition, the number of ACE inhibitors increased substantially.

Enalapril, perindopril, lisinopril and ramipril are some of the more commonly available ACE inhibitors. From treating hypertension, this class of drugs has extended their indication to managing patients with heart attack, heart failure and diminished heart function without overt heart failure. The rates of dying, repeat heart attacks and progression of heart failure was reduced by ACE inhibitors.

Several studies have been conducted to evaluate the efficacy of ACE inhibitors in preventing sudden death for patients with a heart attack. In a review of 15 clinical trials, consisting of 15,104 patients with a recent heart attack, sudden cardiac death was reduced by 20%.[806] Although earlier studies did not show significant reduction of sudden death by administration of ACE inhibitors for patients with heart failure,[807] subsequent clinical trials demonstrated this clinical benefit. The Veterans Administration in the United States enrolled 804 men with heart failure and randomly assigned them to receive enalapril or a combination of two medicines (hydralazine and nitrate) to relax blood vessels.[808] After 30 months, sudden death was 45% lower for those treated with enalapril (14.1% vs. 22.9%). The ability of reducing sudden death was also observed in patients who are at risk for coronary heart disease.[809] A total of 9,297 patients who had some form of vascular disease or diabetes plus one other cardiovascular risk factor such as hypertension and smoking, were followed up for five years. These participants did not have abnormal heart function or heart failure. About half of the patients were randomly assigned to receive an ACE inhibitor, ramipril. Compared with those in the placebo group, the rate of cardiac arrest was lowered by almost 40%, albeit, the absolute reduction was from 1.3% to 0.8%. However, when the occurrence of the combination of sudden death and resuscitated cardiac arrest were considered together, the benefit was only 21% relative reduction, with an event rate of 4.2% in the ramipril group and 3.3% in the placebo group.[810] The mechanism for this benefit is unclear. It may be related to reduction in another heart attack and rhythm disorder which could be fatal.[811] By blocking the action of ACE, other substances may be produced to enhance blood flow to the heart.[812] Blood pressure and plasma noradrenaline increase as a response to a noxious cold stimulus was also blunted.[813]

Certainly, when a patient has a heart attack, particularly those who are suffering from heart failure or at high risk for heart disease, an ACE inhibitor may be administered to prevent sudden death.

Angiotensin Receptor Blockers

After the limelight has shifted away from the catecholamines to the ACE inhibitors, other less desirable effects of ACE inhibitors were increasingly recognised. In particular, cough is not an infrequent occurrence and can be quite irritating. Likely, some of them are due to the fact that ACE is an enzyme with multiple effects. Since inhibiting the function of angiotensin II is the principal mechanism needed to produce benefits, blocking its action is a more direct approach and less likely to induce adverse effects. The development of angiotensin receptor blockers shared common teething challenges with ACE inhibitors. Initially, the agent was made of amino acids. So, it had to be administered by injection. Using computer modelling to simulate the structures of the different molecules, scientists were able to alter the compound to increase the affinity to the angiotensin receptor, provide good oral activity and have adequate duration of action. Eventually, losartan was the first commercially available angiotensin receptor blocker and was launched in the United States in 1995. The names of the medicines in this group end with "sartan."

The first major trial using losartan to treat elderly patients with heart failure was conducted in May 1994.[814] A total of 722 patients were randomly assigned to receiving losartan or captopril. After 48 weeks, 4.8% of the patients treated with losartan died, compared with 8.7% for those treated with captopril. Of note, the occurrence of sudden death was reduced from 3.8% to 1.4%, amounting to 64% risk reduction. Losartan was also better tolerated than captopril. These findings from a moderate-size study was like a dream coming true; a resounding victory for drug discovery. However, when the study was expanded to 3,152 patients, who were followed up for 1.5 years, the results were not only unable to confirm the survival benefit of losartan, they might even appear contradictory.[815]

The proportion of patients who died was 11.7% for the losartan group and 10.4% for the captopril group. Similarly, the rate of sudden death or resuscitated cardiac arrest was marginally higher for those treated with losartan (9.0% vs. 7.3%). This adverse trend for losartan compared with captopril was also observed in another study comparing outcomes of 5,477 high-risk patients after a heart attack (9% vs. 7%).[816] Another clinical trial was conducted in more than 9,000 patients with hypertension and thickening of heart muscle wall. In other words, hypertension has affected the heart.[817] These high-risk hypertensive patients were randomly assigned to losartan-based or atenolol-based, a beta-blocker, treatment regimen. Medicines were administered sequentially to lower their blood pressure. After four years, the reduction of blood pressure was comparable between the two groups of patients. But the chance of suffering from a heart attack, stroke or dying from diseases of the blood vessel was 13% lower for those receiving losartan-based treatment regimen. In the group of 1,195 patients with diabetes, the benefit was amplified to 24%.[818] In fact, in this group of patients, the risk of sudden death was lowered by about 50%.[819]

There were two large-scale international clinical trials evaluating valsartan (Diovan) in the setting of heart failure[820] or heart attack with heart failure or reduced heart function.[821] The first study randomly assigned 5,010 heart failure patients to valsartan or placebo. It is important to note that 93% of them were already receiving an ACE inhibitor. In other words, the findings would have to be interpreted as addition of valsartan to patients who had been treated with an ACE inhibitor compared with those treated with ACE inhibitors alone. Although there was no difference in the likelihood of dying after two years, the occurrence of resuscitated cardiac arrests was marginally lower for those receiving valsartan (0.6% vs. 1.0%). Using valsartan also lowered the chance to be admitted to hospital for heart failure (14% vs. 18%).[820] In the second study, about 15,000 heart attack patients were randomly assigned to 1 of 3 treatment groups; valsartan alone, valsartan plus captopril or captopril alone. After two years, the risk of dying was similar among the three groups, approximately 20% in each category.

Another angiotensin receptor blocker, candesartan (Atacand), was evaluated among patients with heart failure. Within the programme, there were three groups of patients and were followed up for more than three years. The first two categories included those whose heart pump was weakened and either could not tolerate ACE inhibitors or that candesartan was administered together with an ACE inhibitor. The third group consisted of patients with mildly impaired or normal heart function. Overall, 7,599 patients were enrolled and the overall risk of dying was marginally lower, at 10% for those treated with candesartan.[822] Treatment with candesartan was associated with a 15% reduction of sudden death.[823] Not surprisingly, most of the benefit of candesartan was observed in the group of patients who were intolerant to ACE inhibitors (7.9% vs. 11.9%).

A group of Italian researchers hypothesised that the potential harm from angiotensin receptor blockers may be attributed to low doses of the medicine. They analysed 83 patients from the Sant'Andrea Hospital in Rome, in whom an intra-cardiac defibrillator (ICD) has been implanted.[824] Those treated with low doses of an angiotensin blocker were 2.4 times more likely to receive an appropriate discharge. In an international clinical trial of 3,846 patients with heart failure who were unable to tolerate ACE inhibitors, participants were randomly assigned to high- or low-dose losartan.[825] After almost five years, the overall likelihood of dying was lower for those receiving higher doses of the medicine.

Angiotensin receptor blockers probably serve as an alternative to ACE inhibitors for the prevention of sudden death among patients with abnormal heart function or heart failure. The dose should be titrated to the highest amount tolerable.

Aldosterone Antagonists

More than half a century ago, aldosterone was discovered to be a hormone that regulated blood volume by controlling urine output and controlled the concentration of potassium and sodium in the body. It belongs to the steroid family known as mineralocorticoid and its action is mediated via mineralocorticoid receptors.

Aldosterone is secreted mainly from the outer part of the adrenal gland. This organ is located on top of the kidneys. Spironolactone (Aldactone) was the first clinically effective aldosterone antagonist,[826] and was used to treat hypertension and increase urination to get rid of excess water accumulated in the body.[827]

Subsequently, aldosterone is also found to be manufactured and secreted in the heart muscle,[828] brain[829] and blood vessel wall.[830] In 1988, researchers at the Cardiovascular Institute in Chicago evaluated the role of aldosterone in the heart. Raised levels of this hormone were associated with enlargement of the muscle cell and scar formation.[831] It may result in direct injury to blood vessels as well.[832] Aldosterone also impairs the sensors to monitor blood pressure in the body[833] and prolongs the exposure of a signal which stimulates the heart, known as noradrenaline.[834] Preventing the action of aldosterone may prevent scarring and inflammation of the heart muscle[835] and reduce the effect of noradrenaline.[834] Likely, these actions lower the likelihood of potentially lethal rhythm disorder. Of note, their effects are independent of blood pressure and excretion of water plus salt. Spironolactone has also been shown to restore the function of the lining of blood vessels to maintain its normal tone.[836] Although ACE inhibitors lowers the aldosterone level initially, the effect was not sustained,[837] a phenomenon known as "aldosterone escape." Therefore, by preventing its action with an aldosterone antagonist, outcome may be improved.

Clinical trials were conducted to evaluate the usefulness of spironolactone in patients with heart failure. One thousand six hundred and sixty-three patients with moderate to severe heart failure patients receiving optimal medical treatment were randomly assigned to spironolactone or placebo.[838] After two years, the occurrence of dying was 30% lower for those treated with spironolactone. Sudden death was also decreased by about 30% with spironolactone, from 13.1% to 10.0%. However, one of the undesirable effects of spironolactone was that about 10% of men suffered from development of breast tissue. This action is attributed to the reduction of male hormones and increase in the conversion of male to female hormones. Apart from being embarrassed, the man may experience pain in the nipple. Discontinuation of the medicine usually leads to resolution.[839] To overcome this limitation, a new drug, eplerenone (Inspra), was designed by modifying a part of spironolactone so that it would not be metabolised to a substance that act against the male hormone. This new agent retains the specificity to the mineralocorticoid receptor.

As such, a multi-centre study on patients with heart attack, 6,642 patients with heart attack and reduced heart function who have received optimal medical treatment was conducted.[840] The patients were randomly assigned to eplerenone or placebo. After 16 months, the risk of sudden death was lowered by at least 20% for those treated with eplerenone, from 6.1% to 4.9%. Although this medicine was also useful in preventing death in patients with mild heart failure, its benefit was less evident for sudden death[841] among this group of patients. As expected, the incidence of development of breast tissue was substantially lower than spironolactone, at 0.5%, which was comparable to those receiving placebo (0.6%).[840] Since this is a new medicine, eplerenone costs more than spironolactone.

Among patients with heart attack together with significantly reduced heart function and those with heart failure, sudden death may be prevented by using an aldosterone antagonist.

Statins

In 1858, Rudolf Karl Ludwig Virchow, a German pathologist, found that the blood vessels of patients who died from heart attack were thickened and irregular.[842] There was a fatty mass encapsulated by a wall commonly known as a cap. These changes were known as "atheroma" which means "gruel" or "porridge" in Greek. Subsequent researchers demonstrated the excess of cholesterol in the atheroma. In 1913, a young Russian scientist, Nikolai N. Anichkov, fed rabbits with high cholesterol diet, consisting of eggs, milk and brain. On the walls of the aorta, there were changes comparable to those in men.[843] Unlike humans, rabbits are plant-eating animals so the findings may not be applicable to meat-eaters. Subsequently, similar experiments were conducted in various species, including primates,[844,845] and atherosclerosis developed in their blood vessels. However, the response to diet and distribution of disease differed with various primate species. Back in 1889, Lehzen and Kanuss reported a child with multiple lumps at the tendons of the hands and ankles since 3 years old.[846] When the child died suddenly at the age of 11 years, post-mortem examination showed that these lumps were filled with fats and there were also similar deposits in the arteries, including those supplying the heart. Cases of sudden death among children with lumps along tendons were increasingly recognised in the 1950s.[847,848]

As the amount of epidemiological evidence linking cholesterol level and heart disease increased, a young Japanese scientist went to the Albert Einstein College of Medicine in New York to work on an unstable enzyme involved in the formation of bacterial cell wall in 1966.[849] While living in this cosmopolitan city, Akira Endo was amazed at the large number of overweight individuals. The American diet was substantially different from what they ate in his homeland. Within Bronx, Akira often witnessed ambulances fetching elderly persons with heart attack to hospitals. Realising the significance of his experience, he was determined to find a solution to this emerging epidemic on returning to Japan. Based on his study on cell walls, Akira understood that sterols were its key components. These compounds are analogous to steroids in animals since plants and bacteria do not have cholesterol. In 1971, he hypothesised that fungi would produce substances that would inhibit the production of sterols as a form of defence against other microbes. Without a cell wall, the organism dies. After two years and 6,000 microbes, two suitable fungi were identified. A chemical, compactin, was isolated from a fermentation broth containing a blue-green mould, *Penicillium citrinum*, which was obtained earlier from rice belonging to a vendor in Kyoto, and was found to block the action of the enzyme that produces cholesterol. Filled with excitement, the new compound was rapidly tested in the quintessence laboratory animal, the rat. But it did not work as the cholesterol levels did not fall. Instead of falling into despair, they back-tracked and found that compactin induced the enzyme instead of preventing its action. It was the laying hens that saved the day. Compactin reduced cholesterol levels by about 34% in two weeks. From 1976, it was shown to lower cholesterol in rabbits, dogs and monkeys and the programme was revived. In the following year, a doctor from Osaka University, Akira Yamamoto, initiated treatment on an 18-year-old woman with familial hypercholesterolaemia. Finally, clinical trials on compactin were initiated in November 1978. While the results were encouraging, the programme was discontinued in August 1980 because of the development of lymphoma in dogs when the agent was administered in high doses. When the Japanese experience was shared with their colleagues in the United States, mevinolin (the name was later changed to lovastatin) was discovered in autumn 1978. This substance was produced from another fungus, *Asperigillus terreus*, and the chemical structure was fairly similar to compactin with comparable biological properties. As such, clinical trials on humans were postponed initially until its safety was assured by additional animal studies. Investigations on humans were re-initiated in 1983 for patients who were at high risk after a heart attack. Eventually, on 31 August 1987, lovastatin became the first commercially available statin. In 1988, simvastatin was introduced, followed by pravastatin in 1991, fluvastatin in 1994, atorvastatin in 1997, cerivastatin in 1997 and rosuvastatin in 2003.

Numerous high quality clinical trials were conducted to evaluate the safety and efficacy of statin therapy in various categories of patients; those with previous heart attack, bypass surgery, coronary angioplasty, stroke, diabetes and at increased risk for heart disease. The researchers were grouped together by the University of Oxford and formed the Cholesterol Treatment Trialists' Collaborators in November 1994 to unify their data and address key uncertainties of lowering cholesterol.[850] After 14 randomised trials and more than 90,000 participants, they found that total mortality fell by 12% for every mmol/L reduction in low-density lipoprotein (LDL) cholesterol level.[851] Most of the benefits were related to lowering fatal heart attack events (19%). When the adverse outcomes relating to diseased blood vessels were grouped together, such as heart attack, stroke, bypass operation or coronary angioplasty, the relative reduction was 21% for participants receiving statin compared with placebo. They also found that the greater amount of reduction in LDL cholesterol level, the higher the degree of benefit. Due to large number of participants, the researchers also found that outcomes were improved over a wide range of patients. The favourable effects were durable, at least up to five years, which was the average duration of the studies. Importantly, the investigators did not find an increase in the rates of cancer or bleeding in the brain among those treated with statins.

A review was conducted to determine the role of statins on sudden death. A total of 29 trials comprising of 113,568 participants were randomly assigned to treatment with and without statins.[852] Sudden death was lowered by 10% with statin therapy. For other non-sudden death from heart conditions, the reduction was 22%. However, the occurrence of potentially lethal rhythm disorder was not prevented by statins. This finding was in contradistinction from several earlier studies and review,[853] which suggested that abnormal heart rhythm could be suppressed by about a third. In another review, statins prevented sudden death only among patients with coronary heart disease. On the other hand, those with heart failure but without coronary heart disease did not receive any benefit.[854] A major limitation of early studies was that not every heart beat was monitored. With the advent of pacemakers, and more specifically, intra-cardiac defibrillators (ICD) and cardiac resynchronisation therapy with defibrillator (CRT-D), they have been implanted to prevent sudden death. One of the abnormalities among patients with heart failure is that the right and left ventricles do not contract synchronously. In these patients, pacing leads are placed at both ventricles to re-time the contraction of the right and left ventricles to restore normal synchrony as much as possible. This form of treatment is known as cardiac resynchronisation therapy (CRT). When the piece of equipment has a defibrillator function, it is known as CRT-D. These devices are able to record heart beats continuously.

In an international clinical trial evaluating the use of an ICD in 362 patients with coronary heart disease, the investigators found that potentially lethal rhythm disorder was lowered by 40% among those treated with lipid lowering agents.[855] In this study, about 80% of them were treated with statins. Although the proportion of patients dying from heart disease also lowered by about 40% among those receiving lipid lowering therapy, the researchers did not mention about sudden death.

The ability of statin therapy reducing potentially fatal rhythms was also shown in the analysis of a large clinical trial evaluating the usefulness of implantation of an ICD in preventing sudden death.[856] In this study, patients were categorised into three groups, those receiving statins for at least 90% of the duration, 10% or less, and between 10% to 90%. Of 654 American patients in a large international study, the occurrence of these rhythm disorders was 28% lower for those treated with statins consistently compared with patients who received statins occasionally. Correspondingly, the estimated rate of sudden death reduced from 11% to 3% at the end of three years. Due to the benefits of statin therapy among patients with coronary heart disease, there was only a small window of opportunity of conducting a prospective study. A small randomised trial of 106 patients from Belgium and Greece, was conducted from 1 February 2000.[857] The participants had coronary heart disease with potentially lethal heart rhythm disorder and were randomly assigned to receiving atorvastatin 80 mg daily or placebo. Although the study was completed in 2004, it was presented at the Annual Scientific Meeting of the Heart Rhythm Society in Boston, Massachusetts, in May 2006. After one year, the device was appropriately activated in 21% of the patients in the atorvastatin group compared with 38% in the placebo group.

The usefulness of statin therapy was also evaluated among patients with heart failure but without coronary heart disease. In an investigator-initiated trial in the United States, 458 patients with heart failure but without coronary heart disease were enrolled.[858] Although the researchers found that statins reduced the overall chance of dying by almost 80%, there was only a trend to suggest that there was a correspondingly decrease in sudden death. Among the 229 patients who received an ICD in this study, use of statin was not shown to reduce the occurrence of appropriate shock therapy.

The authors attributed the lack of benefit to the small number of participants. In the Multicenter Automatic Defibrillator Implantation Trial with Cardiac Resynchronization Therapy (MADIT-CRT), 821 patients with abnormal heart function but without coronary heart disease were implanted with a CRT-D.[859] Of the 499 who received statins, the risk of potentially fatal rhythm disorder was reduced by 77% compared with non-statin users. Correspondingly, the rate of appropriate discharge of the defibrillator was lowered by 46%.

Several mechanisms may explain the benefits of statins in preventing sudden death. For patients with coronary heart disease, statins have been shown to prevent heart attacks via a variety of possible pathways. They may normalise blood vessel wall function, reduce inflammation, cell movement into blood vessel wall, platelets and clot formation. Since heart attacks are the most common cause of sudden death, this group of medicines could have reduced its occurrence.[860] The improvement of survival observed among patients with heart failure but without coronary heart disease suggest that the benefit was beyond lowering cholesterol.[861]

Like all potential toxins, there are adverse effects from statin therapy. Initially, liver dysfunction and muscle damage were the two most important unwanted actions. Of those in the market, only cerivastatin was withdrawn voluntarily in August 2001 because of 52 deaths attributed to severe injury to the muscle leading to kidney failure.[862] In the United States, there were 31 fatal and 385 non-fatal cases among 700,000 estimated users. Cerivastatin was found to be at least 10 times more likely than other statins to cause fatal muscle damage. Withdrawal of a widely used medicine because of life-threatening side effects has certainly eroded the public confidence in the health care system. The lack of trust in regulatory bodies and the allure of conspiracy between medical and pharmaceutical industries have turned several well-intended individuals to alternative therapeutic approaches, and most of them remained largely untested and unchallenged. Approving drugs for long-term use based on the results of clinical trials of a few thousand patients will continue to challenge the authorities.

Statins are likely to prevent sudden death for patients with heart failure, particularly those with underlying coronary heart disease.

However, the dose and target for treatment have not been clearly established. For those with coronary heart disease, the agent may be administered according to the current guidelines.

Medicines for Rhythm Disorders (Anti-Arrhythmic Agents)

Among the various transactions between the New and Old World, transmission of diseases and healings were brought about by the Spanish conquistadors. Of these, the bark of the South American tree, *Cinchona* (Rubiaceae), was found to be useful for treating fevers in Peru, carried back to Europe by missionaries in 1630.[863] Indeed, it contains quinine, which is a medicine used to treat malaria. Gradually, this compound was found to be helpful in controlling heart rhythm. In 1749, Jean-Baptiste de Sénac reported that it was useful in controlling palpitations[864] in which "long and rebellious palpitations have ceded to this febrifuge."[863] It was not until 1912 that the knowledge of using this bark for treatment of rhythm disorders became more recognised. A 50-year-old stout Dutch merchant went to the clinic of Dr Karel Federik Wenkebach in Vienna, Austria.[865] He wanted to eradicate his episodic attacks of auricular (atrial) fibrillation permanently because it was affecting his work. This is an abnormal heart that affects the atrium or upper chambers of the heart. The patient told him that the irregular heartbeats were aborted 20 to 25 minutes after taking 1 g of quinine. Otherwise, it lasted for 2 to 14 days. Subsequently, Dr Wenkebach tried this medicine with several of his patients and was met with little success. Nonetheless, even for those whose heart rhythm did not normalise, quinine had a "soothing" effect on the rate. Subsequently, Walter von Frey of Berlin discovered that of the four main alkaloids, quinidine was most effective in controlling abnormal heart rhythms. Although this usefulness of this medicine was limited by its severe gastrointestinal symptoms and other adverse effects, quinidine syncope was most fearful. This is due to a potentially lethal rhythm disorder.

Despite substantial improvement in the knowledge of electrical properties of cells and heart muscle, there was little progress in the introduction of new anti-arrhythmic medicines. The Second World War brought about an unusual twist in the development of novel agents. Due to the fall of Indonesia, an important source of quinine was lost. Procainamide, a modification of a local anaesthetic agent, procaine, was discovered in 1951. Subsequently, a common animal model, known as the "Harris dog", was developed. By occluding the coronary artery sequentially, abnormal beats occurred frequently. In humans, electrical activities are generated by movement of charged particles, known as ions, across the cell membrane. There are sodium, potassium and calcium ion channels. Based on the work on animal models, several new drugs were developed to block the sodium ion channels and were found to be effective in suppressing ectopic beats. Potentially fatal rhythm disorders generally consist of rapid runs of ectopic beats for a long duration. During this period, the heart is unable to generate sufficient output to support the body. The presence of ectopic beats after a heart attack has been identified as a marker for sudden death. As such, medicines that reduce these beats would lower the risk of sudden death.

In a pilot trial, three candidates and their therapeutic doses were selected based on the efficacy in preventing ectopic beats.[866] The ultimate challenge came when a large scale randomised clinical trial was conducted. Of the three drugs that were studied in 1,727 patients in the Cardiac Arrhythmia Suppression Trial (CAST), the findings of encainide and flecainide were reported initially.[867] In this investigation, not only did the participants have a heart attack, they also suffered from asymptomatic or mildly symptomatic ectopic beats. Their heart function was on the low side of normal and impaired. After 10 months, the trial was terminated pre-maturely by the Data and Safety Monitoring Committee on 17 April 1989 because of the harmful effects of the study drugs. The proportion that died from abnormal heart rhythm or cardiac arrest was more than 3.5 times higher among those receiving the drugs compared with patients receiving placebo (4.5% vs. 1.2%). Correspondingly, 7.7% of patients taking encainide and flecainide died compared with 3.0% for the placebo group. On 19 April 1989, study sites started to inform patients to discontinue these medicines. Fearing distortions on the information, the United States National Heart, Lung, and Blood Institute made a public announcement at 11 am on 25 April 1989. These counter-intuitive results brought much dismay and apprehension among doctors and patients all over the world. On the day after the announcement, physicians in the United States received the "Dear Doctor" letters from the manufacturers of encainide and flecainide. Distressed patients who were taking these drugs started to call them for advice. The tension and strain during these encounters must be unimaginable. These unwarranted situations would continue to haunt the healthcare industry.

Three years later, the third drug, moricizine, suffered from the same fate.[868] When the data were combined, there were 3,549 patients.[869] At one year, the rate of sudden death or cardiac arrest was higher among those receiving any of the three drugs than placebo (7% vs. 4%). The risk of dying was also correspondingly higher (10% vs. 5%).

The Cardiac Arrhythmia Suppression Trial (CAST) has been an important learning experience for the industry, academics and physicians. It calls for the continual humility and respect in health matters. Despite the best efforts, there are several elements which are largely unknown and could not have accounted for by logic and reasoning. Of the several reasons postulated, the underlying common mechanistic pathway was the promotion of potentially lethal rhythm disorders, a characteristic known as proarrhythmia. For the strict clinical trialists, these findings could only be applied to the study population and drugs.[870] In other words, these medicines should not be administered to patients with heart attack and impaired heart function because of ectopic beats.

Repeatedly, discoveries are made from astute observations by keen and passionate individuals. Dr Gleb von Anreps, born in St Petersburg and trained in England, became a professor in physiology at the King Fouad I University in Cairo, Egypt, in 1931. Since he was interested in circulation of blood to the heart, one of his objectives was to seek a treatment for coronary heart disease. While in Egypt, his technician was administering Khellin for various non-cardiac ailments. He also obtained relief from coronary heart disease. Khellin is an organic compound found in the plant *Ammi visnaga*, a flowering species from the carrot family. As a mixture, Khella, was used in Eygpt for treating kidney stones. In addition, the compound has properties of relaxing blood vessels and ureter. Recognising its potential, the active compound was isolated and amiodarone was discovered in 1961. It was used to treat angina pectoris, chest discomfort or breathlessness due to lack of oxygen supply to heart muscle because of narrowing of blood vessels.

When Bramah Singh, a doctorate candidate at the Oxford University, was studying the mechanistic effects of amiodarone as an anti-anginal agent, he found that there was direct action on the heart muscle as well. There were changes in the electrical properties which were attributed to its action on potassium ion channels. Soon after, Dr Mauricio B. Rosenbaum from Ramos Meija Hospital in Buenos Aires, Argentina, started to use amiodarone to treat patients with rhythm disorders successfully.[871,872] Although amidoarone was available in Canada and Europe since the 1970s, it was not until December 1985 that the United States Food and Drug Administration approved its use. With the development of effective anti-anginal treatment, the use of amiodarone was gradually limited to treatment of rhythm disorders.

Early review of the clinical trials on amiodarone showed that its administration to patients after a recent heart attack, with heart failure, or with clinically evident rhythm disorder, lowered the occurrence of sudden death.[873,874] Subsequent researchers found that amiodarone may not be safe among patients with heart failure.[875,876] The information from more than 3,000 patients participating in a randomised clinical trial on the use of beta-blocker in stable heart failure was re-analysed.[875] They found that those receiving amiodarone were 50% more likely to die, particularly from sudden death after four years. Similarly, when the data from another study — evaluating the use of ACE inhibitors and angiotensin receptor blockers among almost 14,000 patients after a heart attack and with impaired heart function — was analysed again, the researchers found that the risk of dying was significantly higher for those receiving amiodarone.[876] As such, another review of more than 8,500 patients from randomised trials was conducted.[877] Amiodarone reduced the rate of sudden death by more than 25%, and the benefit was observed among patients after a heart attack or with heart failure regardless of use of beta-blocker. But the use of amiodarone was associated with more than 5.5 times increased risk of thyroid disorder and about two times increased risk of lung or liver toxicity. However, the absolute rate of thyroid disorder was 3.6% compared with 0.4% for those not taking amiodarone. The rate of discontinuation of treatment was about 10% for amiodarone (31.6% vs. 21.1%). Despite the controversies associated with the use of this medicine, the researchers suggested that the medicine may be used for patients who were unable to receive an ICD.

Empowering the Rescuer

CPR Training and Advent of Automated External Defibrillator

"When Elisha came into the house, he saw the child lying dead on his bed ... Then he went up and lay on the child, putting his mouth on his mouth, his eyes on his eyes, and his hands on his hands. And as he stretched himself upon him, the flesh of the child became warm. Then he got up again and walked once back and forth in the house, and went up and stretched himself upon him. The child sneezed seven times, and the child opened his eyes."[1]

II Kings 4:32-35

Once a cardiac arrest has occurred, the chance for survival depends substantially on the skill of the rescuer and the available resources. Undoubtedly, the pre-existing condition of the victim also plays a vital role in determining the outcome. Sometimes, miracles do happen. But for several decades, the practice of cardiopulmonary resuscitation in the out-of-hospital setting has remained relatively unchanged. It consisted of a series of actions that support the blood flow and oxygenation of the victim by compressing the chest and blowing air into the lungs at a determined rhythm and order.[878] Among individuals with out-of-hospital cardiac arrest, survival to hospital discharge ranged from 2% to 25% for all cardiac rhythms and 3% to 33% for ventricular fibrillation.[879] In a pooled analysis of three large studies, the survival rate for out-of-hospital cardiac arrest was 6.4%.[880] But for those with ventricular fibrillation, the rate was better at 16.1%. Correspondingly, when a cardiac arrest occurs in a long distance running event, those who received bystander cardiopulmonary resuscitation were more likely to survive.[32] Survivors also received emergency care earlier and were more likely to be in ventricular fibrillation or tachycardia.

Although asystole, or cardiac standstill — which indicates absence of electrical activity, is the most common rhythm for individuals found with sudden cardiac arrest,[880] ventricular fibrillation (Figure 22) is the most frequent abnormal rhythm of a witnessed out-of-hospital sudden cardiac arrest.[881,882] During this episode, the electrical activities of the heart is completely disorganised so that the ventricles (the main heart pump) do not contract normally. This bizarre and chaotic movement was first described by Carl Ludwig and his student, Mauritius Hoffa, in 1849 after exposing the ventricle to an electric current.[883] The term "fibrillation" was first

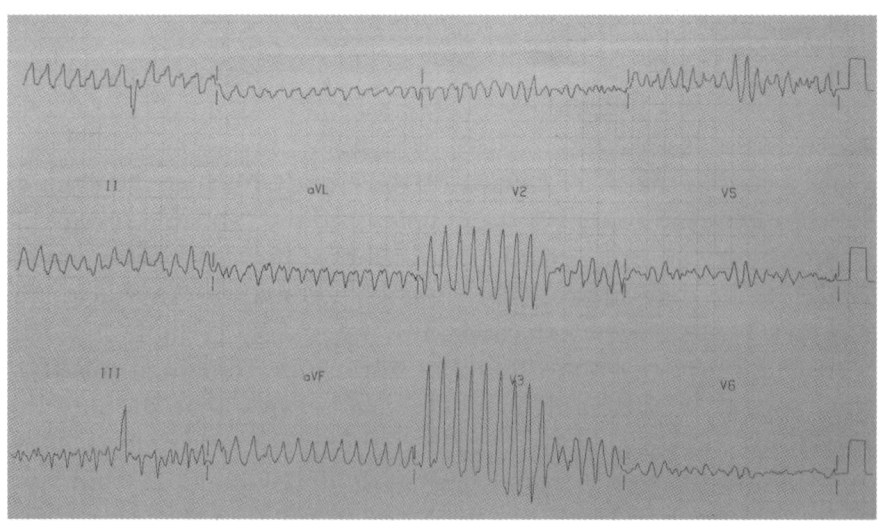

Figure 22.   Electrocardiogram showing ventricular fibirllation.
The pattern on the right end becomes chaotic without any recognisable pattern. This is consistent with a life-threatening rhythm disorder.

used by a French neurophysiologist, Edme Vulpian, who described the origin and sustaining abnormality was derived from the heart.[884] It was not until 1889 that John McWilliam of Aberdeen, Scotland, was the first to suggest that ventricular fibrillation rather than asystole was the underlying mechanism of sudden death in man.[885] He described the condition vividly as chaos across the fibres of the heart, trapping the organ in a helpless quiver and depriving the body of oxygen, bringing death within a matter of minutes.[886] Not unlike a muscle cramp in the leg, the heart is unable to function and pump blood efficiently during ventricular fibrillation. Shortly after the abnormal rhythm has occurred, the victim loses consciousness because of lack of blood supply to the brain. If normal blood flow is not restored within 5 to 10 minutes, the person dies when the heart stops beating altogether.[887] Indeed, within the first 2 minutes of a witnessed collapse, the rhythm was found to be ventricular fibrillation in 64%.[888] Survival rates are estimated to fall by 7% to 10% for every minute after the collapse.[887] When proper cardiopulmonary resuscitation is initiated, outcome has been shown to improve and the decline in survival is reduced to be 3% to 4% per minute from collapse.[881,887,889,890]

The benefit of cardiopulmonary resuscitation was more evident among patients who were responded to by emergency care technicians later than 4 minutes.[891] There were 1,117 persons with out-of-hospital ventricular fibrillation who were attended by the Emergency Medical Services in Seattle, Washington. Among 220 individuals who has collapsed at least 4 minutes and had received about 90 seconds of cardiopulmonary resuscitation, the survival rate was 27%. Conversely, those who did not receive cardiopulmonary resuscitation, the survival rate was only 17%. Over the past three decades, the overall survival from out-of-hospital cardiac arrest remained relatively stable, with an aggregate rate of 7.6%.[892] But survival was more likely if cardiopulmonary resuscitation was performed or if the victim suffered from ventricular tachycardia or fibrillation. Nowadays, there are several organisations, such as the Singapore Heart Foundation, that offer courses to the public on how to perform cardiopulmonary resuscitation.

Fibrillation and Defibrillation

Today, we are well-aware of the deadly power of electricity, and the rather infamous electric chair used for execution. It was as early as in 1775 that electric shocks were systematically delivered to various parts of the body of hens. The bird became lifeless after some shocks to the head. But subsequent shocks that were delivered to the chest could revive the heart.[893] Initially, the hen was stunned and had some difficulty in walking. It did not eat for a day but recovered subsequently and was even able to lay an egg. In 1899, Swiss investigators have shown that a small amount of electric current was able to provoke ventricular fibrillation and a larger electrical shock was able to convert the rhythm to normal.[894] While these experiments were interesting, they had little relevance at that time and were ignored by other investigators. By the end of the 19th century, the miracle of electric power was beginning to be rapidly made available to several people. Nights and winters were brightened. More daily conveniences were invented with the availability of this new source of power. However, it was both a blessing and a curse. There was an increasing number of fatal accidents, especially among power utility line workers, which was due to electrocution. The electric current did not require to be applied on the heart directly, with the chest wall remaining intact. Soon, it was realised that ventricular fibrillation was the most common underlying mechanism for death.[895] Not surprisingly, researchers were keen to search for an effective method to terminate this lethal rhythm.

During one of these experiments, a shock induced ventricular fibrillation in a dog.[896] In 1933, William B. Kouwenhoven, an electrical engineer, accidentally applied a second shock to the animal, and to his surprise, it terminated the abnormal rhythm. Hence, he coined the term countershock. But it was not until 1947 that the first human defibrillation was performed by Claude Beck, a cardiothoracic surgeon at the Case Western Reserve University at Cleveland, Ohio.[897] While closing the surgical incision of a 14-year-old boy after repairing a chest wall deformity of the breast bone ("sunken chest"), his pulse suddenly became absent. So, he re-opened the wound and applied cardiac massage for about 45 minutes. However, the rhythm remained as ventricular fibrillation. Left with no other options, Dr Beck delivered a shock of 1.5 ampere of alternating current derived from 110 volts to the boy. But it failed. After injecting a medicine used to treat abnormal rhythm, a second similar shock was delivered 25 minutes later. Fortunately, it restored the heart to normal rhythm and Richard Heyard did not suffer from any significant brain damage. However, his device was only suitable for use for an exposed heart with silver paddles which looked like large tablespoons. It was built together with his friend, James Rand III. Therefore, it was only used in the operating rooms. Subsequently, in 1952, Naum Gurvich, a physician from Moscow, designed the first commercially available defibrillator that could be used without exposing the heart.[898] In 1955, Dr Paul Zoll was managing a man with recurrent fainting spells. The patient was found to have ventricular fibrillation and Dr Zoll successfully restored him to normal rhythm by applying 710 volts of alternating current for 0.15 seconds.[899]

Indeed, the most efficacious way to treat ventricular fibrillation is electrical defibrillation. This is somewhat similar to a doing a reset when our computers, notebooks, netbooks or hand-held smartphones freeze. By pressing the button, the device stops functioning and then re-starts. During defibrillation, an electrical current is passed through the heart to terminate the potentially lethal disorder. Hopefully, the heart can then re-start with its own normal rhythm. The earlier the procedure, defibrillation, is performed, the higher the likelihood for success and survival.[900] Cardiopulmonary resuscitation increases the chance for successful defibrillation and subsequent survival.[882,887,901] Prolonged periods of ventricular fibrillation may lead to changes of characteristics of the heart as a result of lack of blood supply.[902] Hence, the success of defibrillation diminished. Therefore, cardiopulmonary resuscitation may improve delivery of oxygen to the heart muscle and reduce the accumulation of toxic waste products. As a result, the chance of success with defibrillation may improve.

When defibrillators were first made available, only medical personnel, such as doctors and certain specially-trained intensive care nurses, were initially allowed to use them. This is because there is a critical step of identifying a "shockable" rhythm. Importantly, the approach for treating various rhythm disorders other than ventricular fibrillation differed. As such, there are settings on the machine that the operator needs to adjust before discharging the electrical current. Due to the small number of trained individuals, the time to receive treatment is likely to be delayed.

On the basis that timeliness in defibrillation saves lives, a key strategy is to train first responders to perform the procedure during medical emergency situations. From 1 May 1998 to 31 December 2006, there were 8,782 witnessed out-of-hospital cardiac arrest in the Osaka Prefecture in Japan.[903] Of these, 1,733 (19.7%) of them had ventricular fibrillation. Unfortunately, 392 (22.6%) did not respond to cardioversion. Over the 8 years and 7 months period, the annular occurrence of witnessed ventricular fibrillation increased from 2.0 to 3.3 per 100,000 residents. But the incidence of shock-resistant ventricular fibrillation was unchanged. Mortality at 1-month remained consistently low, at 5.6%. Hence, there is an urgent need to provide more rapid access to defibrillation. The procedure needs to be simplified and made to the public. A greater number of individuals are required to be trained.

Advent of Automated External Defibrillators

Despite its complexities and intricacies, the first external automated defibrillator was invented by Dr Fred Zacouto in Paris in March 1953.[904] The device was known as "Bloc Réanimateur." But as with any prototype, the equipment was bulky. It consisted of two large box-liked apparatus, approximately the size of an old desk-top printer, placed on a two-tier trolley. Using an adaptor-interface, they were attached to the patient who worn a singlet-like clothing. This specialised outfit was probably lined with electrodes and connected by wires. With prohibitively large and heavy equipment, mobility for the patient was understandably limited. Infra-red sensors were attached to various parts of the body, such as fingers and ear lobe, to determine heart rate. When the rate was too slow, the Bloc

Réanimateur would provide electrical impulses to stimulate the heart to beat faster. There were also electrocardiographic leads to detect ventricular fibrillation. An electric shock was delivered once this abnormal rhythm was identified.

The portable monitoring and automated external defibrillator was developed by Archibald W. Diack, Warren S. Welborn and Robert G. Rullman. They filed their patent on 29 December 1975.[905,906] It detects breathing or bodily movement and electrocardiographic signals (electrical activities from the heart) by sensors, microphones and pacing electrodes through an oro-pharyngeal airway and chest-abdominal region. When it senses that there is no electrical activity and there is no bodily motion, the device delivers electrical impulses to stimulate the heart to beat. But when there is electrical activity without bodily motion, an electric shock is delivered for defibrillation. It was first introduced into clinical use in 1979.[906] Subsequently, modestly trained technicians in the United Kingdom were able to use the automated external defibrillator readily.[907] Of 27 individuals with cardiac arrest, successful resuscitation was pre-assessed to be unlikely to be successful in 16 of them and none of them survived despite using the automated external defibrillator. In the remaining 11 patients, 5 survived to hospital discharge. The investigators believed that the widespread use of the device would improve outcome of patients with out-of-hospital cardiac arrest.

The procedure in determining cardiac rhythm could be strengthened. With the advent of better computing power and electronic sophistication, many of the algorithms in recognising various rhythms have been developed. Technological advances have enabled a battery, capacitors and circulatory to analyse electrocardiographic patterns and inform the operator if a shock is indicated to be built into an automated external defibrillator and yet keeping it light-weight and portable. Indeed, the patent for an interactive portable defibrillator was filed on 8 March 1984 by Carlton B. Morgan, Daniel Yerkovich, Thomas D. Lyster and Douglas H. Roberts.[908] This device analyses the heart rhythm and body motion of the patient and determines if an electrical shock could be administered. After placing the electrodes at the appropriate places, it advises the operator on the next step. A response is required in order for the device to proceed. Early evaluation of the automated external defibrillator show high rates of accuracy in determining ventricular fibrillation and delivery of electrical shock.[909] But electrocardiographic tracings differ widely. As such, a library of abnormal rhythms has been developed to evaluate these automated external defibrillators.[910] After testing the efficacy of detection of potentially lethal rhythm disorder using the pre-recorded database of rhythms, it was modified and improved the ascertainment rate from 77% to 94%.[911] Together with these safeguards and improvements, the early experience with automated external defibrillator was encouraging in the 1980s. By 1984, most of the emergency medical units in Seattle, Washington, were equipped with automated external defibrillators. There were 1,287 consecutive patients with out-of-hospital cardiac arrest in the city.[912] The firefighters who arrived at the scene administered treated the victims with automated external defibrillators or cardiopulmonary resuscitation followed by paramedics who carried out standard defibrillation. The rate of survival to hospital discharge for those who received early defibrillation was 30% compared with 19% for those who were treated with defibrillation later. Indeed, early defibrillation was associated with an 80% higher chance of survival. Neurological recovery was also improved.[913]

Soon enough, the initial implementation of automated external defibrillator programme in emergency medical services met with a major setback: device malfunction. On 26 January 1994, the United States Food and Drug Administration issued a Safety Alert to Directors of Emergency Medical Services of Emergency Health Care Provider Organizations. Some of the devices failed to deliver the electrical shock and others administered a second shock even though the rhythm has normalised. There were also problems regarding the power supply and electrode function. The Administration recommended that operators check their equipment at every shift using a prescribed form, perform periodic check by the manufacturer and examine the patient before delivering a second shock. But advocates of this life-saving equipment[914,915] defended its effectiveness fervently and responded robustly to this cautionary statement. In an analysis of published clinical studies, which were performed up to the 1990s, out-of-hospital defibrillation has been shown to improve cardiac survival compared to cardiopulmonary resuscitation.[916] In 1997, the American Heart Association proceeded to make recommendations to enhance the efficacy and safety of automated external defibrillators so that they could be made available in public areas.[917] Thus, the challenge then was to make these devices reliable and easy to operate without fear of misuse and inappropriate electrical discharge.

Recruiting Volunteers

Automated external defibrillators continued to reduce in size, weight, cost and maintenance when they are to be made readily available in public areas. Indeed, modern innovations have simplified the steps and made the equipment smaller and easier to use. Gradually, various lay individuals were taught how to use this device. The initial experience in Minnesota was encouraging when paramedics and police officers were taught how to use the automated external defibrillator.[918] Over the 7-year period, there were 131 patients with ventricular fibrillation. Survival at hospital discharge was 40%, and the rate was comparable between those treated by paramedics and police officers. In Allegheny County, Pennsylvania, the use of automated external defibrillators by police officers improved survival.[919] They were trained to use the equipment and were instructed to apply it to the victim once pulselessness was determined. Compared to the period prior to training of the law enforcement agents, the time to defibrillation for those with ventricular fibrillation was reduced significantly from 11.8 to 8.7 minutes. However, survival until hospital discharge was only marginally higher (14% vs. 6%) and this was probably due to the small number of subjects in the study. When the data was analysed comparing the outcome between those who were treated by police officers with emergency technicians, survival was substantially better for those who were treated by the police (26% vs. 3%).

In contrast, the results of teaching family members to use these devices at home have not been encouraging, with rapid loss of the skills learnt. After three months, their resuscitation proficiency was assessed to be unsatisfactory in about a third of the trainees.[920] While motivation may be high among family members of a patient with heart attack, the lack of regimental practice and refresher sessions could have accounted for the decline. Unexpectedly, the value of re-training at six months was limited, likely because of the complexity and precision required to perform cardiopulmonary resuscitation.[921] The Home Automated External Defibrillator Trial enrolled 7,001 global patients with previous heart attack and who were not candidates for an implantable defibrillator were enrolled to usual care or use of an automated external defibrillator.[922] Family members were randomly assigned to usual care (initiate cardiopulmonary resuscitation and call for emergency medical services) or use of the automated external defibrillator first. Every three months, a video refresher course and an annual hands-on workshop were conducted for those who were in the defibrillator group. Perhaps modern easier-to-operate devices could provide more encouraging findings. After 37 months, there was no difference between the occurrences of death from any cause between the two groups (about 6.5%). The authors attributed their findings to a low rate of mortality, as a result of the extensive use of life-saving medicines. Furthermore, less than half of the sudden death at home was a witnessed event.

A substudy of the Public Access Defibrillation trial, published nine years later, showed that the ability to use the automated external defibrillator by non-medical volunteers remained competent at one year.[923] Although these were not family members, their ability to use the device should also improve correspondingly. On the other hand, despite training and re-training, performance of cardiopulmonary resuscitation deteriorated with 80% maintaining their skill after a year.

The Stake of Your Life

We must have realised that sudden death events occur infrequently. But when it happens, the consequences can be devastating.

Improving outcome for out-of-hospital collapses is extremely challenging, and involves educating and training enormous number of people. Yes, the stakes are high and the odds of winning are low. Despite understanding this axiom, countless number of people visits the casino daily, hoping to win the big one. On 1 July 1997, Thurman Austin hit the biggest jackpot of all. He was a 63-year-old textile worker from China Grove, North Carolina, and was spending his vacation at Stardust Casino in Las Vegas. The casino opened at noon on 2 July 1958. Its fame came from an out-of-the-world sign, showing our solar system with the Earth located at the centre. The beaming neon lights and scintillating electric bulbs must have mesmerised visitors at that time. At about 1:15 pm on that summer afternoon in 1997, Thurman collapsed suddenly. His head hit the dollar slot machine and then he fell on to the floor. Within minutes, the security guards attended to him. Using one of their newly acquired automated external defibrillator, they shocked his heart back to normal rhythm. Fortunately for him, Boyd Gaming Corporation was the first hotel and casino company to be equipped with these devices. After Thurman regained consciousness, he was evacuated to the hospital and made an uneventful recovery. If Thurman was elsewhere, he would have been dead. Indeed, his winning streak also extended to his wife. Gwen, who was at the next machine when he collapsed, had just won almost three hundred dollars. The use of automated external defibrillators continued in Boyd Gaming's properties. For the next six years, another 20 lives were saved.

Indeed, cardiac arrest is not an uncommon situation in Sin City. It has been estimated that cardiac arrest occurred 2 to 3 times more frequently in Las Vegas than other cities of similar size. Visitors are older and tend to eat, drink, smoke and party excessively. The exhaustion from various "fun" activities, together with the stress of gaming, has given rise to the Vegas Syndrome. But what makes it a unique place to suffer from a cardiac arrest is that people in the casinos are constantly and closely watched by security guards with closed circuit cameras. Although their principal task of their constant surveillance is to spot cheaters and trouble-makers, any person who falls in the hall will be noticed immediately. The nearby guards will be notified and rush to attend to the scene. With such close scrutiny and rapid response, some have considered casinos as one of the safest places for a person to survive a cardiac arrest.

The effectiveness of the automated external defibrillator in the casino setting was evaluated in a clinical trial. From 1 March 1997, security officers from 32 casinos in Clark County, Nevada (which includes Las Vegas, Henderson and Laughlin); Lake Tahoe, Nevada; Philadelphia, Mississippi; and Tunica, Mississippi, were trained as a team to handle cardiac arrest and use the device.[924] The goal was to have sufficient number of automated external defibrillators available in each casino so that the victim could be treated within 3 minutes. Over about 32 months, of the 148 cases of cardiac arrest, the initial cardiac rhythm was ventricular fibrillation in 105 (71%) of them. None of those without ventricular fibrillation survived till hospital discharge. On the other hand, 56 (53%) who had ventricular fibrillation survived until hospital discharge. However, it was interesting to note that despite intense surveillance by trained personnel, only 90 (86%) of the 105 cases of ventricular fibrillation were witnessed. About 56% of them received cardiopulmonary resuscitation at about 2.9 minutes after collapse. The mean time to first defibrillation from the time of collapse was 4.4 minutes. Survival was significantly higher for those who received defibrillation within 3 minutes (79% vs. 49%). The authors concluded the defibrillation could be safely and effectively achieved by casino security officers with good survival rates. Indeed defibrillators improve casino odds in cardiac arrest but the fate of the gaming industry is less certain. The rising expectation of visitors of integrated resorts has changed the landscape of the Vegas strip. To make way for a future luxurious complex of hotels, restaurants, ultra-lounges and entertainment, the Stardust Resort and Casino was officially closed at noon on 1 November 2006. Less than a decade ago, a new era in out-of-hospital resuscitation dawned on their gaming floor. An explosive electrical discharge, and in a twinkle of an eye, a life was saved. In the same swift and decisive manner, the iconic structure was unceremoniously demolished by an implosion with accompanying fireworks on 13 March 2007, at 2:33 am. But the legacy of empowering lay persons with automated external defibrillator to rescue lives prevails.

Zapping in the Sky and Beyond

Passengers on long haul flights are kept in a relatively confined area in an uncomfortable and unfamiliar setting, with disruption of circadian rhythm and reduced ambient oxygen (equivalent to 6,050 to 8,450 feet above sea-level when the aircraft is cruising at 29,000 to 37,000 feet[925] and the cabin altitude increases with longer flights[926]). Furthermore, long walks to the gates, queues at immigration and security check-points add to the physical and mental stresses and may result in cardiac arrests. Although there is no systematic reporting of cardiac arrest in the air, the International Airlines Transport Association estimated that there are about 1,000 such events yearly, a number greater than deaths from aircraft accidents.[927] As such, equipping aeroplanes and terminals with automated external defibrillators to save lives was evaluated by Australians in 1991.[928] By August 1992, these devices were installed in all major Australian international terminals and 55 international Qantas aircrafts. Meanwhile, in-flight staff was trained to extricate unconscious passengers, perform cardiopulmonary resuscitation and use the automated external defibrillator. Handling of cardiac arrest has become part of their regular re-training programme and testing and checking the defibrillator as part of their maintenance programme. A helpline was also established between the aircraft and the medical staff at Qantas medical unit in Sydney. Over a 65-month period, these flights carried approximately 31 million passengers. There were only 27 cardiac arrests with six of them suffering from ventricular fibrillation. Cardioversion was successful in five victims and two of them survived more than two years without neurological deficit. Of note, the time from opening the device to defibrillation was only 38 seconds. The heart has stopped or was extremely slow in the remaining 21 passengers. Although cardiopulmonary resuscitation was performed, none of them survived. In contrast, 17 of the

19 cardiac arrests in the terminal were attributed to ventricular fibrillation. Cardioversion was successful in 16 of them and four survived long-term. So, the overall rate of successful restoring normal heart rhythm for those with ventricular fibrillation was 88% (22/25). But among the individuals with 46 cardiac arrests, 6 survived (13%) long-term. Other early adopters of this technology were Virgin Atlantic, Varig, Air Zimbawe and Cathay Pacific Airlines.

In October 1996, the United States Food and Drug Administration approved the use of automated external defibrillator for use in commercial aircrafts. Instead of subscribing to the traditional airline management axiom stating that a fast landing is the most appropriate action for the patient who is severely ill, American Airlines[929] took the lead and bought 300 devices to initiate the cardiac arrest programme in the United States by March 1997.[930] Approximately, 24,000 flight attendants were trained to use the device, including a 3-hour workshop. Despite the enormous initial financial outlay, training, maintenance and commitment, the additional cost to save a life over 5 years was estimated to be only 2 cents per flight.[929,931] On 19 November 1998, an automated external defibrillator which was placed two days earlier in the American Airlines flight 11 from Boston to Los Angeles, saved the life of 62-year-old Michael Tighe. Coincidentally, Michael was the Director of Community Affairs of the Boston Public Health Commission and had just submitted his request for retirement. He was instrumental in placing automated external defibrillators in public buildings, hotels, shopping malls and sports stadium. His wife, Delores, a nurse administrator, was to attend a conference in Los Angeles. Both of them recalled that the weather was fine on that day. Takeoff was smooth and they were looking forward to be in California to visit their daughter as the following week was Thanksgiving Day. After Michael finished watching the movie "Armageddon" and Delores woke up from her sleep, they started to become playful with each other. Suddenly, he became unresponsive and expressionless, and his arm dangled on the side. Thinking that he was play-acting, his wife began to jolt him. But Michael did not respond and Delores began to feel scared. He was not breathing. The gravity of the situation sank into her when

Delores could not feel his pulse. She raised the alarm and must have shouted her lungs out to ask for help. Kevin Dunn, a flight attendant, rushed to her assistance immediately. With aid from some other passengers, they carried him to the aisle. Kevin and Delores started to perform two-man cardiopulmonary resuscitation. Despite his wife pounding on his chest frantically, his pulse did not return. Another flight attendant brought the automated external defibrillator and applied the electrodes on Michael's chest. Shock after shock, he remained lifeless. The fourth attempt finally revived him. As Michael was struggling to catch his breath and regain consciousness, he was disorientated and pushed everyone aside. Gradually, his condition stabilised and the aircraft landed in Denver, Colorado. The ambulance whisked him to the hospital. After an extensive evaluation, Michael was assessed not to have suffered from any significant injury from the episode. He became the first person saved by an automated external defibrillator 35,000 feet in the sky. From 1 June 1997 to 15 July 1999, this device was used on 200 persons, with 191 on the American Airlines flights and 9 in the terminals.[932] But only 99 had lost of consciousness. Due to technical and other reasons, electrocardiograms were available for review in only 185 of them. Of these, 14 showed ventricular fibrillation and were recognised by the device. In all of them, shock was recommended. Except one patient who was terminally ill, it was administered to the remaining 13 patients. Although normal rhythm was restored initially, ventricular fibrillation recurred in 8 of the 13 individuals, and further shocks were required. Some of them succumbed eventually. There were two other patients who received shock but did not survive. Although their electrocardiograms were not available for review, they were presumed to have suffered from ventricular fibrillation. Of these 15 patient with documented or presumed ventricular fibrillation, 6 (55%) survived till hospital discharge. If the 20 patients who lost consciousness were included, the rate for survival with intact neurologic function was 40%. The remaining patients who did not have ventricular fibrillation were found to have normal or other rhythm disorders when they complained of loss of consciousness, chest pain, breathlessness, light-headedness or feeling of one's heart beating hard or fast. While defibrillation was not required, the device was used as a monitor and provided guidance to the crew and other healthcare providers who may be present on board on the management. The investigators felt that the automated external defibrillator was safe and effective in recognising and treating ventricular fibrillation among passengers in the aircraft and terminal. As such, they recommended that such devices should be made standard equipment for all commercial flight. Soon, the proposed legislation was brought up for discussion. By 12 April 2004, the United States Federal Aviation Administration Regulations Part 121 requires aircrafts with payload greater than 7,500 pounds or 3,400 kilogrammes (which is equivalent to a 30-passenger aeroplane) to carry the automated external defibrillation.[933]

Moving Closer to Prime-time

Time is paramount to survival in cardiac arrest. Since delay is inevitable for emergency medical service providers to travel and respond to the scene, bystander intervention is suggested to minimise the time to resuscitation.[934] In Scotland, a clinical study was conducted to determine suitability of sites for placement of automated external defibrillators. Based on the pattern of cardiac arrests over a 7-year period from May 1991, mathematical (statistical) modelling was performed to evaluate the potential impact of public access defibrillators.[935] However, the investigators found that the effect on the overall survival of out-of-hospital cardiac arrest was limited with a programme providing public access automated external defibrillators. At best, the overall survival rate could be improved by 5.0% to 6.3%. They attributed the limited benefit to the fact that most cardiac arrests occurred in sites that were not suitable for locating these devices, with 63% of them occurring at home. Conversely, cardiac arrests occur in obvious sites for placement of these devices already have the shortest ambulance response times and the highest rate of defibrillation. In addition to the challenge of optimising the location of these devices, the authors warned that substantial costs would be incurred with maintenance and re-training of volunteers. Despite these limitations, the British Department of Health planned to spend about £2 million to provide an additional of 400 defibrillators to be placed in public areas and training programmes to teach volunteers how to use them.[936]

In Osaka City in Japan, the situation was different with regards to the location of utilisation of automated external defibrillators.[937] From 1 July 2004 to 31 December 2008, there were 10,375 out-of-hospital cardiac arrests. Of the 908 patients with ventricular fibrillation, 53 (6%) were treated by public-access automated external defibrillators. The majority (34%) were treated at railway stations followed by nursing homes (11%). Most of the shocks were delivered by non-medical personnel (57%) such as railway company employees, teachers and security guards. In one month, neurologically favourable survival (defined as cerebral performance that is good or with moderate disability) increased from 0% in 2005 to 58% in 2008.

The experience in North America was also encouraging. The Resuscitation Outcomes Consortium (ROC) Epistry Cardiac Register involved seven sites in the United States and three Canadian sites from 1 December 2005.[938] These investigators aimed to determine if application of an automated external defibrillator deployed as part of the Public Access Defibrillation programme was associated with better outcome. Information on 13,769 persons with non-traumatic out-of-hospital cardiac arrest and received bystander resuscitation was collected prospectively until 30 April 2007. Of these, more than a third received bystander cardiopulmonary resuscitation. An automated external defibrillator was applied on only 6 of 100 who had assistance from a passer-by. While the proportion was small, it was not unexpected. The rate of ventricular fibrillation or tachycardia has been falling in various parts of the world, accounting for only 10% to 30% of cardiac arrests.[4,939,940]

In the Resuscitation Outcomes Consortium (ROC) Cardiac Registry,[938] the device was placed by a healthcare worker in less than a third. Another third was applied by lay volunteers and the last third was by the police officers together with a small proportion of unknown helpers. The overall survival until hospital discharge was 7% in this population. When the victim received bystander cardiopulmonary resuscitation but not automated external defibrillator, it improved to 9%. Survival improved to 38% when shock was delivered. Application of an automated external defibrillator was associated a 75% chance of higher likelihood of survival. When this information was extended to the population base of 21 million, 474 lives were expected to be saved yearly.

The experience of using the automated external defibrillator in a well-circumscribed area, such as an education institution, has been encouraging. In the general public, the survival rate of sudden cardiac arrest was approximately 5%, even with advanced cardiac life support intervention.[941,942] Sporting and physical activities are frequently conducted in schools and when sudden cardiac death in a young person during an athletic event, it can be especially devastating to the parents, school-mates, friends and teachers. From 2000 to 2006, there were 486 exercise-related sudden cardiac arrests among school-going individuals from the ages of 5 to 22 years in the United States.[943] The survival rate was higher than what was expected, at 11%. Likely, the events were frequently witnessed and that the victims were young. In a cross-sectional survey conducted in the United States from December 2006 to March 2007 to determine the usefulness of the automated external defibrillator among educational institutions. Of 18,974 high schools invited for a survey, 2,084 responded.[944] Among 1,710 of those with automated external defibrillator, there were 36 cases of sudden cardiac arrest. While 14 of them were athletes, the remaining 22 were school employees or spectators. Not surprisingly, 35 (97%) were witnessed and 34 (94%) received bystander cardiopulmonary resuscitation. Electrical cardioversion was administered to 30 (83%) of them. Overall, 23 (64%) survived till hospital discharge, including 9 students (64%) and 14 of the others (64%). These findings suggested that early defibrillation in victims of sudden cardiac arrest in high schools was able to improve survival. Of note, both athletes and older individuals received benefit from the use of an automated external defibrillator.

Using the Automated External Defibrillator

The Public Access Defibrillator Programme[945] is being initiated in several cities. One of the key challenges is optimising the location of an automated external defibrillator (Figure 23). Initially, the

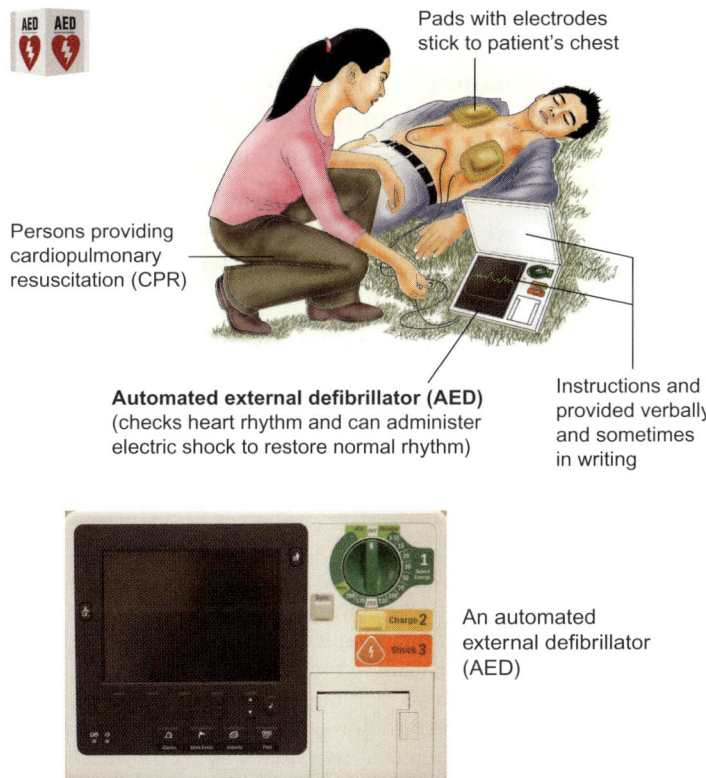

Pads with electrodes
stick to patient's chest

Persons providing
cardiopulmonary
resuscitation (CPR)

Automated external defibrillator (AED)
(checks heart rhythm and can administer
electric shock to restore normal rhythm)

Instructions and
provided verbally
and sometimes
in writing

An automated
external defibrillator
(AED)

Figure 23. Using an Automated External Defibrillator (AED).

When resuscitating a person, always ensure that the site is safe. In particular, when using an AED, check for water around the unconscious person. Since water conducts electricity, delivering electrical energy may result in unnecessary burn or shock to the victim and those around. If necessary, move the individual to a dry and safe area.

Different machines and models may have dissimilar presentation. First, turn on the power. The device will give you step-by-step verbal and visual instructions. Expose the victim's chest. If it is wet, dry it. Excessive chest hair may need to be trimmed. Apply the large sticky pads as shown on the packaging. These pads are

European Resuscitation Council recommended in 2005 that an automated external defibrillator be located places where a witness cardiac arrest occurred once in every two years, such as airports, casinos or sports facilities.[946] On the other hand, the American Heart Association recommended, in 2006, that such a device be placed in the vicinity of at least one cardiac arrest that occurred every five years.[947] Another criterion is that the emergency medical services cannot respond within 5 minutes, highlighting the importance of early access to defibrillation in the public. Using data on all out-of-hospital cardiac arrests in the public in Copenhagen, Denmark, a group of Danish investigators determined the area covered in the city using the European or American guidelines, and the potential to treat them.[948] Based on the assumption of deploying an automated external defibrillator in a 100 m by 100 m of high-incidence area, 125 would be required when the European guidelines were used.[946] This would cover an area of 1.2% of the city and 19.5% of the cardiac arrests. On the other hand, when the American guidelines were complied,[947] 1,104 devices were needed to cover an area of 10.6% of the city and 66.8% of the cardiac arrests. Nonetheless, both approaches were comparably acceptable economically.

Figure 23. (*Continued*) sensors and they are used to deliver the electrical energy. Place one pad on slightly to the right centre of the chest above the nipple. Place the other pad slightly below the other nipple and to the outer aspect of the left of the ribcage. If possible, ensure that the victim is not wearing metallic objects, especially around the pads, such as metal piercings, bracelets, necklaces and underwire brassieres. Metal may result in aberrant flow of electricity causing burns. If there are implanted devices such as a pacemaker, as evident by its outline under the skin below the collar bone or the upper abdomen, place the pads at least 3 cm away.

Ensure the wires from the pads are connected to the AED. When ready to proceed, make sure that no one touches the victim and then press the "analyse" button (rotate on the knob 1 anti-clockwise in this device). During this period, the machine assesses the heart rhythm. If a shock is needed, the AED would inform the rescuer to charge the device (press 2). When it is ready, the machine will instruct everyone to stand clear of the victim. Again, when the rescuer is certain that no one is touching the patient, the "shock" button (3) may be pressed and the energy is delivered. If the victim does not recover, continue cardiopulmonary resuscitation until emergency medical aid arrives. Similarly, when shock is not needed, cardiopulmonary resuscitation should be continued as long as there is no spontaneous pulse or breathing.

Certainly, local or unguided deployment was substantially more costly. Not surprisingly, the revision of the European Resuscitation Council Guidelines in 2010 removed the criterion of a cardiac arrest in two years, and included offices as one of the places where such devices should be placed.[949]

Furthermore, there are legal issues involved in the public use of automated external defibrillator. In the United States, all the 50 states have passed laws and regulations governing the lay rescuer programmes from 1995 to 2000.[947] In 2000, the Cardiac Arrest Survival Act was passed as federal law which provides limited immunity from civil liability for the emergency user of the automated external defibrillator. There are also other initiatives which are required to ensure optimal implementation of such a programme, including training and integration with various emergency and healthcare providers. Several issues on quality also need to be addressed.[950]

With an increasing number of lay individuals having access to these devices, the operator must be certain that the patient is pulseless and not breathing to avoid accidental electrical discharge to a person with normal heart rhythm. Recognising pulse and breathing can be challenging, especially when their presence or absence must be determined within 10 seconds.[951] Surprisingly, this limitation was only observed among lay persons,[952] it was also experienced by various categories of health-care workers.[953–955] From a group of 449 lay volunteers, most of them — who had received training in first-aid — took an average of 9.5 seconds to detect the carotid pulse of young healthy non-obese subjects.[952] More than a quarter of them took more than 10 seconds to identify the carotid pulse. Instead of using mannequins and simulators, the model to evaluate the skill of 206 trained first-aiders, emergency medical technicians in-training, paramedics in-training and certified paramedics was more sophisticated.[953] In this study, patients undergoing coronary artery bypass grafting were used as subjects. During the operation, the heart was stopped when the conduits were being connected. But blood continued to flow in a non-pulsatile manner using a heart-lung machine. At this state, pulselessness was simulated. However, this condition was not identified in 10% of the first responders. About 45% of the examinees were not able to detect the carotid pulse when it was present. Overall, the time to make a diagnosis was 24 seconds. It took twice as long for the first responder to decide that there was no carotid pulse (30 seconds) compared to detecting a pulse (15 seconds). Within 10 seconds, the proportion who made the correct diagnoses was only 15%, and for pulselessness, it was only accurately detected in 2%.

There are several other precautions that would be helpful to minimise injury. Analysis of rhythm should not be carried out when external cardiac massage is being performed or when the patient is having a seizure or being transported in a moving vehicle. The area near the electrodes should be dry and water should be wiped dry. Avoid areas of diseased skin or injury. Remove skin patches, particularly nitroglycerin-eluting ones. Electro-magnetic interference, such as waves discharge from handphones, may affect the performance of these devices. These electromagnetic waves may distort electrical recording and cause the machine to misinterpret the tracing as movement or ventricular fibrillation. Of concern is that shock may be advised when the patient is in sinus rhythm.

Having your Personal ER Team
Intra-Cardiac Defibrillators

"If people do not believe that mathematics is simple, it is only because they do not realize how complicated life is."

János Lajos Neumann (John Louis von Neumann)
Keynote Speaker,
First Meeting of the Association of Machinery Computing, 1947

The intra-cardiac defibrillator is revolutionary in many ways, and has overcome several limitations of the automated external defibrillator. Instead of empowering the rescuer, this "middleman" has been dispensed with. There is no need to look for a defibrillator because it has been implanted in the individual. At least two laboratories were developing this device in the 1960s and 1970s. Of the several scientists, it was the death of his mentor, Professor Harry Heller of Tel Hashomer Hospital in Israel, which inspired him to invent the intra-cardiac defibrillator. Dr Michel Mirowski was determined to seek a way which could have prevented his teacher's death. In 1966, he started to have abnormal rapid rhythm and died two weeks later while having dinner with his family. Similar to the emergence of any disruptive technology, Mirowski faced considerable opposition during the early phases of his work. His papers were initially rejected and funding was challenging to secure. Together with his co-inventor and another cardiologist, Morton Mower, they were supported for two years by a pacemaker company. Failing to recognise the industry application, they were left to seek funding elsewhere. In 1972, Stephen Heilman saw the potential of their invention and began a fruitful partnership. Working with the engineers of Heilman's medical equipment company, Medrad, they successfully developed the intra-cardiac defibrillator.

Initially, the proof-of-concept human studies were conducted among patients undergoing coronary artery bypass grafting.[956] During the procedure, leads were placed by the surgeons through a small cut in the atrium into the right ventricle. The study was conducted when the circulatory function of the patients had been taken over by a heart-lung machine. This equipment was to take over the function of the heart when it was unable to do so. Of the 11 patients, the rhythm in 9 of them was successfully reverted to normal. The investigators attributed the failure in one patient to difficulty in maintaining a good lead position. Due to the long duration of the abnormal rhythm, cardioversion was unsuccessful in the second patient. About five years later, in 1978, the initial implantable system weighed 250 g encased and sealed in titanium and was successfully tested in dogs.[957] A spring-coiled electrode was inserted into the large vein that drained blood from the arms and head. At the tip (apex) of the left ventricle, a patch electrode was placed. From 4 February 1980, the automatic defibrillator (Intec Systems Inc., Pittsburgh, Pennsylvania), weighing 225 g, was implanted in patients by Myron Weisfeldt, a cardiac surgeon, and Philip Reed, a cardiologist with interest in electrical activities of the heart[958] at the Johns Hopkins Hospital in Baltimore, Maryland. By September 1982, 52 patients had received this device from either The Johns Hopkins Hospital or the Stanford University in Palo Alto in California.[959] Based on expected survival rates, the investigators estimated that their device resulted in approximately 50% reduction in mortality in the first year for their patients! Despite the early set-backs, the investigators continued to modify their system. Initially, the procedure was performed by cardiac surgeons. Soon, other doctors began to express interest in this life-saving procedure. With training and experience, cardiologists with clinical interests in electrical disorders of the heart were able to implant these devices with favourable outcomes.[960] Since then, several improvements have been made to make these devices more effective and safer. They are able to detect abnormal rhythms more accurately and equipped with other functions that could terminate the rhythm disorder.

Nowadays, the device is a small battery-operated device, weighing about less than 75 g. It is implanted under the skin but occasionally, the device may be placed under the muscle to camouflage the lump under the skin (Figure 24). The procedure is performed under local anaesthetic and the device is inserted into the area where the incision is made. In the majority of the cases, the device is positioned below the collar bone, usually on the left side. Sometimes, it is placed in the upper abdomen, especially when the wires are placed on the surface of the heart. Young women may prefer the defibrillator to be implanted under the lower abdominal muscle in the "bikini line." Generally, one wire is placed in the lower chamber (right ventricle). Sometimes, two wires are inserted into a vein and positioned in the heart. While one is attached to the upper chamber (right atrium) and the other wire is attached to the lower chamber (right ventricle). During the procedure, X-ray is used to guide the doctor in positioning the wires. Once the wire is in an acceptable stable position, it is tested to ensure that the wire functions normally. If these parameters

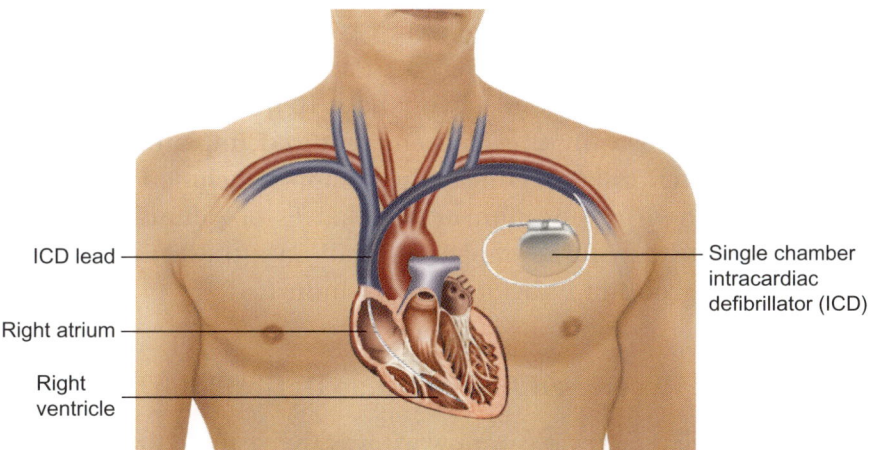

ICD lead

Right atrium

Right ventricle

Single chamber intracardiac defibrillator (ICD)

Figure 24.   Implantable cardiac defibrillator.

indicate a good position, it is secured into the heart muscle by a tiny screw. The other ends of the wires are attached to the device. This device is able to detect, analyse and treat potentially fatal heart rhythm disorders. It can deliver a high-energy electric charge or a brief burst of a series of rapid low-energy pulses to stop or interrupt the rapid rhythms. Alternatively, electrical impulses can also be discharged to stimulate the heart when the rate is too slow. Indeed for those who need the device, it is certainly life-saving.

During the procedure, complications such as bleeding, infection and puncturing the lungs or heart may occur rarely. When any of them occurs, treatment must be instituted immediately. The wound, about 5 cm to 7 cm long, may heal with scars, sometimes with small lumps or an exuberant of tissue (keloid). Pain over the incision site may persist. Rarely, the vein may clot. When it occurs, the arm may be swollen, painful and dusky.

Since high-energy discharges may leave a deep but invisble mental scar, medicines used to treat rhythm disorder may be administered to several patients to modify the disturbance so that it becomes more susceptible to low-energy pacing. However, these medicines may also have side effects and may affect the function of the intra-cardiac defibrillator. Thus, the patient may need to be re-evaluated and the settings may have to be adjusted.

In a regional inherited cardiac conditions clinic in Manchester, there were 193 individuals who were extensively evaluated because someone in their families suffered from a sudden death event.[961] Although they were followed up for about 16 months, none of them died. Importantly, only 2% of them required implantation of an intra-cardiac defibrillator. Hence, the doctors concluded that such a device is needed in the minority of relatives of victims of sudden death. Therefore, routine implantation of an intra-cardiac defibrillator for this group of individuals is not indicated.

Who Should Receive an Intra-Cardiac Defibrillator?

In today's digital age, we can now witness the real-life drama of the amazing work of an intra-cardiac defibrillator. On 7 June 2009, at the 43rd minute of the first half of a Belgian First Division soccer match between K.S.V. (Koninklijke Sport Vereniging) Roeslare and R. (Royal) Antwerp F.C. (Football Club), the entire stadium was stunned and stared in disbelief. Anthony Van Loo, a 20-year-old defender of the K.S.V. Roeslare team, was walking towards an out-of-bound ball when he collapsed on the ground, like a marionette falling when the control bar was released suddenly (http://www.youtube.com/watch?v=DU_i0ZzIV5U). Having landed on his back, his team-mates and trainers rushed to his assistance. While everyone else was confused and probably panicking, the intra-cardiac defibrillator implanted a year ago, recognised the potentially fatal rhythm disorder. He was discovered to have hypertrophic cardiomyopathy. While one of the officials was trying to arouse him, Anthony gave a jerk in about 8 seconds and regained consciousness 5 seconds later. Interestingly, the minder did not appear to have sustained any shock. Fortunately, Anthony survived as intra-cardiac defibrillators may not be designed to withstand the forces of strenuous activities and contact sports.

Overall, survival is improved by 23% to 55% depending on the types of patients enrolled in the studies.[374] Baseline risk for rhythm disorder may impact on all-cause mortality.[962] But clearly, those who have been resuscitated from a sudden cardiac event, and even patients with reversible cause,[963] may benefit from receiving an intra-cardiac defibrillator. In this group, all-cause mortality rate was about 28% lower, and the risk of dying from a rhythm disorder was reduced by 50%.[964] Correspondingly, implantation of the defibrillator is also recommended for those with dilated cardiomyopathy,[965–967] hypertrophy cardiomyopathy[126,968] or arrhythmogenic right ventricular cardiomyopathy[274,293,296,297] and has been resuscitated from a cardiac arrest.

But the decision to implant such a device among patients who have not suffered from a recurrent fainting spells or cardiac arrest is challenging. Several clinical studies were conducted to determine the usefulness of implantation of intra-cardiac defibrillator among patients with abnormal heart function after a heart attack or diseases of heart muscle. However, the recommendations from various internationally well-respected heart colleges, associations, societies and organisations differed in the ejection fraction cut-off value used to recommend implantation of the device.[651] This discrepancy was likely to be attributed to the variation in the entry criteria. Five clinical factors, including age greater than 70 years, New York Heart Association greater than class II, atrial fibrillation, conduction anomaly in the ventricle and blood biochemistry, have been identified to ascertain patients who are more likely to die.[969] Even with impaired left ventricular function after a heart attack, when these factors were absent, mortality risk was low.

How Then Should I Live?

After implantation of the device, the wound is usually covered by a water-proof bandage. Nonetheless, ensure the site is clean and dry. If the defibrillator is implanted in the left upper chest, try not to move the left arm excessively. Notify your doctor as soon as possible if there is excessive pain, redness, discharge, swelling, fever or chills. Generally, the sutures used to close the wound are absorbable so there is no necessity to remove the stitches. Subsequently, the patient should attempt to live as normal a life as possible. This is what the device was intended to do and it is left inside the patient, usually for life. But if definitive treatment, such as heart transplant is performed, the defibrillator may be removed.

A person with such a device must be aware that there are other equipment that may have a strong magnetic field which may interfere with its function. The closer to the apparatus and the longer the duration of exposure would increase the likelihood of adversely affect the function of the intra-cardiac defibrillator. Similar to any electrical device implanted into the body, regular examinations at 3 to 6 months interval are needed to determine who the patient is and whether the device is functioning. A special apparatus, known as a programming wand, is placed on the device and is able to receive and transmit information to and from the intra-cardiac defibrillator. These electromagnetic waves enable an external computer to communicate with the device. Importantly, battery life, pacing and sensing characteristics of the device are ascertained. Disease conditions and certain medicines may alter these parameters and so, during these episodes, it may require more frequent examination. Furthermore, by understanding how the device has been functioning, settings can be changed to optimise its effectiveness. Using data transfer from cell phone networks, remote monitoring can be performed for certain devices. When the amount of energy has reduced to a pre-specified level, the pulse generator may be replaced. If the wires are functioning well, they need not be replaced.

Always carry an identity card for the intra-cardiac defibrillator. There may be other forms of identification, such as a necklace or bracelet. It contains your name, the name of the device and your doctor, the contact details and other important information. Other medical equipment, such as magnetic resonance imaging, extracorporeal shock-wave therapy for kidney stones and electro-cauterisation (an apparatus to arrest bleeding during surgery), can affect the function of the intra-cardiac defibrillator. Recent models of intra-cardiac defibrillator and wires are compatible with magnetic resonance imaging. On the other hand, X-ray-related procedures, including computed tomography, do not interfere with the function of the intra-cardiac defibrillator. However, radiotherapy may damage the circuitry and shielding may be required. Thus, when undergoing magnetic resonance imaging and radiotherapy, the manufacturer needs to be contacted to determine the appropriate course of action. Therefore, all your healthcare providers, including dental surgeons, technicians and nurses, should be informed that a defibrillator has been implanted. Avoid non-emergency potentially "dirty" surgery, such as dental procedures, within three months of implantation. If needed, external defibrillation may be applied. However, the pads should be placed away from on the device.

Similarly, during travel or undergoing any form of security clearance, the corresponding agents should be also informed. Avoid placing hand-held using metal detectors too near the device. Sometimes, especially with older devices, the electronic surveillance systems may briefly inhibit its function. Rarely, the intra-cardiac defibrillator may discharge during long high-altitude flights.

Generally, brief encounters when using household appliances, which include microwave ovens, irons, electric cookers, radios, toasters, television remote controls are acceptable. Caution has to be exercised when using portable telephones and audio players. A cell phone should not be placed near the device, such as the shirt or blouse pocket. Similarly, the cellphone should not be hung near the defibrillator or placed in the arm-band adjacent to the device. When using a cordless or cell telephone, place it on the ear on the opposite side of the defibrillator. Similarly, the portable audio players should be strapped on the other arm away from the device. The device should be at least 15 centimetres or 6 inches from the device. When passing through anti-theft devices in shopping malls, walk briskly by them. Do not use industrial welders, electronic body fat analyzer, any form of equipment that discharges electrical impulses into the body, magnetic rods bars, pads, pillows or mattresses. Stay away, at least 0.5 metres or 2 feet, from electric generators and light-welding equipment. These external electrical or electromagnetic impulses may be mistaken as heart beats and the intra-cardiac defibrillator may be activated leading to inappropriate discharges.

In the first week after the procedure, driving should be avoided. This is to allow the wound to heal. Pain and the swelling over the area may affect the ability to use the steering wheel. In an emergency situation, the delay in response may result in an accident. After a discharge from the device, driving is not recommended for another six months. For the commercial driver, driving may be prohibited permanently.

Physical activity has both psychological and physical benefits. Regular exercises may improve the well-being of a patient with an intra-cardiac defibrillator. But the level of exercise for each individual without requiring a shock needs to be determined. A symptom-limited exercise test helps to ascertain the maximal heart rate and likelihood of rhythm disorder. Of 659 patients from nine studies, there were 14 appropriate shocks (2.1%) during exercise testing.[970] However, there were 13 inappropriate shocks. Nonetheless, one study showed that the chance of receiving a shock was lowered with exercise.[971] A suitable form of physical activity may be chosen based on the patient's interest and physical abilities.

With younger individuals receiving these life-saving devices, the issue of sexual relationship is becoming more relevant. Having sexual intercourse with an individual with a potentially lethal condition and a live electrical device that may discharge can be daunting. Furthermore, the patient may have a weak heart and would further hamper the relationship. Generally, when the wound is healed, by 4 weeks after implantation, sexual intimacy may resume if there are no other outstanding health problems. If the patient can walk up two flights of stairs without undue shortness of breath, chest discomfort or shock should be ready. Alternatively, formal stress testing may be performed by the doctor to determine the health status. However, erectile dysfunction, an over-protective partner, lack of interest in sex, fear of shock from the device during sex and fear of cardiac arrest during sex were some of the major concerns.[971,972] Indeed, shock-related anxiety was more prevalent among 70 young men and women who have received an intra-cardiac defibrillator than 110 individuals who did not. This emotional state was associated with poor sexual function.[974] Although some partners described a "tingle" when the device discharges while the patient may give a "yelp", others may experience a strong jolt or tug. Strangely, some partners seemed to enjoy the stimulation at the peak of passion. Fortunately, almost all of the shocks are not dangerous to the partner. Nonetheless, patients may need encouragement to continue with a fulfilling sex life.

Although the rhythms may be potentially fatal, the electrical discharge may be administered while the individual is fully awake. When it occurs, the patient may experience intense pain. Some described the sensation as being kicked or punched on the chest. The discharge may also stimulate the muscles of the chest wall, diaphragm and vocal cords. Consequently, the muscle may contract producing a spasm and the vocal cord may produce an involuntary "yelp!" which may be interpreted as a call for help. While most of them receive only one shock, the device may deliver more electrical discharges in an attempt to terminate the potentially lethal rhythm disorder. These series of strong impulses can be terrifying. After receiving a "shock", it may sound ridiculous but stay calm. Sit or lie down to rest for a while. Have someone stay close by. If only one shock has occurred, the incident should be reported to the doctor on the next working day. However, if there are three or more shocks or that the shock was felt to be inappropriate, the doctor should be informed as soon as possible. If the person is unwell after a shock, an emergency ambulance should be summoned to fetch the patient to the Emergency Room. Subsequently, the intra-cardiac defibrillator needs to be interrogated to determine if the device or the wires are functioning appropriately and properly or if there is a need to adjust your medicines.

Nonetheless, the patient is likely to be grateful because it was life-saving. But it can be an extremely traumatic experience. The vividness and drama of such an episode may adversely affect the patient psychologically, as well as their family members.[970] This life-or-death situation forms the basis of post-traumatic stress disorder.[975] While the initial response was to disregard their concerns by healthcare providers, the syndrome has been recognised increasingly. Anxiety or depression may creep in because of the fear of recurrent shock or that the device may fail to work when needed. Indeed, anxiety symptoms may occur in 13% to 38% after implantation of an intra-cardiac defibrillator.[976–979] More than half of these patients continued to suffer from chronic anxiety a year after the implantation.[980] About 10% to 46% of patients developed depression after implantation of a defibrillator.[979,981,982] Depression was found to persist in 14% of the patients in up to three months following the procedure.[983] Likely, age, gender, ethnicity, presence of other illnesses and the mode of assessment contributed to the variability in the occurrence of these psychological problems.[984] Hence, psychological support may be useful in helping patients cope with their emotions. Unlike other stress events where relatives can assist in the recovery, implantation of a defibrillator can affect family members adversely.[985] A spouse who has witnessed the cardiac arrest, and especially when participated in the resuscitation, may then be more protective of the patient and impose a higher restriction of activities.[986] The fear of recurrence constantly hovers in the minds of the care-givers. Concerns about finances and other family issues would continue to bother the spouse. Indeed, differences in perceptions and expectations may result in barriers with communication and expression among family members. This complex interplay of sometimes concealed and convoluted factors needs to be clarified candidly so that relationships could return to some form of normality. Although cognitive behavioural therapy has shown promise in improving psychological status, the results of several interventions have been varied.[970]

Quality of life may be affected after a shock. In a multi-centre North American study, it was lower for those receiving the device initially among 905 patients were randomly allocated to an intra-cardiac defibrillator or medicine.[987] By the end of the first year, there was no difference between the two groups of patients. On the other hand, other investigators found that the quality of life, including energy, physical mobility, emotional reactions and sleep disturbance, improved with implantation of a defibrillator.[988,989] But when a shock was delivered to the patient, there was substantial decline in physical function and mental well-being.[987] Others have reported that more than five shocks were needed before the psychological status of the patient would be affected adversely.[988,990–992]

Subcutaneous Defibrillator

Despite the benefits derived by implanting an intra-cardiac defibrillator, there are several limitations. Most importantly, the wires in the veins may break (fracture), cause infection or clotting. To avoid these complications, the totally subcutaneous intra-cardiac defibrillator has been developed so that it does not require any wires to be placed into the veins. The device is placed underneath the left armpit and wires are tunnelled to the side of the breast-bone. Since it does not need to puncture the vein for the wire to be attached to the heart, complications of bleeding, perforating the lung or heart are averted. However, the disadvantages of this novel device are the relatively larger size and inability to send impulses to the heart if it is beating too slowly. Since the device is new, there is limited information on its efficacy in all types of patients who require such a device.

PART IV

The Final Post

*"What we call the beginning is often the end
And to make an end is to make a beginning.
The end is where we start from."*

Thomas Stearns Eliot
Little Gidding
The Four Quartets

Although it may not be apparent, the curse of sudden death certainly hovers over every living individual. While it strikes rarely, the impact is always devastating. For those surviving and who know the victim, the shock continues to grip the very essence of their being. The emotional trauma ranges from grief because someone dear has died, anger that the loved one has left without the opportunity of saying good-bye, fear that the incident may happen again or to someone else in the family, and despair as the event was inexplicable. Even when the story is re-told, the audience would continue to be quietly terrified by the unexpected lost. Hence, whether the encounter is experienced first-hand, or something that is either heard from someone else, read from the magazines or newspaper, it reminds us to begin making a new resolution to live a healthier life. By now, we ought to know that the occurrence and causes of sudden death vary considerably with age (Figure 25).[993] However, not all of the conditions have been described in this book. Abnormalities of heart muscle and electrical stability tend to affect younger patients. However, most of these conditions are relatively uncommon. On the

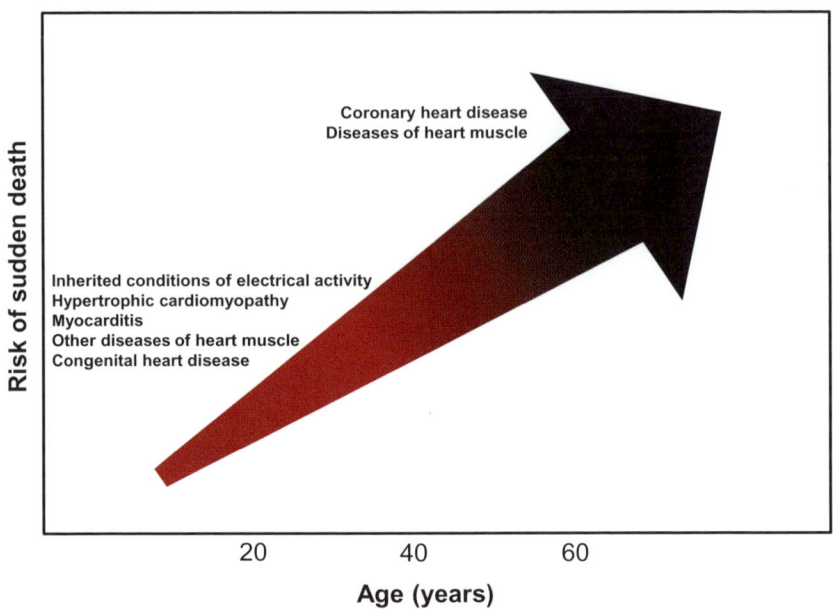

Figure 25.   As the age of a person advances, the risk of sudden death increases correspondingly. However, the causes of sudden death change. In the older individual, coronary heart disease and heart failure are the major causes of sudden death.

other hand, coronary artery disease is the major challenge for older persons.

Indeed, for the majority, living healthily is probably the most effective way of preventing sudden death in the population. A study from the United States provided some insight on the impact of healthy living because these are the factors which an individual can take responsibility for. Among almost 82,000 women in the United States, enrolled from June 1984 to June 2010, and were followed up for 26 years, there were 321 cases of sudden cardiac death.[994] To evaluate the contribution of living a healthy lifestyle in this group of women, the authors defined four low-risk lifestyle characteristics: (1) not currently smoking; (2) body mass index of less than 25 kg/m^2; (3) moderate or vigorous intensity exercise lasting for 30 minutes per day or longer; and (4) top 40% of the alternate

Mediterranean diet score. The components of this score consisted of vegetables (excluding potatoes), fruits, nuts, whole grains, legumes, fish, ratio of monounsaturated to saturated fat, red and processed meats, and alcohol.[995] One point is awarded if the intake of a participant is *above* the median of the cohort for the first seven items. On the other hand, the point is awarded if the consumption of red or processed meat is *below* the median. One point is awarded if alcohol intake is between 5 g to 15 g daily, which approximates to 360 mL of beer, 150 mL of wine or 45 mL of liquor. Up to a maximum of 9 points, the higher the score awarded, the greater the resemblance of the Mediterranean-style diet. They found that with an increasing number of low-risk factors, the likelihood for sudden cardiac death decreased correspondingly. Indeed, the chance of dying suddenly was 92% lower for women with all four low-risk characteristics compared with those that had none of them. This information illustrates the importance of adopting an overall healthy lifestyle strategy. Indeed, the strategy should start with the young and inculcate the habits of regular moderate physical activity and the discipline of proper diet. On the other hand, patients with heart diseases should be regularly reviewed by their doctor. They should adhere to treatment regimens, discuss new symptoms and continue to live healthily.

Within various social circles, very often discussed is what the person was doing prior to dying suddenly. While most individuals associate sudden death with physical activities, a survey on the residents of Multnomah County, Oregon, provided information on the type of activities during a sudden death event.[996] The investigators were able to review the circumstances for those with witnessed attacks, in whom the patients died within an hour of symptoms. Over a 3-year period, there were 304 relatively older individuals. Most of them (63%) were performing light activities, such as bathing, dressing, cooking, cleaning, eating, walking in the house or driving. Importantly, sleep was the second commonest (17%) activity. Only 5% were doing sporting activities, such as tennis, running, jogging, skiing or cycling. Interestingly, 2% were engaged in sexual activity before the event. Most of the events that occurred in a community were during normal activities. However, when taken together with what has been previously described,[659,660,997] those who decide to participate in sports should not suddenly perform high-intensity activities. Instead, there should be a period of training and gradual increase in workload. For older persons starting to engage in physical activities and for those with illnesses, especially heart diseases, their doctors should be consulted.

But for the young who died suddenly, the cause may not be clear after the traditional post-mortem examination, which is based on finding abnormalities detected visually or microscopically. It is estimated to be about 4% among those between the ages of 16 and 64 years. With clinical screening of close relatives, potential conditions that could have caused sudden death were identified in 32% of them.[998] The limitation of medical examination, including the various clinical diagnostic and imaging techniques, may be overcome by evaluation of the molecular constituents. Thus, when genetic analysis was included in the examination, the yield increased to about 40%.[148] A novel strategy, molecular autopsy, has evolved to better detect disease conditions. However, current approaches, focussing on electrical stability of heart muscle cells, could only identify up to 35% of the cases.[999] Newer generation of targeted genetic screening technologies provide cost-effective, comprehensive and accurate means of detecting vulnerable individuals in the near future.[1000]

For decades, the Last Post is the bugle call in uniformed services among Commonwealth nations to signify the completion of activities for the day. At the end of a day, those on night duty would patrol around the parameter of the camp from the first guard post to the last. The familiar and reassuring melody is to inform soldiers that the camp is secured and it is safe for them to rest for the night. Correspondingly, Taps is the musical piece used in the United States. After 1850, both tunes are also played for soldiers going into eternal rest, usually after battles. The bugle call for the end of a day also symbolises the bugle call for the end of a solder's life. Similar to sudden death events, family and friends have to cope with the tragic loss of mostly young active lives. Time has to be set aside for grief and for people to attend to changes generated by the hasty unprepared departure. While helpful, emotional and physical support has to be carefully and thoughtfully provided during this delicate and unpredictable time. In some cases, professional help may be needed to deal with the psychological complexities associated with sudden separation. Much of who we are depends on our relationships with others. So when we lose someone dear, we also lose part of ourselves; the stronger the rapport, the greater the loss. In any case, the personhood has to be re-defined and life has to be rebuilt.

References

1. *The Holy Bible, English Standard Version®*. Wheaton, IL: Crossway, a publishing ministry of Good News Publishers; 2011.

2. Pratt CM, Greenway PS, Schoenfeld MH, Hibben ML, Reiffel JA. Exploration of the precision of classifying sudden cardiac death: Implications for the interpretation of clinical trials. *Circulation*. 1996;**93**:519–524.

3. de Vreede-Swagemakers JJ, Gorgels AP, Dubois-Arbouw WI, van Ree JW, Daemen MJ, Houben LG, Wellens HJ. Out-of-hospital cardiac arrest in the 1990s: A population-based study in the Maastricht area on incidence, characteristics and survival. *J Am Coll Cardiol*. 1997;**30**:1500–1505.

4. Nichol G, Thomas E, Callaway CW, Hedges J, Powell JL, Aufderheide TP, Rea T, Lowe R, Brown T, Dreyer J, Davis D, Indris A, Stiell I, Resuscitation Outcomes Consortium Investigators. Regional variation in out-of-hospital cardiac arrest incidence and outcome. *JAMA*. 2008;**300**:1423–1431.

5. Roger VL, Go AS, Lloyd-Jones DM, Benjamin EJ, Berry JD, Borden WB, Bravata DM, Dai S, Ford ES, Fox CS, Fullerton HJ, Gillespie C, Hailpern SM, Heit JA, Howard VJ, Kissela BM, Kittner SJ, Lackland DT, Lichtman JH, Lisabeth LD, Makuc DM, Marcus GM, Marelli A, Matchar DB, Moy CS, Mozaffarian D, Mussolino ME, Nichol G, Paynter NP, Soliman EZ, Sorlie PD, Sotoodehnia N, Turan TN, Virani SS, Wong ND, Woo D, Turner MB, on behalf of the American Heart Association Statistics Committee and Stroke Statistics Subcommittee. Heart Disease and Stroke Statistics — 2012 Update. A Report from the American Heart Association. *Circulation*. 2012;**125**:e2–e220.

6. Kong MH, Fonarow GC, Peterson ED, Curtis AB, Hernandez AF, Sanders GD, Thomas KL, Hayes DL, Al-Khatib SM. Systemic review of the incidence of sudden cardiac death in the United States. *J Am Coll Cardiol*. 2011;**57**:794–801.

7. Byrne R, Constant O, Smyth Y, Callagy G, Nash P, Daly K, Crowley J. Multiple source surveillance incidence and aetiology of out-of-hospital sudden cardiac death in a rural population in the west of Ireland. *Eur Heart J*. 2008;**29**:1418–1423.

8. Hua W, Zhang LF, Wu YF, Liu XQ, Guo DS, Zhou HL, Gou ZP, Zhao LC, Niu HX, Chen KP, Mai JZ, Chu LN, Zhang Z. Incidence of sudden cardiac death in China: Analysis of 4 regional populations. *J Am Coll Cardiol*. 2009;**54**:1110–1118.

9. Fishman GI, Chugh S, DiMarco JP, Albert CM, Andersen ME, Bonow RO, Buxton AE, Chen P-S, Estes M, Jouven X, Kwong R, Lathrop DA, Mascette AM, Nerbonne JM,

O'Rourke B, Page RL, Roden DM, Rosenbaum DS, Sotoodehnia N, Trayanova NA, Zheng Z-J. Sudden cardiac death prediction and prevention: Report from a National Heart, Lung, and Blood Institute and Heart Rhythm Society Workshop. *Circulation.* 2010;**122**:2335–2348.

10.   Becker LB, Han BH, Meyer PM, Wright FA, Rhodes KV, Smith DW, Barrett J. Racial differences in the incidence of cardiac arrest and subsequent survival. The CPR Chicago Project. *N Engl J Med.* 1993;**329**:600–606.

11.   Kannel WB, Wilson PW, D'Agostino RB, Cobb J. Sudden coronary death in women. *Am Heart J.* 1998;**136**:205–212.

12.   Chugh SS, Jui J, Gunson K, Strcker EC, John BT, Thompson B, Ilias N, Vickers C, Dogra V, Daya M, Kron J, Zheng Z-J, Mensah G, McAnulty J. Current burden of sudden cardiac death: Multiple source surveillance versus retrospective death certificate-based review in a large U.S. community. *J Am Coll Cardiol.* 2004;**44**: 1268–1275.

13.   Albert CM, McGovern BA, Newell JB, Ruskin JN. Sex differences in cardiac arrest survivors. *Circulation.* 1996;**93**:1170–1176.

14.   Thomas AC, Knapman PA, Krikler DM, Davies MJ. Community study of the causes of "natural" sudden death. *Br Med J.* 1988;**297**:1453–1456.

15.   Bowker TJ, Wood DA, Davies MJ, Sheppard MN, Cary NRB, Burton JDK, Chambers DR, Dawling S, Hobson HL, Pyke SDM, Riemersma RA, Thompson SG. Sudden, unexpected cardiac or unexplained death in England: A national survey. *Q J Med.* 2003;**96**:269–279.

16.   Priori SG, Borggrefe M, Camm AJ, Hauer RN, Klein H, Kuck KH, Schwartz PJ, Touboul P, Wellens HJ. Unexplained cardiac arrest. The need for a prospective registry. *Eur Heart J.* 1992;**13**:1445–1446.

17.   Chugh SS, Kelly KL, Titus JL. Sudden cardiac death with apparently normal heart. *Circulation.* 2000;**102**:649–654.

18.   Albert CM, Chae CU, Grodstein F, Rose LM, Rexrode KM, Ruskin JN, Stampfer MJ, Manson JE. Prospective study of sudden cardiac death among women in the United States. *Circulation.* 2003;**107**:2096–2101.

19.   Chugh SS, Uy-Evanado A, Teodorescu C, Reinier K, Mariani R, Gunson K, Jui J. Women have a lower prevalence of structural heart disease as a precursor to sudden cardiac arrest. The Ore-SUS (Oregon Sudden Death Study). *J Am Coll Cardiol.* 2009;**54**:2006–2011.

20.   Zheng ZJ, Croft JB, Giles WH, Mensah GA. Sudden cardiac death in the United States, 1989 to 1998. *Circulation.* 2001;**104**:2158–2163.

21.   Fabre A, Sheppard MN. Sudden adult death syndrome and other non-ischaemic causes of sudden death. *Heart.* 2006;**92**:316–320.

22.   Kitamura T, Iwami T, Nichol G, Nishiuchi T, Hayashi Y, Nishiyama C, Sakai T, Kajino K, Hiraide A, Ikeuchi H, Nonogi H, Kawamura T, Utstein Osaka Project. Reduction in incidence and fatality of out-of-hospital cardiac arrest in females of the reproductive age. *Eur Heart J.* 2010;**31**:1365–1372.

23.   Goldstein S, Bayés de Luna A, Guindo J. *Sudden Cardiac Death.* New York, New York: Futura; 1994.

24.   Bryan CP. *The Papyrus Ebers, translated from the German version.* London: Geoffrey Bles; 1930.

25. Eckart RE, Scoville SL, Campbell CL, Shry EA, Stajduhar KC, Potter RN, Pearse LA, Virmani R. Sudden death in young adults: A 25-year review of autopsies in military recruits. *Ann Intern Med.* 2004;**141**:829–834.

26. Eckart RE, Shry EA, Burke AP, McNear JA, Appel DA, Castillo-Rojas LM, Avedissian L, Pearse LA, Potter RN, Tremaine L, Gentlesk PJ, Huffer L, Reich SS, Stevenson WG, for the Department of Defense Cardiovascular Death Registry Group. Sudden death in young adults. An autopsy-based series of a population undergoing active surveillance. *J Am Coll Cardiol.* 2011;**58**:1254–1261.

27. Tabib A, Miras A, Taniere P, Loire R. Undetected cardiac lesions cause unexpected sudden cardiac death during occasional sport activity. A report of 80 cases. *Eur Heart J.* 1999;**20**:900–903.

28. Wisten A, Forsberg H, Krantz P, Messner T. Sudden cardiac death in 15–35-year olds in Sweden during 1992–99. *J Intern Med.* 2002;**252**:529–536.

29. Huikuri HV, Castellanos A, Myerburg RJ. Sudden death due to cardiac arrhythmias. *N Engl J Med.* 2001;**345**:1473–1482.

30. Myerburg RJ, Mitrani R, Interian Jr A, Castellanos A. Interpretation of outcomes of antiarrhythmic clinical trials: design features and population impact. *Circulation.* 1998; **97**:1514–1521.

31. Bassler T. Jogging deaths. *N Engl J Med.* 1972;**287**:1100.

32. Kim JH, Malhotra R, Chiampas G, d'Hemecourt P, Troyanos C, Cianca J, Smith RN, Wang TJ, Roberts WO, Thompson PD, Baggish AL, for the Race Associated Cardiac Arrest Event Registry (RACER) Study Group. Cardiac arrest during long-distance running races. *N Engl J Med.* 2012;**366**:130–140.

33. Corrado D, Basso C, Pavei A, Michieli P, Shiavon M, Thiene G. Trends in sudden cardiovascular death in young competitive athletes after implementation of a preparticipation screening program. *JAMA.* 2006;**296**:1593–1601.

34. Nishiyama C, Iwami T, Kawamura T, Kitamura T, Tanigawa K, Sakai T, Hayashida S, Nishiuchi T, Hayashi Y, Hiraide A. Prodromal symptoms of out-of-hospital cardiac arrests: A report from a large-scale population-based cohort study. *Resuscitation.* 2013;**84**:558–563.

35. Yearbook of Statistics Singapore, 2011. In: Singapore: Department of Statistics, Ministry of Trade and Industry, Republic of Singapore; 2011:Table 3.9.

36. Myerburg RJ, Kessler KM, Castellanos A. Sudden cardiac death: Epidemiology, transient risk, and intervention assessment. *Ann Intern Med.* 1993;**119**:1187–1197.

37. The GUSTO Investigators. An international randomized trial comparing four thrombolytic strategies for acute myocardial infarction. *N Engl J Med.* 1993;**329**:6 73–682.

38. Finnegan JRJ, Meischke H, Zapka JG, Leviton L, Meshack A, Benjamin-Garner R, Estabrook B, Hall NJ, Schaeffer S, Smith C, Weitzman ER, Raczynski J, Stone E. Patient delay in seeking care for heart attack symptoms: Findings from focus groups conducted in five U.S. regions. *Prev Med.* 2000;**31**:205–213.

39. Drory Y, Turetz Y, Hiss Y, Lev B, Fisman EZ, Pines A, Kramer MR. Sudden unexpected death in persons less than 40 years of age. *Am J Cardiol.* 1991;**68**:1388–1392.

40. Tweet MS, Hayes SN, Pitta SR, Simari RD, Lerman A, Lennon RJ, Gersh BJ, Khambatta S, Best PJM, Rihal CS, Gulati R. Clinical features, management, and prognosis of spontaneous coronary artery dissection. *Circulation.* 2012;**126**:579–588.

41. Nallamothu BK, Bradley EH, Krumholz HM. Time to treatment in primary percutaneous coronary intervention. *N Engl J Med.* 2007;**357**:1631–1638.

42. Solomon SD, Zelenkofske S, McMurray JJ, Finn PV, Velazquez E, Ertl G, Harsanyi A, Rouleau JL, Maggioni A, Kober L, White H, van de Werf F, Pieper K, Califf RM, Pfeffer MA, for the Valsartan in Acute Myocardial Infarction Trial (VALIANT) Investigators. Sudden death in patients with myocardial infarction and left ventricular dysfunction, heart failure, or both. *N Engl J Med.* 2005;**352**:2581–2588.

43. Zijlstra F, Hoorntje JC, de Boer MJ, Reiffers S, Miedema K, Ottervanger JP, van 't Hof AW, Suryapranata H. Long-term benefit of primary angioplasty as compared with thrombolytic therapy for acute myocardial infarction. *N Engl J Med.* 1999;**341**:1413–1419.

44. Hunt SA, Baker DW, Chin MH, Cinquegrani MP, Feldman AM, Francis GS, Ganiats TG, Goldstein S, Gregoratos G, Jessup ML, Noble RJ, Packer M, Silver MA, Stevenson LW, Gibbons RJ, Antman EM, Alpert JS, Faxon DP, Fuster V, Jacobs AK, Hiratzka LF, Russell RO, Smith SC. ACC/AHA guidelines for the evaluation and management of chronic heart failure in the adult: Executive summary: A report of the American College of Cardiology/American Heart Association Task Force on Practice Guidelines (Committee to revise the 1995 guidelines for the evaluation and management of heart failure) developed in collaboration with the International Society for Heart and Lung Transplantation endorsed by the Heart Failure Society of America. *J Am Coll Cardiol.* 2001;**38**:2101–2113.

45. The Multicenter Postinfarction Research Group. Risk stratification and survival after myocardial infarction. *N Engl J Med.* 1983;**309**:331–336.

46. Curtis JP, Sokol SI, Wang Y, Rathore SS, Ko DT, Jadbabaie F, Portnay EL, Marshalko SJ, Radford MJ, Krumholz HZ. The association of left ventricular ejection fraction, mortality, and cause of death in stable outpatients with heart failure. *J Am Coll Cardiol.* 2003;**42**:736–742.

47. Solomon SD, Anavekar N, Skali H, McMurray JJV, Swedberg K, Yusuf S, Granger CB, Michelson EL, Wang D, Pocock S, Pfeffer MA, for the Candesartan in Heart Failure Reduction in Mortality (CHARM) Investigators. Influence of ejection fraction on cardiovascular outcomes in a broad spectrum of heart failure patients. *Circulation.* 2005;**112**:3738–3744.

48. The Criteria Committee of the New York Heart Association. Nomenclature and criteria for diagnosis of diseases of the heart and great vessels. In: 9th ed. Boston, Mass: Little, Brown & Co.; 1994:253–256.

49. Levy WC, Mozaffarian D, Linker DT, Sutradhar SC, Anker SD, Cropp AB, Anand I, Maggioni A, Burton P, Sullivan MD, Pitt B, Poole-Wilson PA, Mann DL, Packer M. The Seattle Heart Failure Model: Prediction of survival in heart failure. *Circulation.* 2006;**113**:1424–1433.

50. Packer DL, Prutkin JM, Hellkamp AS, Mitchell LB, Bernstein RC, Wood F, Boehmer JP, Carlson MD, Frantz RP, McNulty SE, Rogers JG, Anderson J, Johnson GW, Walsh MN, Poole JE, Mark DB, Lee KL, Bardy GH. Impact of implantable cardioverter-defibrillator, amiodarone, and placebo on the mode of death in stable patients with heart failure. Analysis from the Sudden Cardiac Death in Heart Failure Trial. *Circulation.* 2009;**120**:2170–2176.

51. O'Meara E, Solomon S, McMurray J, Pfeffer M, Yusuf S, Michelson E, Granger C, Olofsson B, Young JB, Swedberg K. Effect of candesartan on New York Heart Association

functional class. Results of the Candesartan in Heart failure: Assessment of Reduction in Mortality and morbidity (CHARM) programme. *Eur Heart J.* 2004;**25**:1920–1926.

52. Abdulla J, Køber L, Christensen E, Torp-Pedersen C. Effect of beta-blocker therapy on functional status in patients with heart failure — a meta-analysis. *Eur J Heart Fail.* 2006;**8**:522–531.

53. Bardy GH, Lee KL, Mark DB, Poole JE, Packer DL, Boineau R, Domanski M, Troutman C, Anderson J, Johnson G, McNulty SE, Clapp-Channing N, Davidson-Ray LD, Fraulo ES, Fishbein DP, Luceri RM, Ip JH, Sudden Cardiac Death in Heart Failure Trial (SCD-HeFT) Investigators. Amiodarone or an implantable cardioverter-defibrillator for congestive heart failure. *N Engl J Med.* 2005;**352**:225–237.

54. Smilde TD, Hillege HL, Voors AA, Dunselman PH, van Veldhuisen DJ. Prognostic importance of renal function in patients with early heart failure and mild left ventricular dysfunction. *Am J Cardiol.* 2004;**94**:240–243.

55. Buxton AE, Lee KL, Hafley GE, Pires LA, Fisher JD, Gold MR, Josephson ME, Lehmann MH, Prystowsky EN, for the MUSTT Investigators. Limitations of ejection fraction for prediction of sudden death risk in patients with coronary artery disease: Lessons from the MUSTT study. *J Am Coll Cardiol.* 2007;**50**:1150–1157.

56. Pastore JM, Girouard SD, Laurita KR, Akar FG, Rosenbaum DS. Mechanism linking T-wave alternans to the genesis of cardiac fibrillation. *Circulation.* 1999;**99**:1385–1394.

57. Armoundas AA, Tomaselli GF, Esperer HD. Pathophysiological basis and clinical application of T-wave alternans. *J Am Coll Cardiol.* 2002;**40**:207–217.

58. Gehi AK, Stein RH, Metz LD, Gomes JA. Microvolt T-wave alternans for the risk stratification of ventricular tachyarrhythmic events: A meta-analysis. *J Am Coll Cardiol.* 2005;**46**:75–82.

59. Corrado D, Thiene G, Cocco P, Frescura C. Non-atherosclerotic coronary artery disease and sudden death in the young. *Br Heart J.* 1992;**68**:601–607.

60. Maron BJ, Doerer JJ, Haas TS, Tierney DM, Mueller FO. Sudden deaths in young competitive athletes. Analysis of 1866 deaths in the United States, 1980–2006. *Circulation.* 2009;**119**:1085–1092.

61. Davis JA, Cecchin F, Jones TK, Portman MA. Major coronary anomalies in a pediatric population: Incidence and clinical importance. *J Am Coll Cardiol.* 2001;**37**:593–597.

62. Alexander RW, Griffith GC. Anomalies of the coronary arteries and their clinical significance. *Circulation.* 1956;**14**:800–805.

63. Basso C, Maron BJ, Corrado D, Thiene G. Congenital coronary artery anomalies are an important cause of sudden death in the young. *Cardiol Rev.* 2001;**9**:312–317.

64. Roberts WC. Major anomalies of coronary arterial origins seen in adulthood. *Am Heart J.* 1986;**111**:941–963.

65. Hanzlick RJ, Stivers RR. Sudden death due to anomalous right coronary artery in a 26-year-old marathon runner. *Am J Forens Med.* 1983;**4**:265–268.

66. Cheitlin M, De Castro C, McAllister H. Sudden death as a complication of anomalous left coronary artery origin from the anterior sinus of valsalva: A not-so-minor congenital anomaly. *Circulation.* 1974;**50**:780–787.

67. Mustafa I, Gula G, Radley-Smith R, Durrer S, Yacoub M. Anomalous origin of the left coronary artery from the anterior aortic sinus: A potential cause of sudden death. Anatomic characterization and surgical treatment. *J Thorac Cardiovasc Surg.* 1981;**82**:297–300.

68. Pelliccia A. Congenital coronary artery anomalies in young patients. New perspective for timely identificaiton. *J Am Coll Cardiol.* 2001;**37**:598–600.

69. Angelini P. Coronary artery anomalies: An entity in search of an identity. *Circulation.* 2007;**115**:1296–1305.

70. Basso C, Maron BJ, Corrado D, Thiene G. Clinical profile of congenital coronary artery anomalies with origin from the wrong aortic sinus leading to sudden death in young competitive athletes. *J Am Coll Cardiol.* 2000;**35**:1493–1501.

71. Reyman HC. Dissertatio de vasis cordis propriis. In: von Haller A, Reyman HC, eds. *Bibl Anat.* Göttinger, Germany; 1737:359–379.

72. Geiringer E. The mural coronary. *Am Heart J.* 1951;**41**:359–368.

73. Möhlenkamp S, Hort W, Ge J, Erbel R. Update on myocardial bridging. *Circulation.* 2002;**106**:2616–2622.

74. Morales AR, Romanelli R, Boucek RJ. The mural left anterior descending coronary artery, strenuous exercise and sudden death. *Circulation.* 1980;**62**:230–237.

75. Ishikawa Y, Akasaka Y, Suzuki K, Fujiwara M, Ogawa T, Yamazaki K, Niino H, Tanaka M, Ogata K, Morinaga S, Ebihara Y, Kawahara Y, Sugiura H, Takimoto T, Komatsu A, Shinagawa T, Taki K, Satoh H, Yamada K, Yanagida-Iida M, Shimokawa R, Shimada K, Nishimura C, Ito K, Ishii T. Anatomic properties of myocardial bridge predisposing to myocardial infarction. *Circulation.* 2009;**120**:376–383.

76. Corban MT, Hung OY, Eshtehardi P, Rasoul-Arzrumly E, McDaniel M, Mekonnen G, Timmins LH, Lutz J, Guyton RA, Samady H. Myocardial bridging: Contemporary understanding of pathophysiology with implications for diagnostic and therapeutic strategies. *J Am Coll Cardiol.* 2014;**63**:2346–2355.

77. Hazirolan T, Canyigit M, Karcaaltincaba M, Dagoglu MG, Akata D, Aytemir K, Besim A. Myocardial bridging on MDCT. *Am J Roentgenol.* 2007;**188**:1074–1080.

78. Noble J, Bourassa MG, Petitclerc R, Dyrda I. Myocardial bridging and milking effect of the left anterior descending coronary artery: Normal variant or obstruction. *Am J Cardiol.* 1976;**37**:993–999.

79. Feldman AM, Baughman KL. Myocardial infarctin associated with a myocardial bridge. *Am Heart J.* 1986;**111**:784–787.

80. Faruqui AMA, Maloy WC, Felner JM, Schlant RC, Logan WD, Symbas P. Symptomatic myocardial bridging of coronary artery. *Am J Cardiol.* 1978;**41**:1305–1310.

81. Haager PK, Schwartz ER, vom Dahl J, Klues HG, Reffelmann T, Hanrath P. Long term angiographic and clinical follow up in patients with stent implantation for symptomatic myocardial bridging. *Heart.* 2000;**84**:403–408.

82. Kunamneni PB, Rajdev S, Krishnan P, Moreno PR, Kim MC, Sharma SK, Kini AS. Outcome of intracoronary stenting after failed maximal medical therapy in patients with symptomatic myocardial bridge. *Catheter Cardiovasc Interv.* 2008;**71**:185–190.

83. Tandar A, Whisenant BK, Michaels AD. Stent fracture following stenting of a myocardial bridge: Report of two cases. *Catheter Cardiovasc Interv.* 2008;**71**:191–196.

84. Maron BJ, Towbin JA, Thiene G, Antzelevitch C, Corrado D, Arnett D, Moss AJ, Seidman CE, Young JB. Contemporary definitions and classification of the cardiomyopathies: An American Heart Association Scientific Statement from the Council on Clinical Cardiology, Heart Failure and Transplantation Committee; Quality of Care and Outcomes Research and Functional Genomics and Translational Biology

Interdisciplinary Working Groups; and Council on Epidemiology and Prevention. *Circulation.* 2006;**113**:1807–1816.

85. Franz WM, Muller OJ, Katus HA. Cardiomyopathies: From genetics to the prospect of treatment. *Lancet.* 2001;**358**:1627–1637.

86. Klues HG, Schiffers A, Maron BJ. Phenotypic spectrum and patterns of left ventricular hypertrophy in hypertrophic cardiomyopathy: Morphologic observations and significance as assessed by two-dimensional echocardiography in 600 patients. *J Am Coll Cardiol.* 1995;**26**:1699–1708.

87. Gersh BJ, Maron BJ, Bonow RO, Dearani JA, Fifer MA, Link MS, Naidu SS, Nishimura RA, Ommen SR, Rakowski H, Seidman CE, Towbin JA, Udelson JE, Yancy CW. 2011 ACCF/AHA Guideline for the Diagnosis and Treatment of Hypertrophic Cardiomyopathy: A report of the American College of Cardiology Foundation/American Heart Association Task Force on Practice Guidelines developed in collaboration with the American Society for Thoracic Surgery, American Society of Echocardiography, American Society of Nuclear Cardiology, Heart Failure Society of America, Heart Rhythm Society, Society for Cardiovascular Angiography and Interventions, and Society of Thoracic Surgeons. *J Am Coll Cardiol.* 2011;**58**:e212–e260.

88. Rickers C, Wilke NM, Jerosch-Herold M, Casey SA, Panse P, Panse N, Weil J, Zenovich AG, Maron BJ. Utility of cardiac magnetic resonance imaging in the diagnosis of hypertrophic cardiomyopathy. *Circulation.* 2005;**112**:855–861.

89. Maron BJ. Apical hypertrophic cardiomyopathy: The continuing saga. *J Am Coll Cardiol.* 1990;**15**:91–93.

90. Maron MS, Maron BS, Harrigan C, Buros J, Gibson CM, Olivotto I, Biller L, Lesser JR, Udelson JE, Manning WJ, Appelbaum E. Hypertrophic cardiomyopathy phenotype revisited after 50 years with cardiovascular magnetic resonance. *J Am Coll Cardiol.* 2009;**54**:220–228.

91. Choudhury L, Mahrholdt H, Wagner A, Choi KM, Elliot MD, Klocke FJ, Bonow RO, Judd RM, Kim RJ. Myocardial scarring in asymptomatic or mildly symptomatic patients with hypertrophic cardiomyopathy. *J Am Coll Cardiol.* 2002;**40**:2156–2164.

92. Harris KM, Spirito P, Maron MS, Zenovich AG, Formisano F, Lesser JR, Mackey-Bojack S, Manning WJ, Udelson JE, Maron BJ. Prevalence, clinical profile, and significance of left ventricular remodeling in the end-stage phase of hypertrophic cardiomyopathy. *Circulation.* 2006;**114**:216–225.

93. Watkins H, Ashrafian H, Redwood C. Inherited cardiomyopathies. *N Engl J Med.* 2011;**364**:1643–1656.

94. Marian AJ, Yu QT, Workman R, Greve G, Roberts R. Angiotensin-converting enzyme polymorphism in hypertrophic cardiomyopathy and sudden cardiac death. *Lancet.* 1993;**342**:1085–1086.

95. Van Driest SL, Vasile VC, Ommen SR, Will ML, Tajik AJ, Gersh BJ, Ackerman MJ. Myosin binding protein C mutations and compound heterozygosity in hypertrophic cardiomyopathy. *J Am Coll Cardiol.* 2004;**44**:1903–1910.

96. Maron BJ. Hypertrophic cardiomyopathy: A systematic review. *JAMA.* 2002;**287**:1308–1320.

97. Elliot P, Anderson B, Arbustini E, Bilinska Z, Cecchi F, Charron P, Dubourg O, Kühl U, Maisch B, McKenna WJ, Monserrat L, Pankuweit S, Rapezzi C, Seferovic P, Tavazzi L, Keren A. Classification of the cardiomyopathies: A position statement from the

European Society of Cardiology Working Group on Myocardial and Pericardial Diseases. *Eur Heart J.* 2008;**29**:270–276.

98.   Maron BJ. Hypertrophic cardiomyopathy: An important global disease. *Am J Med.* 2004;**116**:63–65.

99.   Maron BJ, Shirani J, Poliac LC, Mathenge R, Roberts WC, Mueller FO. Sudden death in young competitive athletes: Clinical, demographic, and pathologic profiles. *JAMA.* 1996;**276**:199–204.

100. Basavarajaiah S, Wilson M, Whyte G, Shah A, McKenna W, Sharma S. Prevalence of hypertrophic cardiomyopathy in highly trained athletes. Relevance to pre-participation screening. *J Am Coll Cardiol.* 2008;**51**:1033–1039.

101. Maron BJ, Carney KP, Lever HM, Lewis JF, Barac I, Casey SA, Sherrid MV. Relationship of race to sudden cardiac death in competitive athletes with hypertrophic cardiomyopathy. *J Am Coll Cardiol.* 2003;**19**:974–980.

102. Maron BJ, Olivotto I, Spirito P, Casey SA, Bellone P, Gohman TE, Graham KJ, Burton DA, Cecchi F. Epidemiology of hypertrophy cardiomyopathy-related death: Revisited in a large non-referral-based patient population. *Circulation.* 2000;**102**:858–864.

103. Morrow AG, Braunwald E. Functional aortic stenosis: A malformation characterized by resistance to the left ventricular outflow without anatomic obstruction. *Circulation.* 1959;**20**:181–189.

104. Maron BJ, Epstein SE. Hypertrophic cardiomyopathy: A discussion of nomenclature. *Am J Cardiol.* 1979;**43**:1242–1244.

105. Maron MS, Olivotto I, Zenovich AG, Link MS, Pandian NG, Kuvin JT, Nistri S, Cecchi F, Udelson JE, Maron BJ. Hypertrophic cardiomyopathy is predominantly a disease of left ventricular outflow tract obstruction. *Circulation.* 2006;**114**:2232–2239.

106. Carasso S, Yang H, Woo A, Jamorski M, Wigle ED, Rakowski H. Diastolic myocardial mechanics in hypertrophic cardiomyopathy. *J Am Soc Echocardiogr.* 2010;**23**:164–171.

107. Cannon III RO, Rosing DR, Maron BJ, Leon MB, Bonow RO, Watson RM, Epstein SE. Myocardial ischemia in patients with hypertrophic cardiomyopathy: Contribution of inadequate vasodilator reserve and elevated left ventricular systolic filling pressures. *Circulation.* 1985;**71**:234–243.

108. Wigle ED, Adelman AG, Auger P, Marquis Y. Mitral regurgitation in muscular subaortic stenosis. *Am J Cardiol.* 1969;**24**:698–706.

109. Spirito P, Bellone P. Natural history of hypertrophic cardiomyopathy. *Br Heart J.* 1994;**72**:S10–S12.

110. Maron BJ, Seidman JG, Seidman CE. Proposal for contemporary screening strategies in families with hypertrophic cardiomyopathy. *J Am Coll Cardiol.* 2004;**44**:2125–2132.

111. Adabag AS, Casey SA, Kuskowski MA, Zenovich AG, Maron BJ. Spectrum and prognostic significance of arrhythmias on ambulatory Holter electrocardiogram in hypertrophic cardiomyopathy. *J Am Coll Cardiol.* 2005;**45**:697–704.

112. Sadoul N, Prasad K, Elliot PM, Bannerjee S, Frenneaux MP, McKenna WJ. Prospective prognostic assessment of blood pressure response during exercise in patients with hypertrophic cardiomyopathy. *Circulation.* 1997;**96**:2987–2991.

113. Olivotto I, Maron BJ, Montereggi A, Mazzuoli F, Dolara A, Cecchi F. Blood pressure response during exercise in a community-based patient population with hypertrophic cardiomyopathy. *J Am Coll Cardiol.* 1999;**33**:2044–2051.

114. Dearani JA, Ommen SR, Gersh BJ, Schaff HV, Danielson GK. Surgery insight: Septal myomectomy for obstructive hypertrophic cardiomyopathy — the Mayo Clinic experience. *Nat Rev Cardiol.* 2007;**4**:503–512.

115. Vecht J, Dave R, Vecht R. Alcohol septal ablation: The first patient in 1994. *Br J Cardiol.* 2006;**13**:62–64.

116. Sorajja P, Valeti U, Nishimura RA, Ommen SR, Rihal CS, Gersh BJ, Hodge DO, Schaff HV, Holmes Jr DR. Ouctome of alcohol septal ablation for obstructive hypertrophic cardiomyopasthy. *Circulation.* 2008;**118**:131–139.

117. Sorajja P, Ommen SR, Holmes Jr DR, Dearani JA, Rihal CS, Gersh BJ, Lennon RJ, Nishimura RA. Survival after alcohol septal ablation for obstructive hypertrophic cardiomyopathy. *Circulation.* 2012;**126**:2374–2380.

118. Valeti US, Nishimura RA, Holmes DR, Araoz PA, Glockner JF, Breen JF, Ommen SR, Gersh BJ, Tajik AJ, Rihal CS, Schaff HV, Maron BJ. Comparision of surgical septal myectomy and alcohol septal ablation with cardiac magnetic resonance imaging in patients with hypertrophic obstructive cardiomyopathy. *J Am Coll Cardiol.* 2007;**49**:350–357.

119. Cecchi F, Maron BJ, Epstein SE. Long-term outcome of patients with hypertrophic cardiomyopathy successfully resuscitated after cardiac arrest. *J Am Coll Cardiol.* 1989;**13**:1283–1288.

120. Bos JM, Maron BJ, Ackerman MJ, Haas TS, Sorajja P, Nishimura RA, Gersh BJ, Ommen SR. Role of family history of sudden death in risk stratification and prevention of sudden death with implantable defibrillators in hypertrophic cardiomyopathy. *Am J Cardiol.* 2010;**106**:1481–1486.

121. Elliot PM, Gimeno JR, Tomé MT, Shah J, Ward D, Thaman R, Mogensen J, McKenna WJ. Left ventricular outflow tract obstruction and sudden death risk in piatents with hypertrophic cardiomyopathy. *Eur Heart J.* 2006;**27**:1933–1941.

122. Spirito P, Autore C, Rapezzi C, Bernabo P, Badagliacca R, Maron MS, Bongioanni S, Coccolo F, Estes NNM, Barillà CS, Biagini E, Quarta G, Conte MR, Bruzzi P, Maron BJ. Syncope and risk of sudden death in hypertrophic cardiomyopathy. *Circulation.* 2009;**119**:1703–1710.

123. Elliott PM, Poloniecki J, Dickie S, Sharma S, Monserrat L, Varnava A, Mahon NG, McKenna WJ. Sudden death in hypertrophic cardiomyopathy: Identification of high risk patients. *J Am Coll Cardiol.* 2000;**36**:2212–2218.

124. Moon JC, Reed E, Sheppard MN, Elkington A, Ho S, Burke M, Petrou M, Pennell DJ. The histologic basis of late gadolinium enhancement cardiovascular magnetic resonance in hypertrophic cardiomyopathy. *J Am Coll Cardiol.* 2004;**43**:2260–2264.

125. Chan RH, Maron BJ, Olivotto I, Pencina MJ, Assenza GE, Haas T, Lesser JR, Gruner C, Crean AM, Rakowski H, Udelson JE, Rowin E, Lombardi M, Cecchi F, Tomberli B, Spirito P, Formisano F, Biagini E, Rapezzi C, De Cecco CN, Autore C, Cook EF, Hong SN, Gibson CM, Manning WJ, Appelbaum E, Maron MS. Prognostic value of quantitative contrast-enhanced cardiovascular magnetic resonance for the evaluation of sudden death risk in patients with hypertrophic cardiomyopathy. *Circulation.* 2014;**130**:484–495.

126. Maron BJ, Shen WK, Link MS, Epstein AE, Almquist AK, Daubert JP, Bardy GH, Favale S, Rea RF, Boriani G, Estes III EA, Spirito P. Efficacy of implantable cardioverter-debrillator for the prevention of sudden death in patients with hypertrophic cardiomyopathy. *N Engl J Med.* 2000;**342**:365–373.

127. Maron BJ, Spirito P, Shen WK, Haas TS, Formisano F, Link MS, Epstein AE, Almquist AK, Daubert JP, Lawrenz T, Boriani G, Estes III NA, Favale S, Piccininno M, Winters SL, Santini M, Betocchi S, Arribas F, Sherrid MV, Buja G, Semsarian C, Bruzzi P. Implantable cardioverter-defibrillators and prevention of sudden cardiac death in hypertrophic cardiomyopathy. *JAMA*. 2007;**298**:405–412.

128. Lin G, Nishimura RA, Gersh BJ, Phil D, Ommen SR, Ackerman MJ, Brady PA. Device complications and inappropriate implantatable cardioverter defibrillator shocks in patients with hypertrophic cardiomyopathy. *Heart.* 2009;**95**:709–714.

129. van Rees JB, Borleffs JW, de Bie MK, Stijnen T, van Erven L, Bax JJ, Schalij MJ. Inappropriate implantable cardioverter-defibrillator shocks: Incidence, predictors, and impact on mortality. *J Am Coll Cardiol*. 2011;**57**:556–562.

130. Maron MS, Kalsmith BK, Udelson JE, Li W, DeNofrio D. Survival after cardiac transplantation in patients with hypertrophic cardiomyopathy. *Circ Heart Fail*. 2010;**3**:574–579.

131. Maron BJ, Ackerman MJ, Nishimura RA, Pyeritz RE, Towbin JA, Udelson JE. Task Force 4: HCM and other cardiomyopathies, mitral valve prolapse, myocarditis, and Marfan syndrome. *J Am Coll Cardiol*. 2005;**45**:1340–1345.

132. Pelliccia A, Fagard R, Bjørnstad HH, Anastassakis A, Arbustini E, Assanelli D, Biffi A, Borjesson M, Carrè F, Corrado D, Delise P, Dorwarth U, Hirth A, Heidbuchel H, Hoffmann E, Mellwig KP, Panhuyzen-Goedkoop N, Pisani A, Solberg EE, van-Buuren F, Vanhees L. Recommendations for competitive sports participation in athletes with cardiovascular disease. A consensus document from the Study Group of Sports Cardiology of the Working Group of Cardiac Rehabilitation and Exercise Physiology and the Working Group of Myocardial and Pericardial Diseases of the European Society of Cardiology. *Eur Heart J.* 2005;**26**:1442–1445.

133. Maron BJ, McKenna WJ, Danielson GK, Kappenberger LJ, Kuhn HJ, Seidman CE, Shah PM, Spencer III WH, Spirito P, Ten Cate FJ, Wigle ED. American College of Cardiology Foundation Task Force on Clinical Expert Consensus Documents, European Society of Cardiology Committee for Practice Guidelines; Amercian College of Cardiology/European Society of Cardiology/Clinical Expert Consensus Document on Hypertrophy Cardiomyopathy. A report of the American College of Cardiology Foundation Task Force on Clinical Expert Consensus Documents and the European Society of Cardiology for Practice Guidelines. *Eur Heart J.* 2003;**24**:1963–1991.

134. Corrado D, Pelliccia A, Heidbuchel H, Sharma S, Link M, Basso C, Biffi A, Buja G, Delise P, Gussac I, Anastasakis A, Borjesson M, Bjønstad HH, Carré F, Deligiannis A, Dugmore D, Fagard R, Hoogsteen J, Mellwig KP, Panhuyzen-Goedkoop N, Solberg E, Vanhees L, Drezner J, Estes III NAM, Iliceto S, Mason BJ, Peidro R, Schwartz PJ, Stein R, Thiene G, Zeppilli P, McKenna WJ, on behalf of the Section of Sports Cardiology of the European Association of Cardiovascular Prevention; and the Working Group of Myocardial and Pericardial Disease of the European Society of Cardiology. Recommendations for interpretation of 12-lead electrocardiogram in the athlete. *Eur Heart J.* 2010;**31**:243–259.

135. Rowin EJ, Maron BJ, Appelbaum E, Link MS, Gibson CM, Lesser JR, Haas TS, Udelson JE, Manning WJ, Maron MS. Significance of false negative electrocardiograms in preparticipation screening of athletes for hypertrophic cardiomyopathy. *Am J Cardiol*. 2012;**110**:1027–1032.

136. The Daily Telegraph Reporter. Girl died minutes after first kiss with boyfriend. In: *The Daily Telegraph*; 2011.

137. Puranik R, Chow CK, Duflou JA, Kilborn MJ, McGuire MA. Sudden death in the young. *Heart Rhythm.* 2005;**2**:1277–1282.

138. Stokes P. Schoolgirl dies two weeks after parents not told of school doctor treatment. In: *The Telegraph*. Chatham, Kent; 2008.

139. Schwartz PJ, Stramba-Badiale M, Crotti L, Pedrazzini M, Besana A, Bosi G, Gabbarini F, Goulene K, Insolia R, Mannarino S, Mosca F, Nespoli L, Rimini A, Rosati E, Salice P, Spazzolini C. Prevalence of the congenital long-QT syndrome. *Circulation.* 2009;**120**:1761–1767.

140. Ackerman MJ. The long QT syndrome: Ion channel diseases of the heart. *Mayo Clin Proc.* 1998;**73**:250–269.

141. Moss AJ, Kass RS. Long QT syndrome: From channels to cardiac arrhythmia. *J Clin Invest.* 2005;**115**:2018–2024.

142. Tan HL, Bardai A, Shimizu W, Moss AJ, Schulze-Bahr E, Noda T, Wilde AAM. Genotype-specific onset of arrhythmias in congenital long-QT syndrome: Possible therapy implications. *Circulation.* 2006;**114**:2096–2103.

143. Zareba W, Moss AJ, Schwartz PJ, Vincent GM, Robinson JL, Priori SG, Benhorin J, Locati EH, Towbin JA, Keating MT, Lehmann MH, Hall WJ, for the International Long-QT Syndrome Registry Research Group. Influence of the genotype on the clinical course of the long-QT syndrome. *N Engl J Med.* 1998;**339**:960–965.

144. Goldenberg I, Moss AJ, Bradley J, Polonsky S, Peterson DR, McNitt S, Zareba W, Andrews ML, Robinson JL, Ackerman MJ, Benhorin J, Kaufman ES, Locati EH, Napolitano C, Priori SG, Qi M, Schwartz PJ, Towbin JA, Vincent GM, Zhang L. Long-QT syndrome after age 40. *Circulation.* 2008;**117**:2192–2201.

145. Chugh SS, Reinier K, Singh T, Uy-Evanado A, Socoteanu C, Peters D, Mariani R, Gunson K, Jui J. Determinants of prolonged QT interval and their contribuation to sudden death risk in coronary artery disease. The Oregon Sudden Unexpected Death Study. *Circulation.* 2009;**119**:663–670.

146. Buber J, Mathew J, Moss AJ, Hall WJ, Barsheshet A, McNitt S, Robinson JL, Zareba W, Ackerman MJ, Kaufman ES, Luria D, Eldar M, Towbin JA, Vincent M, Goldenberg I. Risk of recurrent cardiac events after onset of menopause in women with congenital long-QT syndrome types 1 and 2. *Circulation.* 2011;**123**:2784–2791.

147. Tester DJ, Ackerman MJ. Postmortem long QT syndrome genetic testing for sudden unexplained death in the young. *J Am Coll Cardiol.* 2007;**49**:240–246.

148. Tan HL, Hofman N, van Langen IM, van der Wal AC, Wilde AAM. Sudden unexplained death — hereditary and diagnostic yield of cardiological and genertic examination in surviving relatives. *Circulation.* 2005;**112**:207–213.

149. Imboden M, Swan H, Denjoy I, Van Langen IM, Latinen-Forsblom PJ, Napolitano C, Fressart V, Breithardt G, Berthet M, Priori S, Hainque B, Wilde AA, Schulze-Bahr E, Feingold J, Guicheney P. Female predominance and transmission distortion in the long-QT syndrome. *N Engl J Med.* 2006;**355**:2744–2751.

150. Goldenberg I, Moss AJ, Zareba W. QT interval: How to measure it and what is "normal". *J Cardiovasc Electrophysiol.* 2006;**17**:333–336.

151. Schwartz PJ, Periti M, Malliani A. The long Q-T syndrome. *Am Heart J.* 1975;**89**:378–390.

152.   Newton-Cheh C, Guo C-Y, Larson MG, Musone SL, Surti A, Camargo AL, Drake JA, Benjamin EJ, Levy D, D'Agostino Sr RB, Hirschhorn JN, O'Donnell CJ. Common genetic variation in *KCNH2* is associated with QT interval duration. The Framingham Heart Study. *Circulation.* 2007;**116**:1128–1136.

153.   Zhang L, Timothy KW, Vincent GM, Lehmann MH, Fox J, Giuli LC, Shen J, Splawski I, Priori SG, Compton SJ, Yanowitz F, Benhorin J, Moss AJ, Schwartz PJ, Robinson JL, Wang Q, Zareba W, Keating MT, Towbin JA, Napolitano C, Medina A. Spectrum of ST-T-wave patterns and repolarization parameters in congenital long-QT syndrome: ECG findings identify genotypes. *Circulation.* 2000;**102**: 2849–2855.

154.   Takenaka K, Ai T, Shimizu W, Kobori A, Ninomiya T, Otani H, Kubota T, Takaki H, Kamakura S, Horie M. Exercise stress test amplifies genotype-phenotype correlation in the LQT1 and LQT2 forms of the long-QT syndrome. *Circulation.* 2003;**107**: 838–844.

155.   Shimizu W, Noda T, Takaki H, Kurita T, Nagaya N, Satomi K, Suyama K, Aihara N, Kamakura S, Sunagawa K, Echigo S, Nakamura K, Ohe T, Towbin JA, Napolitano C, Priori SG. Epinephrine unmasks latent mutation carriers with LQT1 form of congenital long-QT syndrome. *J Am Coll Cardiol.* 2003;**19**:633–642.

156.   Vyas H, Hejlik J, Ackerman MJ. Epinephrine QT stress testing in the evaluation of congenital long-QT syndrome: Diagnostic accuracy of the paradoxical QT response. *Circulation.* 2006;2006.

157.   Khositseth A, Hejlik J, Shen WK, Ackerman MJ. Epinephrine-induced T-wave notching in congenital long QT syndrome. *Heart Rhythm.* 2005;**2**:141–146.

158.   Struijk JJ, Kanters JK, Andersen MP, Hardahl T, Graff C, Christiansen M, Toft E. Classification of the long-QT syndrome based on discriminant analysis of T-wave morphology. *Med Biol Eng Comput.* 2006;**44**:543–549.

159.   Kanters JK, Fanoe S, Larsen LA, Bloch Thomsen PE, Toft E, Christiansen M. T wave morphology analysis distinguishes between KvLQT1 and HERG mutations in long QT syndrome. *Heart Rhythm.* 2004;**1**:285–292.

160.   Vaglio M, Couderc JP, McNitt S, Xia X, Moss AJ, Zareba W. A quantitative assessment of T-wave morphology in LQT1, LQT2, and healthy individuals based on Holter recording technology. *Heart Rhythm.* 2008;**5**:11–18.

161.   Viskin S, Rosso R, Rogowski O, Belhassen B, Levitas A, Wagshal A, Katz A, Fourey D, Zeltser D, Oliva A, Pollevick GD, Antzelevitch C, Rozovski U. Provocation of sudden heart rate oscillation with adenosine exposes abnormal QT responses in patients with long QT syndrome: A bedside test for diagnosing long QT syndrome. *Eur Heart J.* 2006;**27**:469–475.

162.   Schwartz PJ. Idiopathic long QT syndrome: Progress and questions. *Am Heart J.* 1985;**109**:399–411.

163.   Schwartz PJ, Moss AJ, Vincent GM, Crampton RS. Diagnostic criteria for the long QT syndrome: An update. *Circulation.* 1993;**88**:782–784.

164.   Schwartz PJ. The congenital long QT syndromes from genotype to phenotype: Clinical implications. *J Intern Med.* 2006;**259**:39–47.

165.   Keating M, Atkinson D, Dunn C, Timothy K, Vincent GM, Leppert M. Linkage of a cardiac arrhythmia, the long QT syndrome, and the Harvey ras-1 gene. *Science.* 1991;**252**:704–706.

166. Hofman N, Wilde AAM, Kääb S, van Langen IM, Tanck MWT, Mannens MMAM, Hinterseer M, Beckmann B-M, Tan HL. Diagnostic criteria for congenital long QT syndrome in the era of molecular genetics: Do we need a scoring system? *Eur Heart J.* 2007;**28**:575–580.

167. Al-Khatib SM, LaPointe NMA, Kramer JM, Califf RM. What clinicians should know about the QT interval. *JAMA.* 2003;**289**:2120–2127.

168. Rautaharju PM, Zhou SH, Wong S, Calhoun HP, Berenson GS, Prineas R, Davignon A. Sex differences in the evolution of the electrocardiographic QT interval with age. *Can J Cardiol.* 1992;**8**:690–695.

169. Stramba-Badiale M, Spagnolo D, Bosi G, Schwartz PG. Are gender differences in QTc present at birth? *Am J Cardiol.* 1995;**75**:1277–1278.

170. Merri M, Benhorin J, Alberti M, Locati E, Moss AJ. Electrocardiographic quantitation of ventricular repolarization. *Circulation.* 1989;**80**:1301–1308.

171. Locati EH, Zareba W, Moss AJ, Schwartz PJ, Vincent GM, Lehmann MH, Towbin JA, Priori SG, Napolitano C, Robinson JL, Andrews M, Timothy K, Hall WJ. Age- and sex-related differences in clinical manifestations in patients with congenital long-QT syndrome: Findings from the international LQTS Registry. *Circulation.* 1998;**97**: 2237–2244.

172. Zareba W, Moss AJ, Locati EH, Lehmann MH, Peterson DR, Hall WJ, Schwartz PJ, Vincent GM, Priori SG, Benhorin J, Towbin JA, Robinson JL, Andrews ML, Napolitano C, Timothy K, Zhang L, Medina A, for the International Long QT Syndrome Registry. Modulating effects of age and gender on the clinical course of long QT syndrome by genotype. *J Am Coll Cardiol.* 2003;**42**:103–109.

173. Moss AJ. Molecular genetics and ventricular arrhythmias. *N Eng J Med.* 1992;**327**: 885–887.

174. Roden DM. Drug-induced prolongation of the QT interval. *N Engl J Med.* 2004;**350**:1013–1022.

175. Makkar RR, Fromm RB, Steinman RT, Meissner MD, Lehmann MH. Female gender as a risk factor for torsades de pointes associated with cardiovascular drugs. *JAMA.* 1993;**270**:2590–2597.

176. Ahmed W, Flynn MA, Alpert MA. Cardiovascular complications of weight reduction diets. *Am J Med Sci.* 2001;**321**:280–284.

177. Altun G, Ugur-Altun B, Altun A, Azmak D. Sudden cardiac death in a hunger strike. *Cardiology.* 2003;**100**:107–108.

178. Heist EK, Ruskin JN. Drug-induced arrhythmia. *Circulation.* 2010;**122**:1426–1435.

179. Moss AJ, Zareba W, Benhorin J, Locati EH, Hall WJ, Robinson JL, Schwartz PJ, Towbin JA, Vincent GM, Lehmann MH, Keating MT, MacCluer JW, Timothy KW. ECG T-wave patterns in genetically distinct forms of hereditary long QT syndrome. *Circulation.* 1995;**92**:2929–2934.

180. Goldenberg I, Mathew J, Moss AJ, McNitt S, Peterson DR, Zareba W, Benhorin J, Zhang L, Vincent GM, Andrews ML, Robinson JL, Morray B. Corrected QT variability in serial electrocardiograms in long QT syndrome. The importance of the maximum corrected QT for risk stratification. *J Am Coll Cardiol.* 2006;**48**:1047–1052.

181. Gilmour Jr RF, Riccio ML, Locati EH, Maison-Blanche P, Coumel P, Schwartz PJ. Time- and rate-dependent alterations of the QT interval precede the onset of torsade de pointes in patients with acquired QT prolongation. *J Am Coll Cardiol.* 1997;**30**:209–217.

182. Vincent GM, Timothy KW, Leppert M, Keating M. The spectrum of symptoms and QT intervals in carriers of the gene for the long-QT syndrome. *N Engl J Med.* 1992;**327**: 846–852.

183. Priori SG, Napolitano C, Schwartz PJ. Low penetrance in the long-QT syndrome: Clinical impact. *Circulation.* 1999;**99**:529–533.

184. Goldenberg I, Horr S, Moss AJ, Lopes CM, Barsheshet A, McNitt S, Zareba W, Andrews ML, Robinson JL, Locati EH, Ackerman MJ, Benhorin J, Kaufman ES, Napolitano C, Platonov PG, Priori SG, Qi M, Schwartz PJ, Shimizu W, Towbin JA, Vincent GM, M WAA, Zhang L. Risk for life-threatening cardiac events in patients with genotype-confirmed long-QT syndrome and normal-range correceted QT intervals. *J Am Coll Cardiol.* 2011;**57**:51–59.

185. Priori SG, Schwartz PJ, Napolitano C, Bloise R, Ronchetti E, Grillo M, Vicentini A, Spazzolini C, Nastoli J, Bottelli G, Folli R, Cappelletti D. Risk stratification in the long-QT syndrome. *N Engl J Med.* 2003;**348**:1866–1874.

186. Viskin S, Postema PG, Bhuiyan ZA, Rosso R, Kalman JM, Vohra JK, Guevara-Valdivia ME, Marquez MF, Kogan K, Belhassen B, Glikson M, Strasberg B, Antzelevitch C, Wilde AAM. The response of the QT interval to the brief tachycardia provoked by standing: A bedside test for diagnosing long QT syndrome. *J Am Coll Cardiol.* 2010;**55**: 1955–1961.

187. Sauer AJ, Moss AJ, McNitt S, Petersen DR, Zareba W, Robinson JL, Qi M, Goldenberg I, Hobbs WJ, Ackerman MJ, Benhorin J, Hall WJ, Kaufman ES, Locati EH, Napolitano C, Priori SG, Schwartz PJ, Towbin JA, Vincent GM, Zhang L. Long QT syndrome in adults. *J Am Coll Cardiol.* 2007;**49**:329–337.

188. Napolitano C, Priori SG, Schwartz PJ, Bloise R, Ronchetti E, Nastoli J, Bottelli G, Cerrone M, Leonardi S. Genetic testing in the long QT syndrome. Development and validation of an efficient approach to genotyping in clinical practice. *JAMA.* 2005;**294**: 2975–2980.

189. Vincent GM, Jaiswal D, Timothy KW. Effects of exercise on heart rate, QT, QTc and QT/QS2 in the Romano-Ward inherited long QT syndrome. *Am J Cardiol.* 1991;**68**: 498–503.

190. Chattha IS, Sy RW, Yee R, Gula LJ, Skanes AC, Klein GJ, Bennett MT, Krahn AD. Utility of the recovery electrocardiogram after exercise: A novel indicator for the diagnosis and genotyping of long QT syndrome? *Heart Rhythm.* 2010;**7**:906–911.

191. Schwartz PJ, Priori SG, Locati EH, Napolitano C, Cantù F, Towbin JA, Keating MT, Hammoude H, Brown AM, Chen LS. Long QT syndrome patients with mutations of the *SCN5A* and *HERG* genes have differential responses to Na+ channel blockade and to increases in heart rate: Implications for gene-specific therapy. *Circulation.* 1995;**92**:3381–3386.

192. Swan H, Viitasalo M, Piippo K, Laitinen P, Kontula K, Toivonen L. Sinus node function and ventricular repolarization during exercise stress test in long QT syndrome patients with KvLQT1 and HERG potassium channel defects. *J Am Coll Cardiol.* 1999;**34**:823–829.

193. Sy RW, Chattha IS, Klein GJ, Gula LJ, Skanes AC, Yee R, Bennett MT, Krahn AD. Repolarization dynamics during exercise discriminate between LQT1 and LQT2 genotypes. *J Cardiovasc Electrophysiol.* 2010;**21**:1242–1246.

194. Wong JA, Gula LJ, Klein GJ, Yee R, Skanes AC, Krahn AD. Utility of treadmill testing in identification and genotype prediction in long-QT syndrome. *Circ Arrhythm Electrophysiol.* 2010;**3**:120–125.

195. Horner JM, Horner MM, Ackerman MJ. The diagnostic utility of recovery phase QTc during treadmill exercise stress testing in the evaluation of long QT syndrome. *Heart Rhythm.* 2011;**8**:1698–1704.

196. Sy RW, van der Werf C, Chattha IS, Chockalingam P, Adler A, Healay JS, Perrin M, Gollob MH, Skanes AC, Yee R, Gula LJ, Leong-Sit P, Viskin S, Klein GJ, Wilder AA, Krahn AD. Derivation and validation of a simple exercise-based algorithm for prediciton of genetic testing in relatives of LQTS probands. *Circulation.* 2011;**124**: 2187–2194.

197. Lahiri MK, Kannankeril PJ, Goldberger JJ. Assessment of autonomic function in cardiovascular disease: Physiological basis and prognostic implications. *J Am Coll Cardiol.* 2008;**51**:1725–1733.

198. Webster G, Berul CI. An update on channelopathies: From mechanisms to management. *Circulation.* 2013;**127**:126–140.

199. MacRae CA. Closer look at genetic testing in long-QT syndrome: Will DNA diagnostics ever be enough? *Circulation.* 2009;**120**:1745–1748.

200. Kapa S, Tester DJ, Salisbury BA, Harris-Kerr C, Pungliya MS, Alders M, Wilde AAM, Ackerman MJ. Genertic testing for long-QT syndrome: Distinguishing pathogenic mutations from benign variants. *Circulation.* 2009;**120**:1752–1760.

201. Tester DJ, Will ML, Haglund CM, Ackerman MJ. Effect of clinical phenotype on yield of long QT syndrome genetic testing. *J Am Coll Cardiol.* 2006;**47**:764–768.

202. Tester DJ, Benton AJ, Train L, Deal B, Baudhuin LM, Ackerman MJ. Prevalence and spectrum of large deletions or duplications in the major long QT syndrome — susceptibility genes and implications for long QT syndrome genetic testing. *Am J Cardiol.* 2010;**106**:1124–1128.

203. Ackerman MJ, Priori SG, Willems S, Berul C, Brugada R, Calkins H, Camm AJ, Ellinor PT, Gollob M, Hamilton R, Hershberger RE, Judge DP, Le Marec H, McKenna WJ, Schulze-Bahr E, Semsarian C, Towbin JA, Watkins H, Wilde A, Wolpert C, Zipes DP. HRS/EHRA Expert Consensus Statement on the State of Genetic Testing for the Channelopathies and Cardiomyopathies. *Heart Rhythm.* 2011;**8**:1308–1339.

204. Meulenkamp TM, Tibben A, Mollema ED, van Langen IM, Wiegman A, de Wert GM, de Beaufort ID, Wilde AA, Smets EM. Predictive genetic testing for cardiovascular diseases: Impact on carrier children. *Am J Med Genet A.* 2008;**146A**:3136–3146.

205. Moss AJ, Zareba W, Hall WJ, Schwartz PJ, Crampton RS, Benhorin J, Vincent GM, Locati EH, Priori SG, Napolitano C, Medina A, Zhang L, Robinson JL, Tmothy K, Towbin JA, Andrews ML. Effectiveness and limitations of beta-blocker therapy in congenital long-QT syndrome. *Circulation.* 2000;**101**:616–623.

206. Vincent GM, Schwartz PJ, Denjoy I, Swan H, Bithell C, Spazzolini C, Crotti L, Piippo K, Lupoglazoff J-M, Villain E, Priori SG, Napolitano C, Zhang L. High efficacy of beta-blockers in long-QT syndrome type 1: Contribution of noncompliance and QT-prolonging drugs to the occurrence of beta-blocker treatment "failures". *Circulation.* 2009;**119**:215–221.

207. Etheridge SP, Compton SJ, Tristani-Firouzi M, Mason JW. A new oral therapy for long QT syndrome. Long-term oral potassium improves repolarization in patients with *HERG* mutations. *J Am Coll Cardiol.* 2003;**42**:1777–1782.

208. Schwartz J, Spazzolini C, Priori SG, Crotti L, Vicentini A, Landolina M, Gasparini M, Wilde AAM, Knops RE, Denjoy I, Toivonen L, Mönnig G, Al-Fayyadh M, Jordaens L, Borggrefe M, Holmgren C, Brugada P, De Roy L, Hohnloser SH, Brink PA. Who are

the long-QT syndrome patients who receive an implantable cardioverter-defibrillator and what happens to them? Data from the European Long-QT Syndrome Implantatble Cardioverter-Defibrillator (LQTS ICD) Registry. *Circulation*. 2010;**122**:1272–1282.

209. Moss AJ, McDonald J. Unilateral cervicothoracic sympathetic ganglionectomy for the treatment of long QT interval syndrome. *N Engl J Med*. 1971;**285**:903–904.

210. Odero A, Bozzani A, De Ferrari GM, Schwartz PJ. Left cardiac sympathetic denervation for the prevention of life-threatening arrhythmias: The surgical supraclavicular approach to cervicothoracic sympathetectomy. *Heart Rhythm*. 2010;**7**:1161–1165.

211. Schwartz PJ, Priori SG, Cerrone M, Spazzolini C, Odero A, Napolitano C, Bloise R, De Ferrari GM, Klersy C, Moss AJ, Zareba W, Robinson JL, Hall WJ, Brink PA, Toivonen L, Epstein AE, Li C, Hu D. Left cardiac sympathetic denervation in the management of high-risk patients affected by the long-QT syndrome. *Circulation*. 2004;**109**:1826–1833.

212. Atallah J, Fynn-Thompson F, Cecchin F, DiBardino DJ, Walsh EP, Berul CL. Video-assisted thorascopic cardiac denervation: A potential novel therapeutic option for children with intractable ventricular arrhythmias. *Ann Thorac Surg*. 2008;**86**:1620–1625.

213. Collura CA, Johnson JN, Moir C, Ackerman MJ. Left cardiac sympathetic denervation for the treatment of long QT syndrome and catecholaminergic polymorphic ventricular tachycardia using video-assisted thoracic surgery. *Heart Rhythm*. 2009;**6**:752–759.

214. Silvey J. On the other side of anorexia. In: *The Columbia Daily Tribune*. Columbia, Missouri; 2010:D4.

215. Basso C, Corrado D, Marcus FI, Nava A, Thiene G. Arrhythmogenic right ventricular cardiomyopathy. *Lancet*. 2009;**273**:1289–1300.

216. Marcus FI, Fontaine GH, Guiraudon G, Frank R, Laurenceau JL, Malergue C, Grosgogeat Y. Right ventricular dysplasia: A report of 24 adult cases. *Circulation*. 1982;**65**:384–398.

217. Basso C, Thiene G, Corrado D, Angelini A, Nava A, Valente M. Arrhythmogenic right ventricular cardiomyopathy: Dysplasia, dystrophy, or myocarditis? *Circulation*. 1996;**94**: 983–991.

218. Fontaine G, Frank R, Guiraudon G, Pavie A, Tereau Y, Chomette G, Grosgogeat Y. Signification des troubles de conduction intraventriculaire observes dans la dysplasie ventriculaire droite arhythmogène. *Arc Mal Coeur*. 1984;**77**:872–879.

219. Corrado D, Basso C, Thiene G, McKenna WJ, Davies MJ, Fontaliran F, Nava A, Silvestri F, Blomstrom-Lundqvist C, Wlodarska EK, Fontaine G, Camerini F. Spectrum of clinicopathologic manifestations of arrhythmogenic right ventricular cardiomyopathy/dysplasia: A multicenter study. *J Am Coll Cardiol*. 1997;**30**:1512–1520.

220. Thiene G, Corrado D, Nava A, Rossi L, Poletti A, Boffa GM, Daliento L, Pennelli N. Right ventricular cardiomyopathy: Is there evidence of an inflammatory aetiology? *Eur Heart J*. 1999;**12** (Supp Dl):22–25.

221. Mallat Z, Tedgui A, Fontaliran F, Frank R, Durigon M, Fontaine G. Evidence of apoptosis in arrhythmogenic right ventricualr dysplasia. *N Engl J Med*. 1996;**335**:1190–1196.

222. Valente M, Calabrese F, Thiene G, Angelini A, Basso C, Nava A, Rossi L. *In vivo* evidence of apoptosis in arrhythmogenic right ventricular cardiomyopathy. *Am J Pathol*. 1998;**152**:479–484.

223. Awad MM, Calkins H, Judge DP. Mechanisms of disease: Molecular genetics of arrhythmogenic right ventricular dysplasia/cardiomyopathy. *Nat Clin Prac Cardiovasc Med*. 2008;**5**:258–267.

224. Gerull B, Heuser A, Witchter T, Paul M, Basson CT, McDermott DA, Lerman BB, Markowitz SM, Ellinor PT, MacRae CA, Peters S, Grossmann KS, Drenckhahn J, Michely B, Sasse-Klaassen S, Birchmeier W, Dietz R, Breithardt G, Schulze-Bahr E, Thierfelder L. Mutations in the desmosomal protein plakophilin-2 are common in arrhythmogenic right ventricular cardiomyopathy. *Nat Genet.* 2004;**36**:1162–1164.

225. Basso C, Czarnowska E, Della Barbera M, Bauce B, Beffagna G, Wlodarska EK, Pilichou K, Ramondo A, Lorenzon A, Wozniek O, Corrado D, Daliento L, Danieli GA, Valente M, Nava A, Thiene G, Rampazzo A. Ultrastructural evidence of intercalated disc remodelling in arrhythmogenic right ventricular cardiomyopathy: An electron microscopy investigation on endomyocardial biopsies. *Eur Heart J.* 2006;**27**:1847–1854.

226. Peters S, Trummel M, Meyners W. Prevalence of right ventricular dysplasia-cardiomyopathy in a non-referral hospital. *Int J Cardiol.* 2004;**97**:499–501.

227. Sen-Chowdhry S, Syrris P, Ward D, Asimaki A, Sevdalis E, McKenna WJ. Clinical and genetic characterization of families with arrhythmogenic right ventricular dysplasia/cardiomyopathy provides novel insights into patterns of disease expression. *Circulation.* 2007;**115**:1710–1720.

228. Sen-Chowdhry S, Syrris P, McKenna WJ. Role of genetic analysis in the management of patients with arrhythmogenic right ventricular dyslplasia/cardiomyopathy. *J Am Coll Cardiol.* 2007;**50**:1813–1821.

229. Dalal D, Nasir K, Bomma C, Prakasa K, Tandri H, Piccini J, Roguin A, Tichnell C, James C, Russell SD, Judge DP, Abraham T, Spevak PJ, Bluemke DA, Calkins H. Arrhythmogenic right ventricular dysplasia: A United States experience. *Circulation.* 2005;**112**:3823–3832.

230. Marcus FI, Zareba W, Calkins H, Towbin JA, Basso C, Bluemke DA, Estes III NA, Picard MH, Sanborn D, Thiene G, Wichter T, Cannom D, Wilber DJ, Scheinman M, Duff H, Daubert J, Talajic M, Krahn A, Sweeney M, Garan H, Sakaguchi S, Lerman BB, Kerr C, Kron J, Steinberg JS, Sherrill D, Gear K, Brown M, Severski P, Polonsky S, McNitt S. Arrhythmogenic right ventricular cardiomyopathy/dysplasia clinical presentation and diagnostic evaluation: Results from the North American Multidisciplinary Study. *Heart Rhythm.* 2009;**6**:984–992.

231. Tabib A, Loire R, Chalabreysse L, Meyronnet D, Miras A, Malicier D, Thivolet F, Chevalier P, Bouvagnet P. Circumstances of death and gross and microscopic observations in a series of 200 cases of sudden death associated with arrhythmogenic right ventricular cardiomyopathy and/or dysplasia. *Circulation.* 2003;**108**:3000–3005.

232. Fontaine G, Fornes P. Histology of sudden death in arrhythmogenic right ventricular cardiomyopathy/Dysplasia. *Circulation.* 2004;**110**:e20.

233. Corrado D, Basso C, Schiavon M, Thiene G. Screening for hypertrophic cardiomyopathy in young athletes. *N Engl J Med.* 1998;**339**:364–369.

234. McKenna WJ, Thiene G, Nava A, Fontaliron F, Blomstrom-Lundquist G, Fontaine G, Camerini F, on behalf of the Task Force of the Working Group Myocardial and Pericardial Disease of the European Society of Cardiology and of the Scientific Council on Cardiomyopathies of the International Society and Federation of Cardiology, supported by the Schoepfer Association. Diagnosis of arrhythmogenic right ventricular dysplaisa/cardiomyopathy. *Br Heart J.* 1994;**71**:215–218.

235. Hurst JW. Naming of the waves in the ECG, with a brief account of their genesis. *Circulation.* 1998;**98**:1937–1942.

236.   Jain R, Dalal D, Daly A, Tichnell C, James C, Evenson A, Jain R, Abraham T, Tan BY, Tandri H, Russell SD, Judge D, Calkins H. Electrocardiographic features of arrhythmogenic right ventricular dysplasia. *Circulation.* 2009;**120**:477–487.

237.   Marcus FI, McKenna WJ, Sherrill D, Basso C, Bauce B, Bluemke DA, Calkins H, Corrado D, Cox MGPJ, Daubert JP, Fontaine G, Gear K, Hauer R, Nava A, Picard MH, Protonotarios N, Saffitz JE, Sanborn DMY, Steinberg JS, Tandri H, Thiene G, Towbin JA, Tsatsopoulou A, Wichter T, Zareba W. Diagnosis of arrhythmogenic right ventricular cardiomyopathy/Dysplasia. Proposed modification of the Task Force Criteria. *Circulation.* 2010;**121**:1533–1541.

238.   Cox MG, van der Smagt JJ, Wilde AA, Wiesfeld AC, Atsma DE, Nelen MR, Rodriguez LM, Loh P, Cramer MJ, Doevendans PA, van Tintelen JP, de Bakker JM, Hauer RN. New ECG criteria in arrhythmogenic right ventricular dysplasia/cardiomyopathy. *Circ Arrhythm Electrophysiol.* 2009;**2**:524–530.

239.   Kamath GS, Zareba W, Delaney J, Koneru JN, McKenna W, Gear K, Polonsky S, Sherrill D, Bluemke D, Marcus F, Steinberg JS. Value of the signal-averaged electrocardiogram in arrhythmogenic right ventricular cardiomyopathy/dysplasia. *Heart Rhythm.* 2011;**8**:256–262.

240.   Blomström-Lundqvist C, Olsson SB, Edvardsson N. Follow-up by repeated signal-averaged surface QRS in patients with the syndrome of arrhythmogenic right ventricular dysplasia. *Eur Heart J.* 1989;**10** (Suppl D):54–60.

241.   Leclercq JF, Coumel P. Late potentials in arrhythmogenic right ventricular dysplasia. Prevalence, diagnostic values. *Eur Heart J.* 1993;**14** (Suppl E):80–83.

242.   Turrini P, Angelini A, Thiene G, Buja G, Daliento L, Rizzoli G, Nava A. Late potentials and ventricular arrhythmias in arrhythmogenic right ventricular cardiomyopathy. *Am J Cardiol.* 1999;**83**:1214–1219.

243.   Turrini P, Corrado D, Basso C, Nava A, Bauce B, Thiene G. Dispersion of ventricular depolarization-repolarization: A noninvasive marker for risk stratification in arrhythmogenic right ventricular cardiomyopathy. *Circulation.* 2001;**103**:3075–3080.

244.   Sahu P, Lim PO, Rana BS, Struthers AD. QT dispersion in medicine: Electrophysiological Holy Grail or fool's gold? *Q J Med.* 2000;**93**:425–431.

245.   Perrin MJ, Angaran P, Laksman Z, Zhang H, Porepa LF, Rutberg J, James C, Krahn AD, Judge DP, Calkins H, Gollob MH. Exercise testing in asymptomatic gene carriers exposes a latent electrical substrate of arrhythmogenic right ventricular cardiomyopathy. *J Am Coll Cardiol.* 2013;**62**:1772–1779.

246.   Sen-Chowdhry S, Prasad SK, Syrris P, Wage R, Ward D, Merrifield R, Smith GC, Firmin DN, Pennell DJ, McKenna WJ. Cardiovascular magnetic resonance in arrhythmogenic right ventricular cardiomyopathy revisited. Comparison with Task Force criteria and genotype. *J Am Coll Cardiol.* 2006;**48**:2132–2140.

247.   Tandri H, Saranathan M, Rodriguez R, Martinez C, Bomma C, Nair K, Rosen B, Lima JAC, Calkins H, Bluemke DA. Noninvasive detection of myocardial fibrosis in arrhythmogenic right ventricular cardiomyopathy using delayed-enhancement magnetic resonance imaging. *J Am Coll Cardiol.* 2005;**45**:98–103.

248.   Maceira AM, Prasad SK, Khan M, Pennell DJ. Reference right ventricular systolic and diastolic function normalized to age, gender and body surface area from steady-state free precession cardiovascular magnetic resonance. *Eur Heart J.* 2006;**27**:2879–2888.

249. Burke AP, Farb A, Tashko G, Virmani R. Arrhythmogenic right ventricular cardiomyopathy and fatty replacement of the right ventricular myocardium: Are they different diseases? *Circulation.* 1998;**97**:1571–1580.

250. Bluemke DA, Krupinski EA, Ovitt T, Gear K, Unger E, Axel L, Boxt LM, Casolo G, Ferrari VA, Funaki B, Globbits S, Higgins CB, Julsrud P, Lipton M, Mawson J, Nygren A, Pennell DJ, Stillman A, White RD, Wichter T, Marcus F. MR imaging of arrhythmogenic right ventricular cardiomyopathy: Morphologic findings and interobserver reliability. *Cardiology.* 2003;**99**:153–162.

251. Tandri H, Castillo E, Ferrari VA, Nasir K, Dalal D, Bomma C, Calkins H, Bluemke DA. Magnetic resonance imaging of arrhythmogenic right ventricular dysplasia: Sensitivity, specificity, and observer variability of fat detection versus functional analysis of the right ventricle. *J Am Coll Cardiol.* 2006;**48**:2277–2284.

252. Maintz D, Juergens KU, Grude M, Ozgun M, Fischbach R, Wichter T. Magnetic resonance imaging and computed tomography findings in arrhythmogenic right ventricular cardiomyopathy. *Circulation.* 2006;**113**:673–675.

253. Winkens MHM, Snoep G, Bekkers SCAM. Imaging of arrhythmogenic right ventricular cardiomyopathy. *Circulation.* 2008;**118**:e158–e159.

254. Cox MG, van der Smagt JJ, Noorman M, Wiesfeld AC, Volders PGA, van Langen IM, Atsma DE, Dooijes D, Howeling AC, Loh P, Jordaens L, Arens Y, Cramer MJ, Doevendans PA, van Tintelen JP, Wilde AA, Haude RN. Arrhythmogenic Right Ventricular Dysplasia/Cardiomyopathy Diagnostic Task Force criteria: Impact of new task force criteria. *Circ Arrhythm Electrophysiol.* 2010;**3**:632–638.

255. Vermes E, Strohm O, Otmani A, Childs H, Duff H, Friedrich MG. Impact of the revision of Arrhythmogenic Right Ventricular Cardiomyopathy/Dysplasia Task Force Criteria on its prevalence by CMR criteria. *J Am Coll Cardiol Img.* 2011;**4**:282–287.

256. Sen-Chowdhry S, Syrris P, Prasad SK, Hughes SE, Merrifield R, Ward D, Pennell DJ, McKenna WJ. Left-dominant arrhythmogenic cardiomyopathy: An under-recognized clinical entity. *J Am Coll Cardiol.* 2008;**52**:2175–2187.

257. Basso C, Ronco F, Marcus F, Abudureheman A, Rizzo S, Frigo AC, Bauce B, Maddalena F, Nava A, Corrado D, Grigoletto F, Thiene G. Quantitative assessment of endomyocardial biopsy in arrhythmogenic right ventricular cardiomyopathy/dysplasia: An *in vitro* validation of diagnostic criteria. *Eur Heart J.* 2008;**29**:2760–2771.

258. Asimaki A, Tandri H, Huang H, Halushka MK, Gautam S, Basso C, Thiene G, Tsatsopoulou A, Protonotarios N, McKenna WJ, Calkins H, Saffitz JE. A new diagnostic test for arrhythmogenic right ventricular cardiomyopathy. *N Engl J Med.* 2009;**360**:1075–1084.

259. Bauce B, Frigo G, Benini G, Michieli P, Basso C, Folino AF, Rigato I, Mazzotti E, Daliento L, Thiene G, Nava A. Differences and similarities between arrhythmogenic right ventricular cardiomyopathy and athlete's heart adaptations. *Br J Sports Med.* 2010;**44**:148–154.

260. Lancisi GM. De Motu Cordis et Aneurysmatibus Opus Posthumum In Duas Partes Divisum. In: Naples, Italy; 1736.

261. Segall HN. Parchment heart (Osler). *Am Heart J.* 1950;**40**:948–950.

262. Sugiura M, Hayashi T, Ueno K. Partial absence of the right ventricular muscle in an aged. *Jpn Heart J.* 1970;**11**:582–585.

263. Uhl HS. A previously undescribed congenital malformation of the heart: Almost total absence of the myocardium of the right ventricle. *Bull Johns Hopkins Hosp.* 1952;**91**: 197–205.

264. Gerlis LM, Schmidt-Ott SC, Ho SY, Anderseon RH. Dysplastic conditions of the right ventricular myocardium: Uhl's anomaly *v* arrhythmogenic right ventricular dysplasia. *Br Heart J.* 1993;**69**:142–150.

265. Uhl HSM. Uhl's anomaly revisited. *Circulation.* 1996;**93**:1483–1484.

266. Thiene G, Nava A, Corrado D, Rossi L, Pennelli N. Right ventricular cardiomyopathy and sudden death in young people. *N Engl J Med.* 1988;**318**:129–133.

267. Martini B, Nava A, Thiene G, Buja GF, Canciani B, Scognamiglio R, Daliento L, Dalla Volta S. Ventricular fibrillation without apparent heart disease: Description of six cases. *Am Heart J.* 1989;**118**:1203–1209.

268. Corrado D, Thiene G, Nava A, Rossi L, Pennelli N. Sudden death in young competitive athletes: Clinicopathologic correlation in 22 cases. *Am J Med.* 1990;**89**:588–596.

269. Antzelevitch C, Brugada P, Borggrefe M, Brugada J, Brugada R, Corrado D, Gussak I, LeMarec H, Nademanee K, Riera ARP, Shimizu W, Schulze-Bahr E, Tan H, Wilde A. Brugada Syndrome. Report of the Second Consensus Conference endorsed by the Heart Rhythm Society and the European Heart Rhythm Association. *Circulation.* 2005;**111**:659–670.

270. Krahn AD, Healey JS, Chauhan V, Birnie DH, Simpson CS, Champagne J, Gardner M, Sanatani S, Exner DV, Klein GJ, Yee R, Skanes AC, Gula LJ, Gollob MH. Systematic assessment of patients with unexplained cardiac arrest. Cardiac Arrest Survivors With Preserved Ejection Fraction Registry (CASPER). *Ciruclation.* 2009;**120**:278–285.

271. Basso C, Corrado D, Bauce B, Thiene G. Arrhythmogenic right ventricular cardiomyopathy. *Circ Arrhythm Electrophysiol.* 2012;**5**:1233–1246.

272. Nava A, Bauce B, Basso C, Muriago M, Rampazzo A, Villanova C, Daliento L, Buja G, Corrado D, Danieli GA, Thiene G. Clinical profile and long-term follow-up of 37 families with arrhythmogenic right ventricular cardiomyopathy. *J Am Coll Cardiol.* 2000;**36**: 2226–2233.

273. Lemola K, Brunckhorst C, Helfenstein U, Oechslin E, Jenni R, Duru F. Predictors of adverse outcome in patients with arrhythmogenic right ventricular dysplasia/cardiomyopathy: Long term experience of a tertiary care centre. *Heart.* 2005;**91**:1167–1172.

274. Corrado D, Leoni L, Link MS, Bella PD, Gaita F, Curnis A, Salerno JU, Igidbashian D, Raviele A, Disertori M, Zanotto G, Verlato R, Vergara G, Delise P, Turrini P, Basso C, Naccarella F, Maddalena F, Estes III NAM, Buja G, Thiene G. Implantable cardioverter-defibrillator therapy for prevention of sudden death in patients with arrhythmogenic right ventricular cardiomyopathy/dysplasia. *Circulation.* 2003;**108**:3084–3091.

275. Tabib A, Loire R. Etude anatomo-clinique de 100 cas d'hypoplasie du muscle ventriclaire droit (dont 89 mortis subites inattendues). Parenté avec l'anomalie d'Uhl. *Arch Mal Coeur.* 1992;**85**:1789–1795.

276. Bauce B, Basso C, Rampazzo A, Beffagna G, Daliento L, Frigo G, Malacrida S, Settimo L, Danieli G, Thiene G, Nava A. Clinical profile of four families with arrhythmogenic right ventricular cardiomyopathy caused by dominant desmoplakin mutations. *Eur Heart J.* 2005;**26**:1666–1675.

277. Bauce B, Rampazzo A, Basso C, Mazzotti E, Rigato I, Steriotis A, Beffagna G, Lorenzon A, De Bortoli M, Pilichou K, Marra MP, Corbetti F, Daliento L, Iliceto S, Corrado D,

Thiene G, Nava A. Clinical phenotype and diagnosis of arrhythmogenic right ventricular cardiomyopathy in pediatric patients carrying desmosomal gene mutations. *Heart Rhythm.* 2011;**8**:1686–1695.

278. d'Amati G, di Gioia CR, Giordano C, Gallo P. Myocyte transdifferentiation: A possible pathogenetic mechanism for arrhythmogenic right ventricular cardiomyopathy. *Arch Pathol Lab Med.* 2000;**124**:287–290.

279. Garcia-Gras E, Lombardi R, Giocondo MJ, Willerson JT, Schneider MD, Khoury DS, Marian AJ. Suppression of canonical Wnt/beta-catenin signaling by nuclear plakoglobin recapitulates phenotype of arrhythmogenic right ventricular cardiomyopathy. *J Clin Invest.* 2006;**116**:2012–2021.

280. te Riele ASJM, Bhonsale A, James CA, Rastegar N, Murray B, Burt JR, Tichnell C, Madhavan S, Judge DP, Bluemke DA, Zimmerman SL, Kamel IR, Calkins H, Tandri H. Incremental value of cardiac magnetic resonance imaging in arrhythmic risk stratification of arrhythmogenic right ventricular dysplasia/cardiomyopathy-associated desmosomal mutation carriers. *J Am Coll Cardiol.* 2013;**62**:1761–1769.

281. Saguner AM, Duru F, Brunckhorst CB. Arrhythmogenic right ventricular cardiomyopathy: A challenging disease of the intercalated disc. *Circulation.* 2013;**128**:1381–1386.

282. Kirchhof P, Fabritz I, Zweiener M, Witt H, Schäfers M, Zellerhoff S, Paul M, Athai T, Hiller K-H, Baba HA, Breithardt G, Ruiz P, Wichter T, Levkau B. Age- and training-dependent development of arrhythmogenic plakoglobin-deficient mice. *Circulation.* 2006;**114**:1799–1806.

283. Corrado D, Basso C, Rizzoli G, Schiavon M, Thiene G. Does sports activity enhance the risk of sudden death in adolescents and young adults? *J Am Coll Cardiol.* 2003;**42**:1959–1963.

284. Wichter T, Borggrefe M, Haverkamp W, Chen X, Breithardt G. Efficacy of antiarrhythmic drugs in patients with arrhythmogenic right ventricular disease. Results in patients with inducible and noninducible ventricular tachycardia. *Circulation.* 1992;**86**:29–37.

285. Canu G, Atallah G, Claudel JP, Champagnac D, Desseigne D, Chevalier P, de Zuloaga C, Moncada E, Kirkorian G, Touboul P. Prognosis and long-term development of arrhythmogenic dysplasia of the right ventricle. *Arch Mal Coeur Vaiss.* 1993;**86**:541–548.

286. Marcus FI, Fontaine GH, Frank R, Gallagher JJ, Reiter MJ. Long-term follow-up in patients with arrhythmogenic right ventricular disease. *Eur Heart J.* 1989; **10**(Suppl D): 68–73.

287. Corrado D, Calkins H, Link MS, Leoni L, Favale S, Bevilacqua M, Basso C, Ward D, Boriani G, Ricci R, Piccini JP, Dalal D, Santini M, Buja G, Iliceto S, Estes III M, Wichter T, McKenna WJ, Thiene G, Marcus FI. Prophylactic implantable defibrillator in patients with arrhythmogenic right ventricular cardiomyopathy/dysplasia and no prior ventricular fibrillation or sustained ventricular tachycardia. *Circulation.* 2010;**122**: 1144–1152.

288. Bhonsale A, James CA, Tichnell C, Murray B, Gagarin D, Philips B, Dalal D, Tedford R, Russell SD, Abraham T, Tandri H, Judge DP, Calkins H. Incidence and predictors of implantable cardioverter-defibrillator therapy in patients with arrhythmogenic right ventricular dysplasia/cardiomyopathy undergoing implantable cardioverter-defibrillator implantation for primary prevention. *J Am Coll Cardiol.* 2011;**58**:1485–1496.

289. Hulot JS, Jouven X, Empana JP, Frank R, Fontaine G. Natural history and risk stratification of arrhythmogenic right ventricular dysplasia/cardiomyopathy. *Circulation.* 2004;**110**:1879–1884.

290. Peters S. Long-term follow-up and risk assessment of arrhythmogenic right ventricular dysplasia/cardiomyopathy: Personal experience from different primary and tertiary centres. *J Cardiovasc Med.* 2007;**8**:521–526.

291. Nasir K, Bomma C, Tandri H, Roguin A, Dalal D, Prakasa K, Tichnell C, James C, Spevak PJ, Marcus F, Calkins H. Electrocardiographic features of arrhythmogenic right ventricular dysplasia/cardiomyopathy according to disease severity: A need to broaden diagnostic criteria. *Circulation.* 2004;**110**:1527–1534.

292. Charron P, Arad M, Arbustini E, Basso C, Bilinska Z, Elliott P, Helio T, Keren A, McKenna WJ, Monserrat L, Pankuweit S, Perrot A, Rapezzi C, Ristic A, Seggewiss H, van Langen I, Tavazzi L, European Society of Cardiology Working Group on Myocardial and Pericardial Diseases. Genetic counselling and testing in cardiomyopathies: A position statement of the European Society of Cardiology Working Group on Myocardial and Pericardial Diseases. *Eur Heart J.* 2010;**31**:2715–2726.

293. Hodgkinson KA, Parfrey PS, Bassett AS, Kupprion C, Drenckhahn J, Norman MW, Thierfelder L, Stuckless SN, Dicks EL, McKenna WJ, Connors SP. The impact of implantable cardioverter-defibrillator therapy on survival in autosomal-dominant arrhythmogenic right ventricular cardiomyopathy (ARVD5). *J Am Coll Cardiol.* 2005;**45**:400–408.

294. Piccini JP, Dalal D, Roguin A, Bomma C, Cheng A, Prakasa K, Dong J, Tichnell C, James C, Russell S, Crosson J, Berger RD, Marine JE, Tomaselli G, Calkins H. Predictors of appropriate implantable defibrillator therapies in patients with arrhythmogenic right ventricular dysplasia. *Heart Rhythm.* 2005;**2**:1188–1194.

295. James CA, Tichnell C, Murray B, Daly A, Sears SF, Calkins H. General and disease-specific psychosocial adjustment in patients with arrhythmogenic right ventricular dysplasia/cardiomyopathy with implantable cardioverter defibrillators: A large cohort study. *Circ Cardiovasc Genet.* 2012;**5**:18–24.

296. Wichter T, Paul M, Wollmann C, Acil T, Gerdes P, Ashraf O, Tjan TD, Soeparwata R, Block M, Borggrefe M, Scheld HH, Breithardt G, Böcker D. Implantable cardioverter/defibrillator therapy in arrhythmogenic right ventricular cardiomyopathy: Single-center experience of long-term follow-up and complications in 60 patients. *Circulation.* 2004;**109**:1503–1508.

297. Roguin A, Bomma CS, Nasir K, Tandri H, Tichnell C, James C, Rutberg J, Crosson J, Spevak PJ, Berger RD, Halperin HR, Calkins H. Implantable cardioverter-defibrillators in patients with arrhythmogenic right ventricular dysplasia/cardiomyopathy. *J Am Coll Cardiol.* 2004;**43**:1843–1852.

298. Fontaine G, Cansell A, Tonet JL, Frank R, Gallais Y, Rougier I, Grosgogeat Y. Techniques and methods for catheter endocardial fulguration. *Pacing Clin Electrophysiol.* 1988;**11**:592–602.

299. Fontaine G, Frank R, Rougier I, Tonet J, Gallais Y, Farenq G, Lascault G, Lilamand M, Fontaliran F, Chomette G, Grosgogeat Y. Electrode catheter ablation of resistant ventricular tachycardia in arrhythmogenic right ventricular dysplasia: Experience of 15 patients with a mean follow-up of 45 months. *Heart Vessels.* 1990;**5**:172–187.

300. Fontaine G, Tonet J, Gallais Y, Lascault G, Hidden-Lucet F, Aouate P, Halimi F, Poulain F, Johnson N, Charfeddine H, Frank R. Ventricular tachycardia catheter ablation in

arrhythmogenic right ventricular dysplasia: A 16-year experience. *Curr Cardiol Rep.* 2000;**2**:498–506.

301. Marchlinski FE, Zado E, Dixit S, Gerstenfeld E, Callans DJ, Hsia H, Lin D, Nayak H, Russo A, Pulliam W. Electroanatomic substrate and outcome of catheter ablative therapy for ventricular tachycardia in setting of right ventricular cardiomyopathy. *Circulation.* 2004;**110**:2293–2298.

302. Ellison KE, Friedman PL, Ganz LI, Stevenson WG. Entrainment mapping and radiofrequency catheter ablation of ventricular tachycardia in right ventricular dysplasia. *J Am Coll Cardiol.* 1988;**32**:724–728.

303. Reithmann C, Hahnefeld A, Remp T, Dorwarth U, Dugas M, Steinbeck G, Hoffmann E. Electroanatomic mapping of endocardial right ventricular activation as a guide for catheter ablation in patients with arrhythmogenic right ventricular dysplasia. *Pacing Clin Electrophysiol.* 2003;**26**:1308–1316.

304. Verma A, Kilicaslan F, Schweikert RA, Tomassoni G, Rossillo A, Marrouche NF, Ozduran V, Wazni OM, Elayi SC, Saenz LC, Minor S, Cummings JE, Burkhardt JD, Hao S, Beheiry S, Tchou PJ, Natale A. Short- and long-term success of substrate-based mapping and ablation of ventricular tachycardia in arrhythmogenic right ventricular dysplasia. *Circulation.* 2005;**111**:3209–3216.

305. Dalal D, Jain R, Tandri H, Dong J, Eid SM, Prakasa K, Tichnell C, James C, Abraham T, Russell SD, Sinha S, Judge DP, Bluemke DA, Marine JE, Calkins H. Long-term efficacy of catheter ablation of ventricular tachycardia in patients with arrhythmogenic right ventricular dysplasia/cardiomyopathy. *J Am Coll Cardiol.* 2007;**50**:432–440.

306. Garcia FC, Bazan V, Zado ES, Ren JF, Marchlinski FE. Epicardial substrate and outcome with epicardial ablation of ventricular tachycardia in arrhythmogenic right ventricular cardiomyopathy/dysplasia. *Circulation.* 2009;**120**:366–375.

307. Philips B, Madhavan S, James C, Tichnell C, Murray B, Dalal D, Bhonsale A, Nazarian S, Judge DP, Russell SD, Abraham T, Calkins H, Tandri H. Outcomes of catheter ablation of ventricular tachycardia in arrhythmogenic right ventricular dysplasia/cardiomyopathy. *Circ Arrhythm Electrophysiol.* 2012;**5**:499–505.

308. Coleman MA, Bos JM, Johnson JN, Owen HJ, Deschamps C, Moir C, Ackerman MJ. Videoscopic left cardiac sympathetic denervation for patients with recurrent ventricular fibrillation/malignant ventricular arrhythmia syndromes besides congenital long-QT syndrome. *Circ Arrhythm Electrophysiol.* 2012;**5**:782–788.

309. Tedford RJ, James C, Judge DP, Tichnell C, Bhonsale A, Philips B, Abraham T, Dalal D, Halushka MK, Tandri H, Calkins H, Russell SD. Cardiac transplantation in arrhythmogenic right ventricular dysplasia/cardiomyopathy. *J Am Coll Cardiol.* 2012;**59**:289–290.

310. Bauce B, Daliento L, Frigo G, Russo G, Nava A. Pregnancy in women with arrhythmogenic right ventricular cardiomyopathy/dysplasia. *Eur J Obstet Gynecol Reprod Biol.* 2006;**127**:186–189.

311. Hamid MS, Norman M, Quraishi A, Firoozi S, Thaman R, Gimeno JR, Sachdev B, Rowland E, Elliott PM, McKenna WJ. Prospective evaluation of relatives for familial arrhythmogenic right ventricular cardiomyopathy/dysplasia reveals a need to broaden diagnostic criteria. *J Am Coll Cardiol.* 2002;**40**:1445–1450.

312. Pilichou K, Nava A, Basso C, Beffagna G, Bauce B, Lorenzon A, Frigo G, Vettori A, Valente M, Towbin J, Thiene G, Danielli GA, Rampazzo A. Mutations in desmoglein-2 gene are associated with arrhythmogenic right ventricular cardiomyopathy. *Circulation.* 2006;**113**:1171–1179.

313.   Cox MGPJ, van der Zwaag PA, van der Werf C, van der Smagt JJ, Noorman M, Bhuiyan ZA, Wiesfeld ACP, Volders PGA, van Langen IM, Atsma DE, Dooijes D, van den Wijngaard A, Houweling AC, Jongbloed JDH, Jordaens L, Cramer MJ, Doevendans PA, de Bakker JMT, Wilde AAM, van Tintelen JP, Hauer RNW. Arrhythmogenic right ventricular dysplasia/cardiomyopathy: Pathogenic desmosone mutations in index-patients predict outcome of family screening: Dutch Arrhythmogenic Right Ventricular Dysplasia/Cardiomyopathy Genotype-Phenotype Follow-up Study. *Circulation*. 2011;**123**:2690–2700.

314.   Quarta G, Muir A, Pantazis A, Syrris P, Gehmlich K, Garcia-Pavia P, Ward D, Sen-Chowdhry S, Elliot PM, McKenna WJ. Familial evaluation in arrhythmogenic right ventricular cardiomyopathy: Impact of genetics and revised Task Force criteria. *Circulation*. 2011;**123**:2701–2709.

315.   Kapplinger JD, Landstrom AP, Salisbury BA, Callis TE, Pollevick GD, Tester DJ, Cox MGPJ, Bhuiyan Z, Bikker H, Wiesfeld ACP, Hauer RNW, van Tintelen JP, Jongbloed JDH, Calkins H, Judge DP, Wilde AAM, Ackerman MJ. Distinguishing arrhythmogenic right ventricular cardiomyopathy/dysplasia-associated mutations from background genetic noise. *J Am Coll Cardiol*. 2011;**57**:2317–2327.

316.   Dalal D, Molin LH, Piccini J, Tichnell C, James C, Bomma C, Prakasa K, Towbin JA, Marcus FI, Spevak PJ, Bluemke DA, Abraham T, Russell SD, Calkins H, Judge DP. Clinical features of arrhythmogenic right ventricular dysplasia/cardiomyopathy associated with mutations in plakophilin-2. *Circulation*. 2006;**113**:1641–1649.

317.   van Tintelen JP, Entius MM, Bhuiyan ZA, Jongbloed R, Wiesfeld ACP, Wilde AAM, van der Smagt J, Boven LG, Mannens MMAM, van Langen IM, Hofstra RMW, Otterspoor LC, Doevendans PAFM, Rodriguez L-M, van Gelder IC, Hauer RNW. Plakophilin-2 mutations are the major determinant of familial arrhythmogenic right ventricular dysplasia/cardiomyopathy. *Circulation*. 2006;**113**:1650–1658.

318.   Dalal D, James C, Devanagondi R, Tichnell C, Tucker A, Prakasa K, Spevak PJ, Bluemke DA, Abraham T, Russell SD, Calkins H, Judge DP. Penetrance of mutations in plakophilin-2 among families with arrhythmogenic right ventricular dysplasia/cardiomyopathy. *J Am Coll Cardiol*. 2006;**48**:1416–1424.

319.   Syrris P, Ward D, Asimaki A, Evans A, Sen-Chowdhry S, Hughes SE, McKenna WJ. Desmoglein-2 mutations in arrhythmogenic right ventricular cardiomyopathy: A genotype-phenotype characterization of familial disease. *Eur Heart J*. 2007;**28**:581–588.

320.   Sen-Chowdhry S, Syrris P, Pantazis A, Quarta G, McKenna WJ, Chambers JC. Mutational heterogeneity, modifier genes, and environmental influences contribute to phenotypic diversity of arrhythmogenic cardiomyopathy. *Circ Cardiovasc Genet*. 2010;**3**:323–330.

321.   Lahtinen AM, Lehtonen E, Marjamaa A, Kaartinen M, Heliö T, Porthan K, Oikarinen L, Toivonen L, Swan H, Jula A, Peltonen L, Palotie A, Salomaa V, Kontula K. Population-prevalent desmosomal mutations predisposing to arrhythmogenic right ventricular cardiomyopathy. *Heart Rhythm*. 2011;**8**:1214–1221.

322.   den Haan AD, Tan BY, Zikusoka MN, Lladó LI, Jain R, Daly A, Tichnell C, James C, Amat-Alarcon N, Abraham T, Russell SD, Bluemke DA, Calkins H, Dalal D, Judge DP. Comprehensive desmosome mutation analysis in North Americans with arrhythmogenic right ventricular dysplasia/cardiomyopathy. *Circ Cardiovasc Genet*. 2009;**2**:4 28–435.

323. Christensen AH, Benn M, Bundgaard H, Tybjaerg-Hansen A, Haunso S, Svendsen JH. Wide spectrum of desmosomal mutations in Danish patients with arrhythmogenic right ventricular cardiomyopathy. *J Med Genet.* 2010;**47**:736–744.

324. Bauce B, Nava A, Beffagna G, Basso C, Lorenzon A, Smaniotto G, De Bortoli M, Rigato I, Mazzotti E, Steriotis A, Marra MP, Towbin JA, Thiene G, Danieli GA, Rampazzo A. Multiple mutations in desmosomal proteins encoding genes in arrhythmogenic right ventricular cardiomyopathy/dysplasia. *Heart Rhythm.* 2010;**7**:22–29.

325. Xu T, Yang Z, Vatta M, Rampazzo A, Beffagna G, Pillichou K, Scherer SE, Saffitz J, Kravitz J, Zareba W, Danieli GA, Lorenzon A, Nava A, Bauce B, Thiene G, Basso C, Calkins H, Gear K, Marcus F, Towbin JA. Compound and digenic heterozygosity contributes to arrhythmogenic right ventricular cardiomyopathy. *J Am Coll Cardiol.* 2010;**55**:587–597.

326. Protonotarios N, Tsatsopoulou A, Anastasakis A, Sevdalis E, McKoy G, Stratos K, Gatzoulis K, Tentolouris K, Spiliopoulou C, Panagiotakos D, McKenna W, Toutouzas P. Genotype-phenotype assessment in autosomal recessive arrhythmogenic right ventricular cardiomyopathy (Naxos disease) caused by a deletion in plakoglobin. *J Am Coll Cardiol.* 2001;**38**:1477–1484.

327. van der Zwaag PA, Jongbloed JD, van den Berg MP, van der Smagt JJ, Jongbloed R, Bikker H, Hofstra RM, van Tintelen JP. A genetic variants database for arrhythmogenic right ventricular dysplasia/cardiomyopathy. *Hum Mutat.* 2008;**30**:1278–1283.

328. Marcus FI, Edson S, Towbin JA. Genetics of arrhythmogenic right ventricular cardiomyopathy. A practical guide for physicians. *J Am Coll Cardiol.* 2013;**61**:1945–1948.

329. Corrado D, Basso C, Leoni L, Tokajuk B, Bauce B, Frigo G, Tarantini G, Napodano M, Turrini P, Ramondo A, Daliento L, Nava A, Buja G, Iliceto S, Thiene G. Three-dimensional electroanatomic voltage mapping increases accuracy of diagnosing arrhythmogenic right ventricular cardiomyopathy/dysplasia. *Circulation.* 2005;**111**:3042–3050.

330. Saguner AM, Medeiros-Domingo A, Schwyzer MA, On CJ, Haegeli LM, Wolber T, Hürlimann D, Steffel J, Krasniqi N, S R, Held L, Lüscher TF, Brunckhorst C, Duru F. Usefulness of inducible ventricular tachycardia to predict long-term adverse outcomes in arrhythmogenic right ventricular cardiomyopathy. *Am J Cardiol.* 2013;**111**:250–257.

331. James CA, Bhonsale A, Tichnell C, Murray B, Russell SD, Tandri H, Tedford RJ, Judge DP, Calkins H. Exercise increases age-related penetrance and arrhythmic risk in arrhythmogenic right ventricular dysplasia/cardiomyopathy-associated desmosomal mutatin carriers. *J Am Coll Cardiol.* 2013;**62**:1290–1297.

332. Fabritz L, Fortmüller L, Yu TY, Paul M, Kirchhof P. Can preload-reducing therapy prevent disease progression in arrhythmogenic right ventricular cardiomyopathy? Experimental evidence and concept for a clinical trial. *Prog Biophys Mol Biol.* 2012;**110**:340–346.

333. Wong D. Men who built Singapore: Thai workers in the Construction Industry. In: Chantavanich S, Germershausen A, Beesey A, eds. *Thai migrant workers in East and Southeast Asia 1996–1997.* Bangkok, Thailand: Asia Research Center for Migration, Institute of Asian Studies, Chulalongkorn University; 2000:58–107.

334. Goh KT, Chao TC, Chew CH. Sudden nocturnal deaths among Thai construction workers in Singapore. *Lancet.* 1990;**335**:1154.

335. Kitiarsa P. *Village transnationalism: Transborder identities among Thai-Isan migrant workers in Singapore.* Singapore: Asia Research Institute; 2006.

336. Erlanger S. Singapore Journal; "Nightmare Death" fells Thais, and nations bicker. *The New York Times.* 8 May 1990.

337. Tatsanavivat P, Chiravatkul A, Klungboonkrong V, Chaisiri S, Jarerntanyaruk L, Munger R, Saowakontha S. Sudden and unexplained deaths in sleep (Laitai) of young men in rural northeastern Thailand. *Int J Epidemiol.* 1992;**21**:904–910.

338. Guazon MPH. Algunas notas sobre bangungut. *Revista Filipina de Medicina Y Farmacia.* 1917;**8**:37–42.

339. Majoska AV. Sudden death in Filipino men; an unexplained syndrome. *Hawaii Med J.* 1948;**7**:469–473.

340. Aponte GE. The enigma of "bangungut". *Ann Intern Med.* 1960;**52**:1258–1283.

341. Munger RG, Booton EA. Bangungut in Manila: Sudden and unexplained death in sleep of adult Filipinos. *Int J Epidemiol.* 1998;**27**:677–684.

342. Baron RC, Thacker SB, Gorelkin L, Vernon AA, Taylor WR, Choi K. Sudden death among Southeast Asian refugees. An unexplained nocturnal phenomenon. *JAMA.* 1983;**250**:2947–2951.

343. Centers for Disease Control and Prevention. Update: Sudden unexplained death syndrome among Southeast Asian refugees — United States. *MMWR.* 1988;**37**:568–570.

344. Adler SR. Refugee stress and folk belief: Hmong sudden deaths. *Soc Sci Med.* 1995;**40**:1623–1629.

345. Kirschner RH, Eckner FAO, Baron RC. The cardiac pathology of sudden, unexplained nocturnal death in Southeast Asian refugees. *JAMA.* 1986;**256**:2700–2705.

346. Munger RG, Booton EA. Thiamine and sudden death in sleep of South-East Asian refugees. *Lancet.* 1990;**335**:1154–1155.

347. Munger RG, Jones MP, Prineas RJ, Crow RS, Changbumrung S, Wangsuphachart V, Keane V. Prolonged QT interval and risk of sudden death in South-East Asian men. *Lancet.* 1991;**338**:280–281.

348. Nimmannit S, Malasit P, Chaovakul V, Susaengrat W, Vasuvattakul S, Nilwarangkur S. Pathogenesis of sudden unexplained sudden nocturnal death (lai tai) and endemic distal renal tubular acidosis. *Lancet.* 1991;**338**:930–932.

349. Otto CM, Tauxe RV, Cobb LA, Greene L, Gross BW, Werner JA, Burroughs RW, Samson WE, Weaver WD, Trobaugh GB. Ventricular fibrillation causes sudden death in Southeast Asian immigrants. *Ann Intern Med.* 1984;**100**:45–47.

350. Torjesen I. Pioneers in Cardiology: Pedro Brugada, MD, PhD. Unravelling the genetics of arrhythmia and working to prevent and treat heart failure. *Circulation.* 2008;**117**:f37–f42.

351. Brugada P, Brugada J. Right bundle branch block, persistent ST segment elevation and sudden cardiac death: A distinct clinical and electrocardiographic syndrome. A multicenter report. *J Am Coll Cardiol.* 1992;**20**:1391–1396.

352. Raju H, Papadakis M, Govindan M, Bastiaenen R, Chandra N, O'Sullivan A, Baines G, Sharma S, Behr ER. Low prevalence of risk markers in cases of sudden death due to Brugada syndrome: Relevance to risk stratification in Brugada syndrome. *J Am Coll Cardiol.* 2011;**57**:2340–2345.

353. Miyasaka Y, Tsuji H, Yamada K, Tokunaga S, Saito D, Imuro Y, Matsumoto N, Iwasaka T. Prevalence and mortality of the Brugada-type electrocardiogram in one city in Japan. *J Am Coll Cardiol.* 2001;**38**:771–774.

354. Nademanee K, Veerakul G, Nimmannit S, Chaowakul V, Bhuripanyo K, Likittanasombat K, Tunsanga K, Kuasirikul S, Malasit P, Tansupasawadikul S, Tatsanavivat P. Arrhythmogenic marker for the sudden unexplained death syndrome in Thai Men. *Circulation.* 1997;**96**:2595–2600.

355. Vatta M, Dumaine R, Varghese G, Richard TA, Shimizu W, Aihara N, Nademanee K, Brugada R, Brugada J, Veerakul G, Li H, Bowles NE, Brugada P, Antzelevitch C, Towbin JA. Genetic and biophysical basis of sudden unexplained nocturnal death syndrome (SUNDS), a disease allelic to Brugada syndrome. *Hum Mol Genet.* 2002;**11**:337–345.

356. Kapplinger JD, Tester DJ, Alders M, Benito B, Berthet M, Brugada J, Brugada P, Fressart V, Guerchicoff A, Harris-Kerr C, Kamakura S, Kyndt F, Koopmann TT, Miyamoto Y, Pfeiffer R, Pollevick GD, Probst V, Zumhagen S, Vatta M, Towbin JA, Shimizu W, Schulze-Bahr E, Antzelevitch C, Salisbury BA, Guicheney P, Wilde AA, Brugada R, Schott JJ, Ackerman MJ. An international compendium of mutations in the SCN5A-encoded cardiac sodium channel in patients referred for Brugada syndrome genetic testing. *Heart Rhythm.* 2009;**7**:33–46.

357. Kapplinger JD, Tester DJ, Alders M, Benito B, Berthet M, Brugada J, Brugada P, Fressart V, Guerchicoff A, Harris-Kerr C, Kamakura S, Kyndt F, Koopmann TT, Miyamoto Y, Pfeiffer R, Pollevick GD, Probst V, Zumhagen S, Vatta M, Towbin JA, Shimizu W, Schulze-Bahr E, Antzelevitch C, Salisbury BA, Guicheney P, Wilde AA, Brugada R, Schott JJ, Ackerman MJ. An international compendium of mutations in the SCN5A-encoded cardiac sodium channel in patients referred for Brugada syndrome genetic testing. *Heart Rhythm.* 2010;**7**:33–46.

358. Hu D, Barajas-Martínez H, Pfeiffer R, Dezi F, Pfeiffer J, Buch T, Betzenhauser MJ, Belardinelli L, Kahlig KM, Rajamani S, DeAntonio HJ, Myerburg RJ, Ito H, Deshmukh P, Marieb M, Nam G-B, Bhatia A, Hasdemir C, Haïssaguerre M, Veltmann C, Schimpf R, Borggrefe M, Viskin S, Antzelevitch C. Mutations in *SCN10A* are responsible for a large fraction of cases of Brugada syndrome. *J Am Coll Cardiol.* 2014;**64**:66–79.

359. Nogami A, Nakao M, Kubota S, Sugiyasu A, Doi H, Yokoyama K, Yumoto K, Tamaki T, Kato K, Hosokawa N, Sagai H, Nakamura H, Nitta J, Yamauchi Y, Aonuma K. Enhancement of J-ST-elevation by glucose and insulin test in Brugada syndrome. *Pacing Clin Electrophysiol.* 2003;**26**:332–337.

360. Mizumaki K, Fujiki A, Nishida K, Iwamoto J, Sakamoto T, Sakabe M, Tsuneda T, Sugao M, Inoue H. Postprandial augmentation of bradycardia-dependent ST elevation in patients with Brugada syndrome. *J Cardiovasc Electrophysiol.* 2007;**18**:839–844.

361. Antzelevitch C, Brugada R. Fever and Brugada syndrome. *Pacing Clin Electrophysiol.* 2002;**25**:1537–1539.

362. Miyazaki T, Mitamura H, Miyoshi S, Soejima K, Aizawa Y, Ogawa S. Autonomic and antiarrhythmic drug modulation of ST segment elevation in patients with Brugada syndrome. *J Am Coll Cardiol.* 1996;**27**:1061–1070.

363. Batchvarov VN, Govindan M, Macfarlane P, Camm AJ, Behr ER. Diagnostic utility of bipolar precordial leads during ajmaline testing for suspected Brugada syndrome. *Heart Rhythm.* 2010;**7**:208–215.

364. Veltmann C, Schimpf R, Echternach C, Eckardt L, Kuschyk J, Streitner F, Sphehl S, Borggrefe M, Wolpert C. A prospective study on spontaneous fluctuations between diagnostic and non-diagnostic ECGs in Brugada syndrome: Implications for correct phenotyping and risk stratification. *Eur Heart J.* 2006;**27**:2544–2552.

365. Hong K, Brugada J, Oliva A, Berruezo-Sanchez A, Potenza D, Pollevick GD, Guerchicoff A, Matsuo K, Burashnikov E, Dumaine R, Towbin JA, Nesterenko V, Brugada P, Antzelevitch C, Brugada R. Value of electrocardiographic parameters and ajmaline test in the diagnosis of Brugada syndrome caused by SCN5A mutation. *Circulation.* 2004;**110**:3023–3027.

366. Matsuo K, Akahoshi M, Nakashima E, Suyama A, Seto S, Hayano M, Yano K. The prevalence, incidence and prognostic value of the Brugada-type electrocardiogram. A population-based study of four decades. *J Am Coll Cardiol.* 2001;**38**:765–770.

367. Sakabe M, Fujiki A, Tani M, Nishida K, Mizumaki K, Inoue H. Proportion and prognosis of healthy people with coved or saddle-back type ST segment elevation in the right precordial leads during 10 years follow-up. *Eur Heart J.* 2003;**24**:1488–1493.

368. Priori SG, Napolitano C, Gasparini M, Pappone C, Della Bella P, Giordano U, Bloise R, Giustetto C, De Nardis R, Grillo M, Ronchetti E, Faggiano G, Nastoli J. Natural history of Brugada syndrome: Insights for risk stratification and management. *Circulation.* 2002;**105**:1342–1347.

369. Priori SG, Gasparini M, Napolitano C, Bella PD, Ottonelli AG, Sassone B, Giordano U, Pappone C, Mascioli G, Rossetti G, De Nardis R, Colombo M. Risk stratification in Brugada syndrome. Results of the PRELUDE (PRogrammed ELectrical stimUlation preDictive valuE) Registry. *J Am Coll Cardiol.* 2011;**59**:37–45.

370. Sarkozy A, Sorgente A, Boussy T, Casado R, Paprella G, Capulzini L, Chierchia G-B, Yazaki Y, De Asmundis C, Coomans D, Brugada J, Brugada P. The value of a family history of sudden death in patients with diagnostic type I Brugada ECG pattern. *Eur Heart J.* 2011;**32**:2153–2160.

371. Benito B, Sarkozy A, Mont L, Henkens S, Berruezo A, Tamborero D, Arzamendi D, Berne P, Brugada R, Brugada P, Brugada J. Gender differences in clinical manifestations of Brugada syndrome. *J Am Coll Cardiol.* 2008;**52**:1567–1577.

372. Probst V, Veltmann C, Eckardt L, Meregalli PG, Gaita F, Tan HL, Babuty D, Sacher F, Giustetto C, Schulze-Bahr E, Borggrefe M, Haissaguerre M, Mabo P, Le Marec H, Wolpert C, Wilde AAM. Long-term prognosis of patients diagnosed with Brugada syndrome. Results of the FINGER Brugada Syndrome Registry. *Circulation.* 2010;**121**: 635–643.

373. Tsuji H, Sato T, Morisaki K, Iwasaka T. Prognosis of subjects with Brugada-type electro-cardiogram in a population of middle-aged Japanese diagnosed during a health examination. *Am J Cardiol.* 2008;**102**:584–587.

374. Zipes DP, Camm JA, Borggrefe M, Buxton AE, Chaitman B, Fromer M, Gregoratos G, Klein G, Moss AJ, Myerburg RJ, Priori SG, Quinones MA, Roden DM, Silka MJ, Tracy C. ACC/AHA/ESC 2006 Guidelines for management of patients with ventricular arrhythmias and the prevention of sudden death. A report of the American College of Cardiology/American Heart Association Task Force and the European Society of Cardiology Committee for Practice Guidelines (Writing Committee to develop guidelines for management of patients with ventricular arrhythmias and the prevention of sudden cardiac death) developed in collaboration with the European

Heart Rhythm Association and the Heart Rhythm Society. *Circulation*. 2006;**114**: 385–484.

375. Paul M, Gerss J, Schulze-Bahr E, Wichter T, Vahlhaus C, Wilde AAM, Breithardt G, Eckardt L. Role of programmed ventricular stimuation in patients with Brugada syndrome: A meta-analysis of worldwide published data. *Eur Heart J*. 2007;**28**: 2126–2133.

376. Morita H, Kusano KF, Miura D, Nagase S, Nakamura K, Morita ST, Ohe T, Zipes DP, Wu J. Fragmented QRS as a marker of conduction abnormality and a predictor of prognosis of Brugada syndrome. *Circulation*. 2008;**118**:1697–1704.

377. Fish JM, Antzelevitch C. Role of sodium and calcium channel block in unmasking the Brugada syndrome. *Heart Rhythm*. 2004;**1**:210–217.

378. Brugada J, Brugada R, Brugada P. Right bundle-branch block and ST-segment elevation in leads V1 through V3: A marker for sudden death in patients without demonstrable structural heart disease. *Circulation*. 1998;**97**:457–460.

379. Hermida J-S, Denjoy I, Clerc J, Extramiana F, Jarry G, Milliez P, Guicheney P, Di Fusco S, Rey J-L, Cauchemez B, Leenhardt A. Hydroquinidine therapy in Brugada syndrome. *J Am Coll Cardiol*. 2004;**43**:1853–1860.

380. Belhassen B, Glick A, Viskin S. Efficacy of quinidine in high-risk patients with Brugada syndrome. *Circulation*. 2004;**110**:1731–1737.

381. Tsuchiya T, Ashikaga K, Honda T, Arita M. Prevention of ventricular fibrillation by cilostazol, an oral phosphodiesterase inhibitor, in a patient with Brugada syndrome. *J Cardiovasc Electrophysiol*. 2002;**13**:698–701.

382. Nademanee K, Veerakul G, Chandanamattha P, Chaothawee L, Ariyachaipanich A, Jirasirirojanakorn K, Likttanasombat K, Bhuripanyo K, Ngarmukos T. Prevention of ventricular fibrillation episodes in Brugada syndrome by catheter ablation over ther anterior right ventricular outflow tract epicardium. *Circulation*. 2011;**123**: 1270–1279.

383. Richardson P, McKenna W, Bristow M, Maisch B, Mautner B, O'Connell J, Olsen E, Thiene G, Goodwin J, Gyafas I, Martin I, Nordet P. Report of the 1995 World Health Organization/International Society and Federation of Cardiology Task Force on the Definition and Classification of Cardiomyopathies. *Circulation*. 1996;**93**:841–842.

384. Kindermann I, Barth C, Mahfoud F, Ukena C, Lenski M, Yilmaz A, Klingel K, Kandolf R, Sechtem U, Cooper LT, Böhm M. Update on myocarditis. *J Am Coll Cardiol*. 2012;**59**:779–792.

385. Corvisart JN. Essai sur les maladies et les lésions organisque du coeur. *Gast J MMSS*. 1812;**182**:299–303.

386. Dennert R, Crijns HJ, Heymans S. Acute viral myocarditis. *Eur Heart J*. 2008;**29**: 2073–2082.

387. Mason JW, O'Connell JB, Herskowitz A, Rose NR, McManus BM, Billingham ME, Moon TE. A clinical trial of immunosuppressive therapy for myocarditis. The Myocarditis Treatment Trial Investigators. *N Engl J Med*. 1995;**333**:269–275.

388. Mavrogeni S, Spargias K, Bratis C, Kolovou G, Papadopoulou E, Pavlides G. EBV infection as a cause of VT: Evaluation by CMR. *J Am Coll Cardiol Img*. 2011;**4**:561–562.

389. Bratincsák A, El-Said HG, Bradley JS, Shayan K, Grossfeld PD, Cannavino CR. Fulminant myocarditis associated with pandemic H1N1 influenza A virus in children. *J Am Coll Cardiol*. 2010;**55**:928–929.

390.   Mavrogeni S, Bratis C, Kitsiou A, Kolovou G, Manoussakis MN, Papadopoulou E, Magoutas A, Pavlides G. CMR assessment of myocarditis in patients with cardiac symptoms during H1N1 viral infection. *J Am Coll Cardiol Img.* 2011;**4**:307–309.

391.   Bültmann BD, Klingel K, Sotlar K, Bock CT, Baba HA, Sauter M, Kandolf R. Fatal parvovirus B19-associated myocarditis clinically mimicking ischemic heart dieasea: An endothelial cell-mediated disease. *Hum Pathol.* 2003;**34**:92–95.

392.   Ventéo L, Bourlet T, Renois F, Douche-Aourik F, Mosnier J-F, De la Grand Maison GL, Pluot M, Pozzetto B, Andreoletti L. Enterovirus-related activation of the cardiomyocyte mitochondrial apoptotic pathway in patients with acute myocarditis. *Eur Heart J.* 2010;**31**:728–736.

393.   Caforio ALP, Pankuweit S, Arbustini E, Basso C, Gimeno-Blanes J, Felix SB, Fu M, Heliö T, Heymans S, Jahns R, Klingel K, Linhart A, Maisch B, McKenna W, Mogensen J, Pinto YM, Ristic A, Schulthesis H-P, Seggewiss H, Tavazzi L, Thiene G, Yilmaz A, Charron P, Elliot PM. Current state of knowledge on aetiology, diagnosis, management, and therapy of myocarditis: A position statement of the European Society of Cardiology Working Group on Myocardial and Pericardial Diseases. *Eur Heart J.* 2013;**34**:2636–2648.

394.   Freimuth P, Philipson L, Carson SD. The coxsackievirus and adenovirus receptor. *Curr Top Microbiol Immunol.* 2008;**323**:67–87.

395.   Shi Y, Chen C, Lisewski U, Wrackmeyer U, Radke M, Westermann D, Sauter M, Tschöpe C, Poller W, Klingel K, Gotthardt M. Cardiac deletion of the Coxsackievirus-Adenovirus Receptor abolishes coxackievirus B3 infection and prevents myocarditis in vivo. *J Am Coll Cardiol.* 2009;**53**:1219–1226.

396.   Caforio AL, Mahon NJ, Tona F, McKenna WJ. Circulating cardiac autoantibodies in dilated cardiomyopathy and myocarditis: Pathogenetic and clinical significance. *Eur J Heart Fail.* 2002;**4**:411–417.

397.   Lee GH, Badorff C, Knowlton KU. Dissociation of sarcoglycans and the dystrophin carboxyl terminus from the sarcolemma in enteroviral cardiomyopathy. *Circ Res.* 2000;**87**:887–893.

398.   Phillips M, Robinowitz M, Higgins JR, Boran KJ, Reed T, Virmani R. Sudden cardiac death in Air Force recruits: A 20-year review. *JAMA.* 1986;**256**:2696–2699.

399.   Caforio ALP, Calabrese F, Angelini A, Tona F, Vinci A, Bottaro S, Ramondo A, Carturan E, Illiceto S, Thiene G, Daliento L. A prospective study of biopsy-proven myocarditis: Prognostic relevance of clinical and aetiopathogenetic features at diagnosis. *Eur Heart J.* 2007;**28**:1326–1333.

400.   Woodruff JF. Viral myocarditis: A review. *Am J Pathol.* 1980;**101**: 425–484.

401.   Smith WG. Coxsackie B myopericarditis in adults. *Am Heart J.* 1970;**80**:34–46.

402.   Mahrholdt H, Wagner A, Deluigi CC, Kispert E, Hager S, Meinhardt G, Vogelsberg H, Fritz P, Dippon J, Bock C-T, Klingel K, Kandolf R, Sechtem U. Presentation, patterns of myocardial damage, and clinical course of viral myocarditis. *Circulation.* 2006;**114**:1 581–1590.

403.   Abdel-Aty H, Boyé P, Zagrosek A, Wassmuth R, Kumar A, Messroghli D, Bock P, Dietz R, Friedrich MG, Schulz-Menger J. Diagnostic performance of cardiovascular magnetic resonance in patients with suspected acute myocarditis. *J Am Coll Cardiol.* 2005;**45**: 1815–1822.

404.   Francone M, Chimenti C, Galea N, Scopelliti F, Verardo R, Galea R, Carbone I, Catalano C, Fedele F, Frustaci A. CMR sensitivity varies with clinical presentation and

extent of cell necrosis in biopsy-proven acute myocarditis. *J Am Coll Cardiol Img.* 2014;**7**:254–263.

405. Zagrosek A, Abdel-Aty H, Boyé P, Wassmuth R, Messroghli D, Utz W, Rudolph A, Bohl S, Dietz R, Schulz-Menger J. Cardiac magnetic resonance monitors reversible and irreversible myocardial injury in myocarditis. *J Am Coll Cardiol Img.* 2009;**2**:131–138.

406. Mahrholdt H, Goedecke C, Wagner A, Meinhardt G, Athanasiadis A, Vogelsberg H, Fritz P, Klingel K, Kandolf R, Sechtem U. Cardiovascular magnetic resonance assessment of human myocarditis: A comparison to histology and molecular pathology. *Circulation.* 2004;**109**:1250–1258.

407. Friedrich MG, Sechtem U, Schulz-Menger J, Holmvang G, Alakija P, Cooper LT, White JA, Abdel-Aty H, Gutberlet M, Prasad S, Aletras A, Laissy JP, Paterson I, Filipchuk NG, Kumar A, Pauschinger M, Liu P, International Consensus Group on Cardiovascular Magnetic Resonance in Myocarditis. Cardiovascular magnetic resonance in myocarditis: A JACC White Paper. *J Am Coll Cardiol.* 2009;**53**:1475–1487.

408. Leone O, Veinot JP, Angelini A, Baandrup UT, Basso C, Berry G, Bruneval P, Burke M, Butany J, Calabrese F, d'Amati G, Edwards WD, Fallon JT, Fishbein MC, Gallagher PJ, Halushka MK, McManus B, Pucci A, Rodriguez ER, Saffitz JE, Sheppard MN, Steenbergen C, Stone JR, Tan C, Thiene G, van der Wal AC, Winters GL. 2011 Consensus statement on endomyocardial biopsy from the Association for European Cardiovascular Pathology and the Society for Cardiovascular Pathology. *Cardiovasc Pathol.* 2012;**21**:245–274.

409. Chow LH, Radio SJ, Sears TD, McManus BM. Insensitivity of right ventricular endomyocardial biopsy in the diagnosis of myocarditis. *J Am Coll Cardiol.* 1989;**14**:915–920.

410. Hauck AJ, Kearney DL, Edwards WD. Evaluation of postmortem endomyocardial biopsy specimens from 38 patients with lymphocytic myocarditis: Implications for role of sampling error. *Mayo Clin Proc.* 1989;**64**:1235–1245.

411. Lurz P, Eitel I, Adam J, Steiner J, Grothoff M, Desch S, Fuernau G, de Waha S, Sareban M, Luecke C, Klingel K, Kandolf R, Schuler G, Gutberlet M, Thiele H. Diagnostic performance of CMR imaging compared with EMB in patients with suspected myocarditis. *J Am Coll Cardiol Img.* 2012;**5**:513–524.

412. Mahfoud F, Gärtner B, Kindermann M, Ukena C, Gadomski K, Klingel K, Kandolf R, Böhm M, Kindermann I. Virus serology in patients with suspected myocardiitis: Utility or futility? *Eur Heart J.* 2011;**32**:897–903.

413. Asaumi Y, Yasuda S, Morii I, Kakuchi H, Otsuka Y, Kawamura A, Sasako Y, Nakatani T, Nonogi H, Miyazaki S. Favourable clinical outcome in patients with cardiogenic shock due to fulminant myocarditis supported by percutaneous extracorporeal membrane oxygenation. *Eur Heart J.* 2005;**26**:2185–2192.

414. Frustaci A, Russo MA, Chimenti C. Randomized study on the efficacy of immunosuppressive therapy in patients with virus-negative inflammatory cardiomyopathy: The TIMIC study. *Eur Heart J.* 2009;**30**:1995–2002.

415. Basso C, Carturan E, Corrado D, Thiene G. Myocarditis and dilated cardiomyopathy in athletes: Diagnosis, management, and recommendations for sport activity. *Cardiol Clin.* 2007;**25**:423–429.

416. Cocker MS, Abdel-Aty H, Strohm O, Friedrich MG. Age and gender effects on the extent of myocardial involvement in acute myocarditis: A cardiovascular magnetic resonance study. *Heart.* 2009;**95**:1925–1930.

417. Amabile N, Fraisse A, Bouvenot J, Chetaille P, Ovaert C. Outcome of acute fulminant myocarditis in children. *Heart.* 2006;**92**:1269–1273.

418. Kindermann I, Kindermann M, Kandolf R, Klingel K, Bültmann B, Müller T, Lindinger A, Böhm M. Predictors of outcome in patients with suspected myocarditis. *Circulation.* 2008;**118**:639–648.

419. Fuse K, Kodama M, Okura Y, Ito M, Hirono S, Kato K, Hanawa H, Aizawa Y. Predictors of disease course in patients with acute myocarditis. *Circulation.* 2000;**102**:2829–2835.

420. Billingham ME, Tazelaar HD. The morphological progression of viral myocarditis. *Postgrad Med J.* 1986;**62**:581–584.

421. Quigley PJ, Richardson PJ, Meany BT, Olsen EGJ, Monaghan MJ, Jackson G, Jewitt DE. Long-term follow-up of acute myocarditis. Correlation of ventricular function and outcome. *Eur Heart J.* 1987;**8** (Suppl J):39–42.

422. Heymans S, Pauschinger M, De Palma A, Kallwellis-Opara A, Rutschow S, Swinnen M, Vanhoutte D, Gao F, Torpai R, Baker AH, Padalko E, Neyts J, Schultheiss HP, Van de Werf F, Carmeliet P, Pinto YM. Inhibition of urokinase-type plasminogen activator or matrix metalloproteinases prevents cardiac injury and dysfunction during viral myocarditis. *Circulation.* 2006;**114**:565–573.

423. Hurst D. The hidden heart timebomb: After Fabrice Muamba's collapse, how thousands are in danger from undetected heart problems. In: *The Daily Mail.* London, United Kingdom; 2012.

424. Hershberger RE, Siegfried JD. Update 2011: Clinical and genetic issues in familial dilated cardiomyopathy. *J Am Coll Cardiol.* 2011;**57**:1641–1649.

425. Ogle R. Swindon photographer repatriation images praised. In: *Swindon Link.* Swindon, United Kingdom; 2010.

426. Bowles NE, Richardson PJ, Olsen EG, Archard LC. Detection of Coxsackie-B-virus-specific RNA sequences in myocardial biopsy samples from patients with myocarditis and dilated cardiomyopathy. *Lancet.* 1986;**1**:1120–1123.

427. Fujioka S, Kitaura Y, Ukimura A, Deguchi H, Kawamura K, Isomura T, Suma H, Shimizu A. Evaluation of viral infection in the myocardium of patients with idiopathic dilated cardiomyopathy. *J Am Coll Cardiol.* 2000;**36**:1920–1926.

428. Packer DL, Bardy GH, Worley SJ, Smith MS, Cobb FR, Coleman RE, Gallagher JJ, German LD. Tachycardia-induced cardiomyopathy: A reversible form of left ventricular dysfunction. *Am J Cardiol.* 1986;**57**:563–570.

429. Feiker GM, Thompson RE, Hare JM, Hruban RH, Clemetson DE, Howard DL, Baughman KL, Kasper EK. Underlying causes and long-term survival in patients with initially unexplained cardiomyopathy. *N Engl J Med.* 2000;**342**:1077–1084.

430. Oakley C. Aetiology, diagnosis, investigation, and management of the cardiomyopathies. *Br Med J.* 1997;**315**:1520–1524.

431. Anderson KP, Freedman RA, Mason JW. Sudden death in idiopathic dilated cardiomyopathy. *Ann Intern Med.* 1987;**107**:104–106.

432. Jefferies JL, Towbin JA. Dilated cardiomyopathy. *Lancet.* 2010;**375**:752–762.

433. Likoff MJ, Chandler SL, Kay HR. Clinical determinants of mortality in chronic heart failure secondary to idiopathic dilated or to ischemic cardiomyopathy. *Am J Cardiol.* 1987;**59**:634–638.

434. Franciosa JA, Wilen M, Ziesche S, Cohn JN. Survival in men with severe chronic left ventricular failure due to either coronary artery disease or idiopathic dilated cardiomyopathy. *Am J Cardiol.* 1987;**59**:831–836.

435. Unverferth DV, Magorien RD, Moeschberger ML, Baker PB, Fetters JK, Leier CV. Factors influencing the one-year mortality of dilated cardiomyopathy. *Am J Cardiol.* 1984;**54**:147–152.

436. Pasotti M, Klersy C, Pilotto A, Marziliano N, Rapezzi C, Serio A, Mannarino S, Gambarin F, Favalli V, Grasso M, Agozzino M, Campana C, Gavazzi A, Febo O, Marini M, Landolina M, Mortara A, Piccolo G, Viganò M, Tavazzi L, Arbustini E. Long-term outcome and risk stratification in dilated cardiolaminopathies. *J Am Coll Cardiol.* 2008;**52**:1250–1260.

437. Lowes BD, Gilbert EM, Abraham WT, Minobe WA, Larrabee P, Ferguson D, Wolfel EE, Lindenfeld J, Tsvetkova T, Robertson AD, Quaife RA, Bristow MR. Myocardial gene expression in dilated cardiomyopathy treated with beta-blocking agents. *N Engl J Med.* 2002;**346**:1357–1365.

438. Packer M, Coats AJS, Fowler MB, Katus HA, Krum H, Mohacsi P, Rouleau JL, Tendera M, Castaigne A, Roecker EB, Schultz MK, DeMets DL, for the Carvedilol Prospective Randomized Cumulative Survival Study Group. Effect of carvedilol on survival in severe chronic heart failure. *N Engl J Med.* 2001;**344**:1651–1658.

439. Tuunanen H, Engblom E, Naum A, Någren K, Scheinin M, Hesse B, Airaksinen J, Nuutila P, Iozzo P, Ukkonen H, Opie LH, Knuuti J. Trimetazidine, a metabolic modulator, has cardiac and extracardiac benefits in idiopathic dilated cardiomyopathy. *Circulation.* 2008;**118**:1250–1258.

440. Prospective Studies Collaboration. Blood cholesterol and vascular mortality by age, sex, and blood pressure: A meta-analysis of individual data from 61 prospective studies with 55 000 vascular deaths. *Lancet.* 2007;**370**:1829–1839.

441. Ridker PM, Danielson E, Fonseca FAH, Genest J, Gotto Jr AM, Kastelein JJP, Koenig W, Libby P, Lorenzatti AJ, MacFadyen JG, Nordestgaard BG, Shepherd J, Willerson JT, Glynn RJ, on behalf of the JUPITER Trial Study Group. Reduction in C-reactive protein and LDL cholesterol and cardiovascular event rates after initiation of rosuvastatin: A prospective study of the JUPITER trial. *Lancet.* 2009;**373**: 1175–1182.

442. Goldberger JJ, Subacius H, Schaechter A, Howard A, Berger R, Shalaby A, Levine J, Kadish AH, for the DEFINITE Investigators. Effects of statin therapy on arrhythmic events and survival in patients with nonischemic dilated cardiomyopathy. *J Am Coll Cardiol.* 2006;**48**:1228–1233.

443. Folkers K, Vadhanavikit S, Mortensen SA. Biochemical rationale and myocardial tissue data on the effective therapy of cardiomyopathy with coenzyme Q10. *Proc Natl Acad Sci USA.* 1985;**82**:901–904.

444. Desai AS, Fang JC, Maisel WH, Baughman KL. Implantable defibrillators for the prevention of mortality in patients with nonischemic cardiomyopathy: A meta-analysis of randomized controlled trials. *JAMA.* 2004;**292**:2874–2879.

445. Bänsch D, Antz M, Boczor S, Volkmer M, Tebbenjohanns J, Seidl K, Block M, Gietzen F, Berger J, Kuck KH, for the CAT Investigators. Primary prevention of sudden cardiac death in idiopathic dilated cardiomyopathy. The Cardiomyopathy Trial (CAT). *Circulation.* 2002;**105**:1453–1458.

446. Stecker EC, Vickers C, Waltz J, Socoteanu C, John BT, Mariani R, McAnulty JH, Gunson K, Jui J, Chugh SS. Population-based analysis of sudden cardiac death with and without left ventricular systolic dysfunction. Two-year findings from the Oregon Sudden Unexpected Death Study. *J Am Coll Cardiol.* 2006;**47**:1161–1166.

447. Goldberger JJ, Subacius H, Patel T, Cunnane R, Kadish AH. Sudden cardiac death risk stratification in patients with nonischemic dilated cardiomyopathy. *J Am Coll Cardiol.* 2014;**63**:1879–1889.

448. Salerno-Uriarte JA, De Ferrari GM, Klersy C, Pedretti RFE, Tritto M, Sallusti L, Libero L, Pettinati G, Molon G, Curnis A, Occhetta E, Morandi F, Ferrero P, Accardi F, for the ALPHA Study Group Investigators. Prognostic value of T-wave alternans in patients with heart failure due to nonischemic cardiomyopathy. Results of the ALPHA Study. *J Am Coll Cardiol.* 2007;**50**:1896–1904.

449. Smith JM, Clancy E, Valeri C, Ruskin J, Cohen R. Electrical alternans and cardiac electrical instability. *Circulation.* 1988;**77**:110–121.

450. Kalter HH, Schwartz ML. Electrical alternans. *N Y State J Med.* 1948;**1**:1164–1166.

451. Floré V, Van Wijngaerden E, Willems R. A marker of mayhem: Macrovolt T-wave alternans preceding polymorphic ventricular tachycardia. *Eur Heart J.* 2011;**32**:2488.

452. Adam DR, Powell AO, Gordon H, Cohen RJ. Ventricular fibrillation and fluctuations in the magnitude of the repolarization vector. *IEEE Comput Cardiol.* 1982;241–244.

453. Bloomfield DM, Hohnloser SH, Cohen RJ. Interpretation and classification of microvolt T-wave alternans tests. *J Cardiovasc Electrophysiol.* 2002;**13**:502–512.

454. Narayan SM. T-wave alternans and the susceptibility to ventricular arrhythmias. *J Am Coll Cardiol.* 2006;**47**:269–281.

455. Hohnloser SH, Ikeda T, Bloomfield DM, Dabbous OH, Cohen RJ. T-wave alternans negative coronary patients with low ejection and benefit from defibrillator implantation. *Lancet.* 2003;**362**:125–126.

456. Chow T, Kereiakes DJ, Bartone C, Booth T, Schloss EJ, Waller T, Chung ES, Menon S, Nallamothu BK, Chan PS. Prognostic utility of microvolt T-wave alternans in risk stratification of patients with ischemic cardiomyopathy. *J Am Coll Cardiol.* 2006;**47**: 1820–1827.

457. Rosenbaum DS, Jackson LE, Smith JM, Garan H, Ruskin JN, Cohen RJ. Electrical alternans and vulnerability to ventricular arrhythmias. *N Engl J Med.* 1994;**330**:235–241.

458. Gold MR, Bloomfield DM, Anderson KP, El-Sherif NE, Wilber DJ, Groh ES, Estes III NAM, Kaufman ES, Greenberg ML, Rosenbaum DS. A comparison of T-wave alternans, signal averaged electrocardiography and programmed ventricular stimuation for arrhythmia risk stratification. *J Am Coll Cardiol.* 2000;**36**:2247–2253.

459. Costantini O, Hohnloser SH, Kirk MM, Lerman BB, Baker II JH, Sethuraman B, Dettmer MM, Rosenbaum DS, for the ABCD Trial Investigators. The ABCD (Alternans Before Cardioverter Defibrillator) Trial. Strategies using T-wave alternans to improve efficiency of sudden cardiac death prevention. *J Am Coll Cardiol.* 2009;**53**:471–479.

460. Cantillon DJ, Stein KM, Markowitz SM, Mittal S, Shah BK, Morin DP, Zacks ES, Janik M, Ageno S, Mauer AC, Lerman BB, Iwai S. Predictive value of microvolt T-wave alternans in patients wiht left ventricular dysfunction. *J Am Coll Cardiol.* 2007;**50**:166–173.

461. Gold MR, Ip JH, Costantini O, Poole JE, McNulty S, Mark DB, Lee KL, Bardy GH. Role of microvolt T-wave alternans in assessment of arrhythmia vulnerability among patients with heart failure and systolic dysfunction. Primary results from the T-wave Alternans Sudden Cardiac Death in Heart Failure Trial substudy. *Circulation.* 2008;**118**: 2022–2028.

462. Rosenbaum DS. T-wave alternans in the sudden cardiac death in heart failure trial population. Signal or noise? *Circulation.* 2008;**118**:2015–2018.

463. Chow T, Kereiakes DJ, Onufer J, Woelfel A, Gursoy S, Peterson BJ, Brown ML, Pu W, Benditt DG, on behalf of the MASTER Trial Investigators. Does microvolt T-wave alternans testing predict ventricular tachyarrhythmias in patients with ischemic cardiomyopathy and prophylactic defibrillators? the MASTER (Microvolt T Wave Alternans Testing for Risk Stratification of Post-myocardial Infarction Patients) Trial. *J Am Coll Cardiol.* 2008;**52**:1607–1615.

464. Huikuri HV, Raatikainen MJP, Moerch-Joergensen R, Hartikainen J, Virtanen V, Boland J, Anttonen O, Hoest N, Boersma LVA, Platou ES, Messier MD, Bloch-Thomsen P-E, for the Cardiac Arrhythmias and Risk Stratification after acute myocardial infarction (CARISMA) study group. Prediction of fatal or near-fatal cardiac arrhythmia events in patients with depressed left ventricular function after an acute myocardial infarction. *Eur Heart J.* 2009;**30**:689–698.

465. Swerdlow C, Chow T, Das M, Gillis AM, Zhou X, Abeyratne A, Ghanem RN. Intracardiac electrogram T-wave alternans/variability increases before spontaneous ventricular tachyarrhythmias in implantable cardioverter-defibrillator patients: A prospective, multi-center study. *Circulation.* 2011;**123**:1052–1060.

466. Goldberger JJ, Cain ME, Hohnloser SH, Kadish AH, Knight BP, Lauer MS, Maron BJ, Page RL, Passman RS, Siscovick D, Stevenson WG, Zipes DP. American Heart Association/American College of Cardiology Foundation/Heart Rhythm Society Scientific Statement on noninvasive risk stratification techniques for identifying patients at risk for sudden cardiac death. A scientific statement from the American Heart Association Council on Clinical Cardiology Committee on Electrocardiology and Arrhythmias and Council on Epidemiology and Prevention. *J Am Coll Cardiol.* 2008;**52**:1179–1199.

467. Verrier RL, Klingenheben T, Malik M, El-Sherif N, Exner DV, Hohnloser SH, Ikeda T, Martínez JP, Narayan SM. Microvolt T-wave alternans. Physiological basis, methods of measurement and clinical utility — Consensus Guideline by International Society for Holter and Noninvasive Electrocardiology. *J Am Coll Cardiol.* 2011;**58**: 1309–1324.

468. Nieminen T, Lethimäki T, Viik J, Lehtinen R, Nikus K, Kööbi T, Niemelä K, Turjanmaa V, Kaiser W, Huhtala H, Verrier RL, Huikuri H, Kähönen M. T-wave alternans predicts mortality in a population undergoing a clinically indicated exercise test. *Eur Heart J.* 2007;**28**:2332–2337.

469. Wolff L, Parkinson J, White PD. Bundle-branch block with short P-R interval in healthy young people prone to paroxysmal tachycardia. *Am Heart J.* 1930;685–704.

470. Kurland GS. Louis Wolff: 1898–1972. *Clin Cardiol.* 1989;**12**:301–302.

471. Waktare JEP. Atrial fibrillation. *Circulation.* 2002;**106**:14–16.

472. Cohn AE, Fraser FR. Paroxysmal tachycardia and the effect of stimuatlion of the vagus nerve by pressure. *Heart.* 1913;**5**:93–105.

473. Zipes DP, Cobb Jr LA, Garson Jr A, Gillette PC, James TN, Lazzara R, Rink L. 16th Bethesda Conference: Cardiovascular Abnormalities in the Athlete: Recommendations Regarding Eligibility for Competition: Task Force VI: Arrhythmias. *J Am Coll Cardiol.* 1985;**6**:1225–1232.

474. Wiedermann CJ, Becker AE, Hopferwieser T, Mühlberger V, Knapp E. Sudden death in a young competitive athlete with Wolff-Parkinson-White syndrome. *Eur Heart J.* 1987;**8**:651–655.

475. Wood FC, Wolferth CC, Geckeler GD. Histologic demonstration of accessory muscular connections between auricle and ventricle in a case of short P-R interval and prolonged QRS complex. *Am Heart J.* 1943;**25**:454–462.

476. Kent AFS. Researches on the structure and function of the mammalian heart. *J Physiol.* 1893;**14**:i233–254.

477. Kent AFS. Observations on the auriculo-ventricular juncton of the mammalian heart. *Q J Exper Physiol.* 1913;**7**:193–195.

478. Tawara S. Eine anatomischhistologische Studie uder das atrio-ventrikularbundle und die Purkinjeschen faden. In: *Des reizleitungsystem des Saugetierherzens.* Jena, Germany: Verlag von Gustav Fischer; 1906.

479. Mahaim I. Kent's fibers and the A-V paraspecific conduction through the upper connections of the bundle of His-Tawara. *Am Heart J.* 1947;**33**:651–653.

480. Mines GR. On dynamic equilibrium in the heart. *J Physiol.* 1913;**46**:349–383.

481. Mines GR. On circulating excitiations in heart muscles and their possible relationship to tachycardia and fibrillation. *Trans R Soc Can (third series).* 1914;**8**:43–52.

482. DeSilva RA. George Ralph Mines, Ventricular fibrillation and the discovery of the vulnerable period. *J Am Coll Cardiol.* 1997;**29**:1397–1402.

483. Holzmann M, Scherf D. Uber elektrokardiogramme mit verkurzter Vorhof-Kammerdiztanz und P-Zacken. *Z Klin Med.* 1932;**121**:404–423.

484. Wolferth CC, Wood FC. The mechanism of production of short P-R interval and prolonged QRS complexes in patients with presumably undamaged hearts; hypothesis of an accessory pathway of auriculo-ventricular conduction (bundle of Kent). *Am Heart J.* 1933;**8**:297–311.

485. James TN. The Wolff-Parkinson-White syndrome. *Ann Intern Med.* 1969;**71**:399–406.

486. Öhnell RF. Pre-excitation, a cardiac abnormality. *Acta Med Scand.* 1944;**118**:9–167.

487. Segers PM, Lequime J, Denolin H. L'activation ventriculaire précoce de certains coeurs hyperexcitables: Etude de l'onde? de l'électrocardiogramme. *Cardiologia.* 1944;**8**:113–167.

488. Hiss RG, Lamb LE. Electrocardiographic findings in 122,043 individuals. *Circulation.* 1962;**25**:947–961.

489. Averill KH, Fosmoe RJ, Lamb LE. Electrocardiogrpahic findings in 67,375 asymptomatic subjects. IV. Wolff-Parkinson-White syndrome. *Am J Cardiol.* 1961;**6**:108–129.

490. Munger TM, Packer DL, Hammill SC, Feldman BJ, Bailey KR, Ballard DJ, Holmes Jr DR, Gersh BJ. A population study of the natural history of Wolff-Parkinson-White syndrome in Olmsted County, Minnesota, 1953–1989. *Circulation.* 1993;**87**:866–873.

491. Goudevenos JA, Katsouras CS, Graekas G, Argiri O, Giogiakas V, Sideris DA. Ventricular pre-excitation in the general population: A study on the mode of presentation and clinical course. *Heart.* 2000;**83**:29–34.

492. Fitzsimmons PJ, McWhirter PD, Peterson DW, Kruyer WB. The natural history of Wolff-Parkinson-White syndrome in 228 military aviators: A long-term follow-up of 22 years. *Am Heart J.* 2001;**142**:530–536.

493. Klein GJ, Bashore TM, Sellers TD, Pritchett EL, Smith WM, Gallagher JJ. Ventricular fibrillation in the Wolff-Parkinson-White syndrome. *N Engl J Med.* 1979;**301**:1080–1085.

494. Vidaillet Jr HJ, Pressley JC, Henke E, Harrell Jr FE, German LD. Familial occurrence of accessory atrioventricular pathways (preexcitation syndrome). *N Engl J Med.* 1987;**317**:65–69.

495. Obeyesekere MN, Leong-Sit P, Massel D, Manlucu J, Modi S, Krahn AD, Skanes AC, Yee R, Gula LJ, Klein GJ. Risk of arrhythmia and sudden death in patients with asymptomatic preexcitation. A meta-analysis. *Circulation.* 2012;**125**:2308–2315.

496. Pappone C, Vicedomini G, Manguso F, Baldi M, Pappone A, Petretta A, Vitale R, Saviano M, Ciaccio C, Giannelli L, Calovic Z, Tavazzi L, Santinelli V. Risk of malignant arrhythmias initially symptomatic patients with Wolff-Parkinson-White syndrome: Results of a prospective long-term electrophysiological follow-up study. *Circulation.* 2012;**125**:661–668.

497. Timmermans C, Smeets JL, Rodriguez LM, Vrouchos G, van den Dool A, Wellens HJ. Aborted sudden death in the Wolff-Parkinson-White syndrome. *Am J Cardiol.* 1995;**76**:492–494.

498. Schwartz SP, Jezer A. Studies on transient ventricular fibrillation. I. Observations on the alterations in the rhythm of the heart preceding syncopal seizures in a patient with normal sinus rhythm. *Am J Med Sci.* 1934;**187**:469–477.

499. Fox TT, Weaver J, March HW. On the mechanism of the arrhythmias in aberrant atrioventricular conduction (Wolff-Parkinson-White). *Am Heart J.* 1951;**43**:507–520.

500. Dreifus LS, Haiat R, Watanabe Y, Arriaga J, Reitman N. A possible mechanism of sudden death in patients with Wolff-Parkinson-White syndrome. *Circulation.* 1971;**43**:520–527.

501. Basso C, Corrado D, Rossi L, Thiene G. Ventricular preexcitation in children and young adults: Atrial myocarditis as a possible trigger of sudden death. *Circulation.* 2001;**103**:269–275.

502. Montoya PT, Brugada P, Smeets J, Talajic M, Della Bella P, Lezaun R, vd Dool A, Wellens HJ, Bayés de Luna A, Oter R, Breithardt G, Borggrefe M, Klein H, Kuck KH, Kunze K, Coumel P, Leclercq JF, Chouty F, Frank R, Fontaine G. Ventricular fibrillation in the Wolff-Parkinson-White syndrome. *Eur Heart J.* 1991;**12**:144–150.

503. Beckman KJ, Gallastegui JL, Bauman JL, Hariman RJ. The predictive value of electrophysiologic studies in untreated patients with Wolff-Parkinson-White syndrome. *J Am Coll Cardiol.* 1990;**15**:640–647.

504. Auricchio A, Klein H, Trappe H-J, Wenzlaff P. Lack of prognostic value of syncope in patients with Wolff-Parkinson-White syndrome. *J Am Coll Cardiol.* 1991;**17**:152–158.

505. Attoyan C, Haissaguerre M, Dartigues JF, Le Metayer P, Warin JF, Clementy J. Ventricular fibrillation in Wolff-Parkinson-White syndrome. Predictive factors [in French]. *Arch Mal Coeur Vaiss.* 1994;**87**:889–897.

506. Wellens HJ. When to perform catheter ablation in asymptomatic patients with a Wolff-Parkinson-White electrocardiogram. *Circulation.* 2005;**112**:2201–2207.

507. Wellens HJJ, Brugada P, Roy D, Weiss J, Bar FW. Effect of isoproterenol on the antegrade refractory period of the accessory pathway in patients with the WPW syndrome. *Am J Cardiol.* 1981;**50**:180–184.

508. Bricker JT, Porter CJ, Garson Jr A, Gillette PC, McVey P, Traweek M, McNamara DG. Exercise testing in children with Wolff-Parkinson-White syndrome. *Am J Cardiol.* 1985;**55**:1001–1004.

509. Pappone C, Stantinelli V, Rosanio S, Vicedomini G, Nardi S, Pappone A, Tortoriello V, Manguso F, Mazzone P, Gulletta S, Oreto G, Alfieri O. Usefulness of invasive electrophysiologic testing to stratify the risk of arrhythmic events in asymptomatic patients with Wolff-Parkinson-White pattern. Results from a large prospective long-term follow-up study. *J Am Coll Cardiol.* 2003;**41**:239–244.

510. Santinelli V, Radinovic A, Manguso F, Vicedomini G, Gulletta S, Paglino G, Mazzone P, Ciconte G, Sacchi S, Sala S, Pappone C. The natural history of asymptomatic ventricular pre-excitation: A long-term prospective follow-up study of 184 asymptomatic children. *J Am Coll Cardiol.* 2009;**53**:275–280.

511. Pappone C, Santinelli V, Manguso F, Augello G, Santinelli O, Vicedomini G, Gulletta S, Mazzone P, Tortoriello V, Pappone A, Dicandia C, Rosanio S. A randomized study of prophylactic catheter ablation in asymptomatic patients with the Wolff-Parkinson-White syndrome. *N Engl J Med.* 2003;**349**:1803–1811.

512. Pappone C, Santinelli V. Catheter ablation should be performed in asymptomatic patients with Wolff-Parkinson-White syndrome. *Circulation.* 2005;**112**:2207–2215.

513. Blomström-Lundqvist C, Scheinman MM, Aliot EM, Alpert JS, Calkins H, Camm AJ, Campbell WB, Haines DE, Kuck KH, Lerman BB, Miller DD, Shaeffer CW, Stevenson WG, Tomaselli GF. ACC/AHA/ESC guidelines for the management of patients with supraventricular arrhythmias — executive summary: A report of the American College of Cardiology/American Heart Association Task Force on Practice Guidelines, and the European Society of Cardiology Committee for Practice Guidelines (Writing Committee to Develop Guidelines for the Management of Patients With Supraventricular Arrhythmias.). *J Am Coll Cardiol.* 2003;**42**:1493–1531.

514. Wellens HJJ, Bar FW, Gorgels AP, Vanagt EJ. Use of ajmaline in identifying patients with the Wolff-Parkinson-White syndrome and a short refractory period of their accessory pathway. *Am J Cardiol.* 1980;**45**:130–133.

515. Wellens HJJ, Braat SH, Brugada P, Gorgels AP, Bar FW. Use of procainamide in patients with the Wolff-Parkinson-White syndrome to disclose a short refractory period of the accessory pathway. *Am J Cardiol.* 1982;**50**:921–925.

516. Chimienti M, Moizi M, Klersy C. A modified ajmaline test for prediction of the effective refractory period of the accessory pathway in the Wolff-Parkinson-White syndrome. *Am J Cardiol.* 1987;**59**:164–165.

517. Fananapazir L, Packer DL, German LD, Greer SG, Gallagher JJ, Presley JC, Prystowsky EN. Procainamide infusion tests: Inability to identify patients with Wolff Parkinson White syndrome who are potentially at risk of sudden death. *Circulation.* 1988;**77**: 1291–1296.

518. Gaita F, Giustetto C, Ricardi R, Mangiardi L, Brusca A. Stress and pharmacological tests as message to identify patients with Wolff-Parkinson-White syndrome at risk of sudden death. *Am J Cardiol.* 1989;**64**:487–490.

519. Klein GJ, Yee R, Sharma AD. Longitudinal electrophysiologic assessment of asymptomatic patients with the Wolff-Parkinson-White electrocardiographic pattern. *N Engl J Med.* 1989;**320**:1229–1233.

520. Leitch JW, Klein GJ, Yee R, Murdock C. Prognostic value of electrophysiology testing in asymptomatic patients with Wolff-Parkinson-White pattern. *Circulation.* 1990;**82**: 1718–1723.

521. Cobb FR, Blumenschein SD, Sealy WC, Boineau JP, Wagner GS, Wallace AG. Successful surgical interruption of the Bundle of Kent in a patient with Wolff-Parkinson-White syndrome. *Circulation.* 1968;**38**:1018–1029.

522. Cox JL. The status of surgery for cardiac arrhythmias. *Circulation.* 1985;**71**:413–417.

523. Weber H, Schmitz L. Catheter technique for closed-chest ablation of an accessory atrioventricular pathway. *N Engl J Med.* 1983;**308**:653–654.

524. Calkins H, Sousa J, el-Atassi R, Rosenheck S, de Buitleir M, Kou WH, Kadish AH, Langberg JJ, Morady F. Diagnosis and cure of the Wolff-Parkinson-White syndrome or paroxysmal supraventricular tachycardias during a single electrophysiologic test. *N Engl J Med.* 1991;**324**:1612–1618.

525. Jackman WM, Beckman KJ, McClelland JH, Wang X, Friday KJ, Roman CA, Moulton KP, Twidale N, Hazlitt HA, Prior MI, Oren J, Overholt ED, Lazzara R. Treatment of supraventricular tachycardia due to atrioventricular nodal reentry by radiofrequency catheter ablation of slow-pathway conduction. *N Engl J Med.* 1992;**327**:313–318.

526. Pappone C, Radinovic A, Santinelli V. Sudden death and ventricular preexcitation: Is it necessary to treat the asymptomatic patients? *Curr Pharm Des.* 2008;**14**:762–765.

527. Mezzani A, Giovannini T, Michelucci A, Padeletti L, Resina A, Cupelli V, Musante R. Effects of training on the electrophysiologic properties of atrium and accessory pathway in athletes with Wolff-Parkinson-White syndrome. *Cardiology.* 1990;**77**:295–302.

528. Zipes DP, Ackerman MJ, Estes III NAM, Grant AO. Task Force 7: Arrhythmia. In: Maron BJ, Zipes DP, eds. *36th Bethesda Conference: Eligibility Recommendations for Competitive Athletes with Cardiovascular Abnormalities.* New Orleans, Louisiana: *J Am Coll Cardiol;* 2005:1354–1363.

529. Corrado D, Pelliccia A, Bjørnstad HV, Vanhees L, A B, Borjesson M, Panhuyzen-Goedkoop N, Deligiannis A, Solborg E, Dugmore D, Mellwig KP, Assanelli D, Delise P, van-Buuren F, Anastasakis A, Heidbuchel H, Hoffman E, Fagard R, Priori SG, Basso C, Arbustini E, Blomstrom-Lundqvist C, McKenna WJ, Thiene G. Cardiovascular pre-participation screening of young competitive athletes for prevention of sudden death: Proposal for a common European protocol: Consensus statement of the Study Group of Sport Cardiology of the Working Group of Cardiac Rehabilitation and Exercise Physiology and the Working Group of Myocardial and Pericardial Diseases of the European Society of Cardiology. *Eur Heart J.* 2005;**26**:516–524.

530. Cohen MI, Triedman JK, Cannon AM, Davis AM, Drago F, Janousek J, Klein GJ, Law IH, Morady FJ, Paul T, Perry JC, Sanatani S, Tanel RE. PACES/HRS Expert Consensus Statement on the Management of the Asymptomatic Young Patient with a Wolff-Parkinson-White (WPW, Ventricular Preexcitation) Electrocardiographic Pattern. Developed in partnership between the Pediatric and Congenital Electrophysiology Society (PACES) and the Heart Rhythm Society (HRS). Endorsed by the governing bodies of PACES, HRS, the American College of Cardiology Foundation (ACCF), the American Heart Association (AHA), the American Academy of Pediatrics (AAP), and the Canadian Heart Rhythm Society (CHRS). *Heart Rhythm.* 2012;**9**:1006–1024.

531. Deal BJ, Keane JF, Gillette PC, Garson Jr A. Wolff-Parkinson-White syndrome and supra-ventricular tachycardia during infancy: Management and follow-up. *J Am Coll Cardiol.* 1985;**5**:130–135.

532. Khoo JCM, Kwa CG, Khoo LY. The death of Sir Thomas Stamford Raffles (1781–1826). *Singapore Med J.* 1998;**39**:564–565.

533. Al-Shahi R, Bhattacharya JJ, Currie DG, Papanastassiou V, Ritchie V, Roberts RC, Sellar RJ, Warlow CP. Prospective, population-based detection of intracranial vascular mal-formations in adults: The Scottish Intracranial Vascular Malformation Study (SIVMS). *Stroke.* 2003;**34**:1163–1169.

534. Hillman J. Population-based analysis of arteriovenous malformation treatment. *J Neurosurg.* 2001;**95**:633–637.

535. Stapf C, Mast H, Sciacca RR, Berenstein A, Nelson PK, Gobin YP, Pile-Spellman J, Mohr JP. The New York Islands AVM Study: Design, study progress, and initial results. *Stroke.* 2003;**34**:e29–e33.

536. Gabriel RA, Kim H, Sidney S, McCulloch CE, Singh V, Johnston C, Ko NU, Achrol AS, Zaroff JG, Young WL. Ten-year detection rate of brain arteriovenous malformations in a large, multiethnic, defined population. *Stroke.* 2010;**41**:21–26.

537. Al-Shahi R, Fang JSY, Lewis SC, Warlow CP. Prevalence of adults with brain arteriovenous malformations: A community based study in Scotland using capture-recapture analysis. *J Neurol Neurosurg Psychiatry.* 2002;**73**:547–551.

538. Morris Z, Whiteley WN, Jongstreth Jr WT, Weber F, Lee Y-C, Tsushima Y, Alphs H, Ladd SC, Warlow C, Wardlaw JM, Salman RA. Incidental findings on brain magnetic resonance imaging: Systematic review and meta-analysis. *Br Med J.* 2009;**339**:b3016.

539. Hofmeister C, Stapf C, Hartmann A, Sciacca RR, Mansmann U, terBrugge K, Lasjaunias P, Mohr JP, Mast H, Meisel J. Demographic, morphological, and clinical characteristics of 1289 patients with brain arteriovenous malformation. *Stroke.* 2000;**31**:1307–1310.

540. Korja M, Lehto H, Juvela S. Lifelong rupture risk of intracranial aneurysms depends on risk factors: A prospective Finnish cohort study. *Stroke.* 2014;**45**:1958–1963.

541. Juvela S, Porras M, Poussa K. Natural history of unruptured intracranial aneurysms: Probability and risk factors for aneurysm rupture. *J Neurosurg.* 2000;**93**:378–387.

542. Rinkel GJ, Djibuti M, Algra A, van Gijn J. Prevalence and risk of rupture of intracranial aneurysms: A systematic review. *Stroke.* 1998;**29**:251–256.

543. Korja M, Silventoinen K, Laatikainen T, Jousilahti P, Salomaa V, Kaprio J. Cause-specific mortality of 1-year survivors of subarachnoid hemorrhage. *Neurology.* 2013;**80**:481–486.

544. Vernooij MW, Ikram MA, Tanghe HL, Vincent AJPE, Hofman A, Krestin GP, Niessen WJ, Breteler MMB, van der Lugt A. Incidental findings on brain MRI in the general population. *N Engl J Med.* 2007;**357**:1821–1828.

545. Inagawa T, Hirano A. Autopsy study of unruptured incidental intracranial aneurysms. *Surg Neurol.* 1990;**34**:361–365.

546. Vlak MH, Algra A, Brandengurg R, Rinkel GJ. Prevalence of unruptured intracranial aneurysms, with emphasis on sex, age, comorbidity, country, and time period: A systematic review and meta-analysis. *Lancet Neurol.* 2011;**10**:626–636.

547. Schievink WI, Wijdicks EF, Parisi JE, Piepgras DG, Whisnant JP. Sudden death from aneurysmal subarachnoid hemorrhage. *Neurology.* 1995;**45**:871–875.

548. Matschke J, Lockermann U, Schulz F. Intracranial arteriovenous malformations presenting as sudden unexpected death: A report of 3 cases and review of the literature. *Am J Forensic Med Pathol.* 2007;**28**:173–176.

549. Crawford PM, West CR, Chadwick DW, Shaw MDM. Arteriovenous malformations of the brain: Natural history in unoperated patients. *J Neurol Neurosurg Psychiatry.* 1986;**49**:1–10.

550. Ondra SL, Troupp H, George ED, Schwab K. The natural history of symptomatic arteriovenous malformations of the brain: A 24-year follow-up assessment. *J Neurosurg.* 1990;**73**:387–391.

551. Spetzler RF, Martin NA. A proposed grading system for ateriovenous malformations. *J Neurosurg.* 1986;**65**:476–483.

552. Stapf C, Mast H, Sciacca RR, Choi JH, Khaw AV, Connolly ES, Pile-Spellman J, Mohr JP. Predictors of hemorrhage in patients with untreated brain arteriovenous malformation. *Neurology*. 2006;**66**:1350–1355.

553. da Costa L, Wallace MC, ter Grugge KG, O'Kelly C, Willinksy RA, Tymianski M. The natural history and predictive features of hemorrhage from brain arteriovenous malformations. *Stroke*. 2009;**40**:100–105.

554. Mast H, Young WL, Koennecke HC, Sciacca RR, Osipov A, Pile-Spellman J, Hacein-Bey L, Duong H, Stein BM, Mohr JP. Risk of spontaneous haemorrhage after diagnosis of cerebral arteriovenous malformation. *Lancet*. 1997;**350**:1065–1068.

555. Mohr JP, Parides MK, Stapf C, Moquete E, Moy CS, Overbey JR, Al-Shahi S, Vicaut E, Young WL, Houdart E, Cordonnier C, Stefani MA, Hartmann A, von Kummer R, Biondi A, Berkefeld J, Klijn CJ, Harkness K, Libman R, Barreau X, Moskowitz AJ, for the International ARUBA Investigators. Medical treatment with or without interventional therapy for unruptured brain arteriovenous malformations (ARUBA): A multicentre, non-blinded, randomised trial. *Lancet*. 2014;**383**:614–621.

556. van Beijnum J, van der Worp HB, Buis DR, Salman RA, Kappelle LJ, Rinkel GJE, van der Sprenkel JWB, Vandertop WP, Algra A, Klijn CJM. Treatment of brain arteriovenous malformations. A systematic review and meta-analysis. *JAMA*. 2011;**306**: 2011–2019.

557. Al-Shahi Salman RA, White PM, Counsell CE, de Plessis J, van Beijnum J, Josephson CB, Wilkinson T, Wedderburn CJ, Chandy Z, St George J, Sellar RJ, Warlow CP, for the Scottish Audit of Intracranial Vascular Malformations. Outcome after conservative management or intervenion for unruptured brain arteriovenous malformations. *JAMA*. 2014;**311**:1661–1669.

558. Symington IS, Stack BH. Pulmonary thromboembolism after travel. *Br J Dis Chest*. 1977;**71**:138–140.

559. Select Committee on Science and Technology. Air Travel and Health, Session 1999–2000 5th Report. In: London: The Stationary Office: House of Lords; 2000: 6.1–6.31.

560. Simpson K. Shelter deaths from pulmonary embolism. *Lancet*. 1940;**236**:744.

561. Chandra D, Parisini E, Mozaffarian D. Meta-analysis: Travel and risk for venous thromnboembolism. *Ann Intern Med*. 2009;**151**:180–190.

562. Kakkar VV, Howe CT, Flanc C, Clarke MB. Natural history of postoperative deep-vein thrombosis. *Lancet*. 1969;**2**:230–232.

563. Flanc C, Kakkar VV, Clarke MB. The detection of venous thrombosis of the legs using 125-I-labelled fibrinogen. *Br J Surg*. 1968;**55**:742–747.

564. Kearon C. Natural history of venous thromboembolism. *Circulation*. 2003;**107**:I-22–I-33.

565. Anderson Jr FA, Wheeler HB, Goldberg RJ, Hosmer DW, Patwardhan NA, Jovanovic B, Forcier A, Dalen JE. A population-based perspective of the hsopital incidence and case-fatality rates of deep vein thrombosis and pulmonary embolism. The Worcester DVT Study. *Arch Intern Med*. 1991;**151**:933–938.

566. Cushman M, Tsai AW, White RH, Heckbert SR, Rosamond WD, Enright P, Folsom AR. Deep vein thrombosis and pulmonary embolism in two cohorts: The longitudinal investigation of thromboembolism etiology. *Am J Med*. 2004;**117**:19–25.

567. Rathbun S. The Surgeon General's call to action to prevent deep vein thrombosis and pulmonary embolism. *Circulation*. 2009;**119**:e480–e482.

568.   Silverstein MD, Heit JA, Mohr DN, Petterson TM, O'Fallon WM, Melton III LJ. Trends in the incidence of deep vein thrombosis and pulmonary embolism: A 25-year population-based study. *Arch Intern Med.* 1998;**158**:585–593.

569.   White RH, Zhou H, Murin S, Harvey D. Effect of ethnicity and gender on the incidence of venous thromboembolism in a diverse population in California in 1996. *Thromb Haemost.* 2005;**93**:298–305.

570.   Heit JA, Silverstein MD, Mohr DN, Petterson TM, Lohse CM, O'Fallon WM, Melton III LJ. The epidemiology of venous thromboembolism in the community. *Thromb Haemost.* 2001;**86**:452–463.

571.   Lucena J, Rico A, Vázquez R, Marín R, Martínez C, Salguero M, Miguel L. Pulmonary embolism and sudden-unexpected death: Prospective study on 2477 forensic autopsies performed at the Institute of Legal Medicine in Seville. *J Forensic Leg Med.* 2009;**16**: 196–201.

572.   Tang Y, Sampson B, Pack S, Shah K, Um SY, Wang D, Wang T, Prinz M. Ethnic differences in out-of-hospital fatal pulmonary embolism. *Circulation.* 2011;**123**:2219–2225.

573.   Coady MA, Rizzo JA, Elefteriades JA. Pathologic variants of thoracic aortic dissections. Penetrating atherosclerotic ulcers and intramural haematomas. *Cardiol Clin.* 1999;**17**:637–657.

574.   Masumura JS, Cambria RP, Dake MD, Moore RD, Svensson LG, Snyder S, TX2 Clinical Trial Investigators. International controlled clinical trial of thoracic endovascular aneurysm repair with the Zenith TX2 endovascular graft: 1-year results. *J Vasc Surg.* 2008;**47**:247–257.

575.   Hagan PG, Nienaber CA, Isselbacher EM, Bruckman D, Karavite DJ, Russman PL, Evangelista A, Fattori R, Suzuki T, Oh JK, Moore AG, Malouf JF, Pape LA, Gaca C, Sechtem U, Lenferink S, Deutsch HJ, Diedrichs H, Marcos y Robles J, Llovet A, Gilon D, Das SK, Armstrong WF, Deeb GM, Eagle KA. The International Registry of Acute Aortic Dissection (IRAD): New insights into an old disease. *JAMA.* 2000;**283**:897–903.

576.   Hirst Jr AE, Johns Jr VJ, Kime Jr SW. Dissecting aneurysms of the aorta: A review of 505 cases. *Medicine (Baltimore).* 1958;**37**:217–279.

577.   Sweeting MJ, Thompson SG, Brown LC, Powell JT, RESCAN collaborators. Meta-analysis of individual patient data to examine factors affecting growth and rupture of small abdominal aortic aneurysms. *Br J Surg.* 2012;**99**:655–665.

578.   Cosford PA, Leng GC. Screening for abdominal aortic aneurysm. *Cochrane Database Syst Rev.* 2007;**18**:CD002945.

579.   Kim LG, Scott RAP, Ashton HA, Thompson SG, for the Multicentre Aneurysm Screening Study Group. A sustained mortality benefit from screening for abdominal aortic aneurysm. *Ann Intern Med.* 2007;**146**:699–706.

580.   Guirguis-Blake JM, Beil TL, Sun X, Senger CA, Whitlock EP. Primary care screening for abdominal aortic aneurysm: An evidence update for the U.S. Preventive Services Task Force. Evidence Synthesis No. 109. AHRQ Publication No. 14–05202-EF-1. In: Rockville, MD: Agency for Healthcare Research and Quality; 2014.

581.   Shores J, Berger KR, Murphy EA, Pyeritz RE. Progression of aortic dilatation and the benefit of long-term beta-adrenergic blockade in Marfan's syndrome. *N Engl J Med.* 1994;**330**:1335–1341.

582.   Lindholt JS, Henneberg EW, Juul S. Impaired results of a randomised double blinded clinical trial of propranolol versus placebo on the expansion rate of small abdominal aortic aneurysms. *Int J Angiol.* 1999;**18**:52–57.

583. Ahimastos AA, Aggarwal A, D'Orsa KM, Formosa MF, White AJ, Savarirayan R, Dart AM, Kingwell BA. Effect of perindopril on large artery stiffness and aortic root diameter in patients with Marfan syndrome: A randomized controlled trial. *JAMA.* 2007;**298**:1539–1547.

584. Brooke BS, Habashi JP, Judge DP, Patel N, Loeys B, Dietz III HC. Angiotensin II blockade and aortic-root dilation in Marfan's syndrome. *N Engl J Med.* 2008;**358**:2787–2795.

585. Takagi H, Mizuno Y, Yamamoto H, Goto SN, Umemoto T, ALICE (All-Literature Investigation of Cardiovascular Evidence) Group. Alice in Wonderland of statin therapy for small abdominal aortic aneurysm. *Int J Cardiol.* 2013;**166**:252–255.

586. Meijer CA, Stijnen T, Wasser MNJM, Hamming JF, van Bockel J, Lindeman JHN, for the Pharmaceutical Aneurysm Stabilisation Trial Study Group. Doxycycline for stabilization of abdominal aortic aneurysms. A randomized trial. *Ann Intern Med.* 2013;**59**:815–823.

587. Freed LA, Levy D, Levine RA, Larson MG, Evans JC, Fuller DL, Lehman B, Benjamin EJ. Prevalence and clinical outcome of mitral-valve prolapse. *N Engl J Med.* 1999;**341**:1–7.

588. Jeresaty RM. Mitral valve prolapse: An update. *JAMA.* 1985;**254**:793–795.

589. Nishimura RA, McGoon MD, Shub C, Miller Jr FA, Ilstrup DM, Tajik AJ. Echocardiographically doucmented mitral-valve prolapse. Long-term follow-up of 237 patients. *N Engl J Med.* 1985;**313**:1305–1309.

590. Duren DR, Becker AE, Dunning AJ. Long-term follow-up of idiopathic mitral valve prolapse in 300 patients: A prospective study. *J Am Coll Cardiol.* 1988;11.

591. Chesler E, King RA, Edwards JE. The myxomatous mitral valve and sudden death. *Circulation.* 1983;**67**:632–639.

592. Avierinos J-F, Gersh BJ, Melton III LJ, Bailey KR, Shub C, Nishimura RA, Tajik AJ, Enriquez-Sarano M. Natural history of asymptomatic mitral valve prolapse in the community. *Circulation.* 2002;**106**:1355–1361.

593. Sriram CS, Syed FF, Ferguson ME, Johnson JN, Enriquez-Sarano M, Cetta F, Cannon BC, Asirvatham SJ, Ackerman MJ. Malignant bileaflet mitral valve prolapse syndrome in patients with otherwise idiopathic out-of-hospital cardiac arrest. *J Am Coll Cardiol.* 2013;**62**:222–230.

594. Grigioni F, Enriquez-Sarano M, Ling LH, Bailey KR, Seward JB, Tajik AJ, Frye RL. Sudden death in mitral regurgitation due to flail leaflet. *J Am Coll Cardiol.* 1999;**34**:2078–2085.

595. Hoffman JIE, Kaplan S. The incidence of congenital heart disease. *J Am Coll Cardiol.* 2002;**39**:1890–1900.

596. Rosenhek R, Binder T, Porenta G, Lang I, Christ G, Schemper M, Maurer G, Baumgartner H. Predictors of outcome in severe, asymptomatic aortic stenosis. *N Engl J Med.* 2000;**343**:611–617.

597. Pellikka PA, Sarano ME, Nishimura RA, Maulouf JF, Bailey KR, Scott CG, Barnes ME, Tajik AJ. Outcome of 622 adults with asymptomatic hemodynamically significant aortic stenosis during prolonged follow-up. *Circulation.* 2005;**111**:3290–3295.

598. Carabello BA, Paulus WJ. Aortic stenosis. *Lancet.* 2009;**373**:956–966.

599. Jaster JH, Ottaviani G, Matturri L, Lavezzi AM, Zamecnik J, Smith TW. Sudden unexpected death related to medullary brain lesions. *Am J Forensic Med Pathol.* 2008;**29**: 371–374.

600. Langan Y, Nashef L, Sander JWAS. Sudden unexpected death in epilepsy: A series of witnessed deaths. *J Neurol Neurosurg Psychiatry.* 2000;**68**:211–213.

601. Leestma JE, Walczak T, Hughes JR, Kalelkar MB, Teas SS. A prospective study on sudden unexpected death in epilepsy. *Ann Neurol.* 1989;**26**:195–203.

602. Walczak TS, Leppik IE, D'Amelio M, Rarick J, So E, Ahman P, Ruggles K, Cascino GD, Annegers JF, Hauser WA. Incidence and risk factors in sudden unexpected death in epilepsy: A prospective cohort study. *Neurology.* 2001;**56**:519–525.

603. Hesdorffer DC, Tomson T, Benn E, Sander JW, Nilsson L, Langan Y, Walczak TS, Beghi E, Brodie MJ, Hauser WA, for the ILAE Commission on Epidemiology (Subcommission on Mortality). Do antiepileptic drugs or generalized tonic-clonic seizure frequency increase SUDEP risk? A combined analysis. *Epilepsia.* 2011;**53**:249–252.

604. Natelson BH, Farahmand B, Persson P-G, Thiblin I, Tomson T. Risk factors for sudden unexpected death in epilepsy: a case-control study. *Lancet.* 1999; **353**:888-893.

605. Opeskin K, Harvey AS, Cordner SM, Berkovic SF. Sudden unexpected death in epilepsy in Victoria. *J Clin Neurosci.* 2000;**7**:34–37.

606. Earnest MP, Thomas GE, Eden RA, Hossack KF. The sudden unexplained death syndrome in epilepsy: Demographic, clinical, and postmortem features. *Epilepsia.* 1992;33.

607. Natelson BH, Suarez RV, Terrence CF, Turizo R. Patients with epilepsy who die suddenly have cardiac disease. *Arch Neurol.* 1998;**55**:857–860.

608. Nei M, Ho RT, Abou-Khalil BW, Drislane FW, J L, Romeo A, Sperling MR. EEG and ECG in sudden unexplained death in epilepsy. *Epilepsia.* 2004;**45**:338–345.

609. Rugg-Gunn FJ, Simister RJ, Squirrell M, Holdright DR, Duncan JS. Cardiac arrhythmia in focal epilepsy: A prospective long-term study. *Lancet.* 2004;**364**:2212–2219.

610. Langan Y, Nashef L, Sander JW. Case-control study of SUDEP. *Neurology.* 2005;**64**: 1131–1133.

611. Nilsson L, Ahlbom A, Farahmand BY, Tomson T. Mortality in a population-based cohort of epilepsy surgery patients. *Epilepsia.* 2003;**44**:575–581.

612. Seymour N, Granbichler CA, Polkey CE, Nashef L. Mortality after temporal lobe epilepsy surgery. *Epilepsia.* 2012;**53**:267–271.

613. Hussein AA, Gottdiener JS, Bartz TM, Sotoodehnia N, deFilippi C, Dickfeld T, Deo R, Siscovick D, Stein PK, Lloyd-Jones D. Highly sensitive troponin assay sudden cardiac death in the community. The Cardiovascular Health Study. *J Am Coll Cardiol.* 2013;**62**:2112–2120.

614. Emerson H. Periodic medical examinations of apparently health persons. *JAMA.* 1923;**80**:1376–1381.

615. Hayward RSA, Steinberg EP, Ford DE, Roizen MF, Roach KW. Preventive Care Guidelines: 1991. *Ann Intern Med.* 1991;**114**:758–783.

616. Marteau TM, Kinmonth AL. Screening for cardiovascular risk: Public health imperative or matter for individual informed choice. *Br Med J.* 2002;**325**:78–80.

617. Krogsbøll LT, Jørgensen KJ, Larsen CG, Gøtzsche PC. General health checks in adults for reducing morbidity and mortality from disease: Cochrane systematic review and meta-analysis. *Br Med J.* 2012;**345**:e7191.

618. Van Camp SP, Bloor CM, Mueller FO, Cantu RC, Olson HG. Non-traumatic sports death in high school and college athletes. *Med Sci Sports Exerc.* 1995;**27**:641–647.

619. Maron BJ. Sudden death in young athletes. *N Engl J Med.* 2003;**349**:1064–1075.

620. Maron BJ, Thompson PD, Ackerman MJ, Balady G, Berger S, Cohen D, Dimeff R, Douglas PS, Glover DW, Roberts WO, Puffer JC. Recommendations and considerations

related to preparticipation screening for cardiovascular abnormalities in competitive athletes: 2007 update: A scientific statement from the American Heart Association Council on Nutrition, Physical Activity, and Metabolism: Endorsed by the American College of Cardiology Foundation. *Circulation.* 2007;**115**:1643–1655.

621. Maron BJ, Thompson PD, Puffer JC, McGrew CA, Strong WB, Douglas PS, Clark LT, Mitten MJ, Carwford MH, Atkins DL, Driscoll DJ, Epstein AE. Cardiovascular preparticipation screening of competitive athletes: A statement for health professional from the Sudden Cardiac Death Committee (Clinical Cardiology) and Congenital Cardiac Defects Committee (Cardiovascular Disease in the Young), American Heart Association. *Circulation.* 1996;**94**:850–856.

622. Pelliccia A, Maron BJ. Preparticipation cardiovascular evaluation of competitive athlete: Perspectives from the 30-year Italian experience. *Am J Cardiol.* 1995;**75**:827–829.

623. Maron BJ, Pelliccia A. The heart of trained athletes: Cardiac remodeling and the risks of sports, including sudden death. *Circulation.* 2006;**114**:1633–1644.

624. Oswald MD, Dvorak J, Corrado D, Brenner J, Hoogsteen J, McKenna W, Meijboom F, Thiene G, Kappenberger L, Zorzoli M, Rivier L, Sangenis P, Schamasch P, Greinig S, Meijboom E, Bille K, Figueiras D, Sprumont D. Sudden cardiovascular death in sport. Lausanne Recommendations for preparticipation cardiovascular screening. In: Lausanne, Switzerland: International Olympic Council Medical Commission; 2004.

625. Roberts WO, Stovitz S. Incidence of sudden cardiac death in Minnesota high school athletes 1993–2012 screened with a standardized pre-participation evaluation. *J Am Coll Cardiol.* 2013;**62**:1298–1301.

626. Harmon KG, Asif IM, Klossner D, Drezner JA. Incidence of sudden cardiac death in National Collegiate Athletic Association athletes. *Circulation.* 2011;**123**:1594–1600.

627. Montgomery JV, Harris KM, Casey SA, Zenovich AG, Maron BJ. Relation of electrocardiographic patterns to phenotypic expression and clinical outcome in hypertrophic cardiomyopathy. *Am J Cardiol.* 2005;**96**:270–275.

628. Baggish AL, Wood MJ. Athlete's heart and cardiovascular care of the athlete. Scientific and clinical update. *Circulation.* 2011;**123**:2723–2735.

629. Maron BJ, Bodison SA, Wesley YE, Tucker E, Green KJ. Results of screening a large group of intercollegiate competitive athletes for cardiovascular disease. *J Am Coll Cardiol.* 1987;**10**:1214–1221.

630. Tasaki H, Hamasaki Y, Ichimaru T. Mass screening for heart disease of school children in Saga city: 7-year follow up study. *Jpn Circ J.* 1987;**51**:1415–1420.

631. Haneda N, Mori C, Nishio T, Saito M, Kajino Y, Watanabe K, Kijima Y, Yamada K. Heart diseases discovered by mass screening in the schools of Shimane Prefecture over a period of 5 years. *Jpn Circ J.* 1986;**50**:1325–1329.

632. Pelliccia A, Di Paolo FM, Corrado D, Buccolieri C, Quattrini FM, Pisicchio C, Spataro A, Biffi A, Granata M, Maron BJ. Evidence for efficacy of the Italian national pre-participation screening programme for identification of hypertrophic cardiomyopathy in competitive athletes. *Eur Heart J.* 2006;**27**:2196–2200.

633. Fuller CM, McNulty CM, Spring DA, Arger KM, Bruce SS, Chryssos BE, Drummer EM, Kelley FP, Newmark MJ, Whipple GH. Prospective screening of 5,615 high school athletes for risk of sudden cardiac death. *Med Sci Sports Exerc.* 1997;**29**:1131–1138.

634. Baggish AL, Hutter Jr AM, Wang F, Yared K, Weiner RB, Kupperman E, Picard MH, Wood MJ. Cardiovascular screening in college athletes with and without electrocardiography. *Ann Intern Med.* 2010;**152**:269–275.

635. Steinvil A, Chundadze T, Zeltser D, Rogowski O, Halkin A, Galily Y, Perluk H, Viskin S. Mandatory electrocardiographic screening of athletes to reduce their risk for sudden death. Proven fact or wishful thinking? *J Am Coll Cardiol.* 2011;**57**:1291–1296.

636. Chandra N, Bastiaenen, R, Papadakis M, Panoulas VF, Ghani S, Duschl J, Foldes D, Raju H, Osborne R, Sharma S. Prevalence of electrocardiographic anomalies in young individuals: Relevance to a Nationwide Cardiac Screening Program. *J Am Coll Cardiol.* 2014;**63**:2028–2034.

637. Chandra N, Bastiaenen R, Papdakis M, Sharma S. Sudden cardiac death in young athletes. Practical challenges and diagnostic dilemmas. *J Am Coll Cardiol.* 2013;**61**: 1027–1040.

638. Bianco M, Bria S, Gianfelici A, Sanna N, Palmieri V, Zeppilli P. Does early repolarisation in the athelete have analogies with the Brugda syndrome? *Eur Heart J.* 2001;**22**:504–510.

639. Wheeler MT, Heldenreich PA, Froelicher VF, Hlatky MA, Ashley EA. Cost-effectiveness of preparticipation screening for prevention of sudden cardiac death in young athletes. *Ann Intern Med.* 2010;**152**:276–286.

640. Halkin A, Steinvil A, Rosso R, Adler A, Rozovski U, Viskin S. Preventing sudden death of athletes with electrocardiographic screening. What is the absolute benefit and how much will it cost? *J Am Coll Cardiol.* 2012;**60**:2271–2276.

641. Harris KM, Sponsel A, Hutter Jr AM, Maron BJ. Cardiovascular screening practices of major North American professional sports teams. *Ann Intern Med.* 2006;**145**: 507–511.

642. Sofi F, Capalbo A, Pucci N, Giuliattini J, Condino F, Alessandri F, Abbate R, Gensini GF, Califano S. Cardiovascular evaluation, including resting and exercise electrocardiography, before participation in competitive sports: Cross sectional study. *Br Med J.* 2008;**337**:a346.

643. Thompson PD. Preparticipation screening of competitive athletes: Seeking simple solutions of a complex problem. *Circulation.* 2009;**119**:1072–1074.

644. Marijon E, Tafflet M, Celermajer DS, Dumas F, Perier M-C, Mustafic H, Tousaaint J-F, Desnos M, Rieu M, Benameur N, Le Heuzey J-Y, Empana J-P, Jouven X. Sports-related sudden death in the general population. *Circulation.* 2011;**124**:672–681.

645. Pilote L, Pashkow F, Thomas JD, Snader CE, Harvey SA, Marwick TH, Lauer MS. Clinical yield and cost of exercise treadmill testing to screen for coronary artery disease in asymptomatic adults. *Am J Cardiol.* 1998;**81**:219–224.

646. La Gerche A, Baggish AL, Knuuti J, Prior DL, Sharma S, Heidbuchel H, Thompson PD. Cardiac imaging and stress testing asymptomatic athletes to identify those at risk of sudden cardiac death. *J Am Coll Cardiol Img.* 2013;**6**:993–1007.

647. Maron BJ, Pelliccia A, Spirito P. Cardiac disease in young trained athletes. Insights into methods of distinguishing athlete's heart from structural heart disease, with particular emphasis on hypertrophic cardiomyopathy. *Circulation.* 1995;**91**:1596–1601.

648. Sharma S, Elliott PM, Whyte G, Mahon N, Virdee MS, Mist B, McKenna WJ. Utility of metabolic exercise testing in distinguishing hypertrophic cardiomyopathy from physiologic left ventricular hypertrophy in athletes. *J Am Coll Cardiol.* 2000;**36**:864–870.

649. Jouven X, Schwartz PJ, Escolano S, Straczek C, Tafflet M, Desnos M, Empana JP, Ducimetière P. Excessive heart rate increase during mild mental stress in preparation for exercise predicts sudden death in the general population. *Eur Heart J.* 2009;**30**: 1703–1710.

650. La Rovere MT, Bigger Jr JT, Marcus FI, Mortara A, Schwartz PJ, for the ATRAMI (Autonomic Tone and Reflexes After Myocardial Infarction) Investigators. Baroreflex sensitivity and heart-rate variability in prediction of total cardiac mortality after myocardial infarction. *Lancet.* 1998;**351**:478–484.

651. Epstein AE, DiMarco JP, Ellenbogen KA, Estes III NAM, Freedman RA, Gettes LS, Gillinov AM, Gregoratos G, Hammill SC, Hayes DL, Hlatky MA, Newby LK, Page RL, Schoenfeld MH, Silka MJ, Stevenson LW, Sweeney MO. ACC/AHA/HRS 2008 Guidelines for device-based therapy of cardiac rhythm abnormalities. A report of the American College of Cardiology/American Heart Association Task Force on Practice Guidelines (Writing Committee to revise the ACC/AHA/NASPE 2002 Guideline Update for Implantation of Cardiac Pacemakers and Antiarrhythmia Devices) developed in collaboration with the American Association for Thoracic Surgery and Society of Thoracic Surgeons. *J Am Coll Cardiol.* 2008;**51**:e1–e62.

652. Wagner A, Mahrholdt H, Holly TA, Elliott MD, Regenfus M, Parker M, Klocke FJ, Bonow RO, Kim RJ, Judd RM. Contrast-enhanced MRI and routine single photon emission computed tomography (SPECT) perfusion imaging for detection of subendocardial myocardial infarcts: An imaging study. *Lancet.* 2003;**361**:374–379.

653. Dawson DK, Hawlisch K, Prescott G, Roussin I, Di Pietro E, Deac M, Wong J, Frenneaux MP, Pennell DJ, Prasad SK. Prognostic role of CMR in patients presenting with ventricular arrhythmias. *J Am Coll Cardiol Img.* 2013;**6**:335–344.

654. Klem I, Weinsaft JW, Bahnson TD, Hegland D, Kim HW, Hayes B, Parker MA, Judd RM, Kim RJ. Assessment of myocardial scarring improves risk stratification in patients evaluated for cardiac defibrillator implantation. *J Am Coll Cardiol.* 2012;**60**:408–420.

655. Gao P, Yee R, Gula L, Krahn AD, Skanes A, Leong-Sit P, Klein GJ, Stirrat J, Fine N, Pallaveshi L, Wisenberg G, Thompson TR, Prato F, Drangova M, White JA. Prediction of arrhythmic events in ischemic and dilated cardiomyopathy patients referred for implantable cardiac defibrillator: Evaluation of multiple scar quantification measures for late gadolinium enhancement magnetic resonance imaging. *Circ Cardiovasc Imaging.* 2012;**5**:448–456.

656. Aljaroudi WA, Flamm SD, Saliba W, Wilkoff BL, Kwon D. Role of CMR imaging in risk stratification for sudden cardiac death. *J Am Coll Cardiol Img.* 2013;**6**:392–406.

657. Morris JN, Heady JA, Raffle PA, Robert CG, Parks JW. Coronary artery disease and physical activity of work. *Lancet.* 1953;**265**:1111–1120.

658. Morris JN, Chave SPW, Adam C, Sirey C, Epstein L, Sheehan DJ. Vigorous exercise in leisure-time and the incidence of coronary heart-disease. *Lancet.* 1973;**301**: 333–339.

659. Siscovick DS, Weiss NS, Fletcher RH, Lasky T. The incidence of primary cardiac arrest during vigorous exercise. *N Engl J Med.* 1984;**311**:874–877.

660. Albert CM, Mittleman MA, Chae CU, Lee I-M, Hennekens CH, Manson JE. Triggering of sudden death from cardiac causes by vigorous exertion. *N Engl J Med.* 2000;**343**: 1355–1361.

661. Whang W, Manson JE, Hu FB, Chae CU, Rexrode KM, Willett WC, Stampfer MJ, Albert CM. Physical exertion, exercise, and sudden cardiac death in women. *JAMA.* 2006;**295**:1399–1403.

662. Burke AP, Farb A, Malcolm GT, Liang Y, Smialek JE, Virmani R. Plaque rupture and sudden death related to exertion in men with coronary artery disease. *JAMA.* 1999;**281**:921–926.

663. Neilan TG, Yoerger DM, Douglas PS, Marshall JE, Halpern EF, Lawlor D, Picard MH, Wood MJ. Persistent and reversible cardiac dysfunction among amateur marathon runners. *Eur Heart J.* 2006;**27**:1079–1084.

664. Neilan TG, Januzzi JL, Lee-Lewandrowski E, Ton-Nu T-T, Yoerger DM, Jassal DS, Lewandrowski KB, Siegel AJ, Marshall JE, Douglas PS, Lawlor D, Picard MH, Wood MJ. Myocardial injury and ventricular dysfunction related to training levels among non-elite participants in the Boston Marathon. *Circulation.* 2006;**114**:2325–2333.

665. Pelliccia A, Kinoshita N, Pisicchio C, Quattrini F, DiPaolo FM, Ciardo R, Di Giacinto B, Guerra E, De Blasiis E, Casaco M, Culasso F, Maron BJ. Long-term clinical consequences of intense, uninterrupted endurance training in Olympic athletes. *J Am Coll Cardiol.* 2010;**55**:1619–1625.

666. Abergel E, Chatellier G, Hagege AA, Oblak A, Linhart A, Ducardonnet A, Menard J. Serial left ventricular adaptations in world-class professional cyclists. Implications for disease screening and follow-up. *J Am Coll Cardiol.* 2004;**44**:144–149.

667. Laukkanen JA, Mäkikallio TH, Rauramaa R, Kiviniemi V, Ronkainen K, Kurl S. Cardiorespiratory fitness is related to the risk of sudden cardiac death. A population-based follow-up study. *J Am Coll Cardiol.* 2010;**56**:1476–1483.

668. Goraya TY, Jacobsen SJ, Pellikka PA, Miller TD, Khan A, Weston SA, Gersh BJ, Roger VL. Prognostic value of treadmill exercise testing in elderly persons. *Ann Intern Med.* 2000;**132**:862–870.

669. Myers J, Prakash M, Froelicher V, Do D, Partington S, Atwood JE. Exercise capacity and mortality among men referred for exercise testing. *N Engl J Med.* 2002;**346**:793–801.

670. Laukkanen JA, Kurl S, Salonen R, Rauramaa R, Salonen JT. The predictive value of cardiorespiratory fitness for cardiovascular events in men with various risk profiles: A prospective population-based cohort study. *Eur Heart J.* 2004;**25**:1428–1437.

671. Tulppo MP, Mäkikallio TH, Seppänen T, Laukkanen RT, Huikuri HV. Vagal modulation of heart rate during exercise: Effects of age and physical fitness. *Am J Physiol.* 1988;**274**:H424–429.

672. Bouchard C, Sarzynski MA, Rice TK, Kraus WE, Church TS, Sung YJ, Rao DC, Rankinen T. Genomic predictors of the maximal O_2 uptake response to standardized exercise training programs. *J Appl Physiol.* 2011;**110**:1160–1170.

673. Berry JD, Willis B, Gupta S, Barlow CE, Lakoski SG, Khera A, Rohatgi A, de Lemos JA, Haskell W, Lloyd-Jones DM. Lifetime risks for cardiovascular disease mortality by cardiorespiratory fitness levels measured at ages 45, 55, and 65 years in men. The Cooper Center Longitudinal Study. *J Am Coll Cardiol.* 2011;**57**:1604–1610.

674. Caspersen CJ, Powell KE, Christenson GM. Physical activity, exercise, and physical fitness: Definitions and distinctions for health-related research. *Public Health Rep.* 1985;**100**:126–131.

675. U.S. Department of Health and Human Services. *2008 Physical activity guidelines for Americans (Publication No. U0036)*. Washington, D.C.: Office of Disease Prevention and Health Promotion, U.S. Department of Health and Human Services; 2008.

676. Sattelmair J, Pertman J, Ding EL, Kohl III HW, Haskell W, Lee I-M. Dose response between physical activity and risk of coronary heart disease: A meta-analysis. *Circulation.* 2011;**124**:789–795.

677. Church TS, Thomas DM, Tudor-Locke C, Katzmarzyk PT, Earnest CP, Rodarte RQ, Martin CK, Blair SN, Bouchard C. Trends over 5 decades in U.S. occupation-related physical activity and their associations with obesity. *PLoS One.* 2011;**6**:e19657.

678. Schoenborn CA, Adams PE. Health behaviors of adults: United States, 2005–2007. *Vital Health Stat.* 2010;**10**(245):1–132.

679. Epidemiology and Disease Control Division. National Health Surveillance Survey 2007. In: Singapore: Ministry of Health, Singapore; 2007:7–14.

680. Paffenbarger Jr RS, Hyde RT, Wing AL, Lee I-M, Jung DL, Kampert JB. The association of changes in physical activity level and other lifestyle characteristics with mortality among men. *N Engl J Med.* 1993;**328**:538–545.

681. Lee CD, Folsom AR, Blair SN. Physical activity and stroke risk: A meta-analysis. *Stroke.* 2003;**34**:2475–2481.

682. Diabetes Prevention Program Research Group. Reduction in the incidence of type 2 diabetes with lifestyle intervention or metformin. *N Engl J Med.* 2002;**346**:393–403.

683. Thompson PD, Buchner D, Piña IL, Balady GJ, Williams MA, Marcus BH, Berra K, Blair SN, Costa F, Franklin B, Fletcher GF, Gordon NF, Pate RR, Rodriguez BL, Yancey AK, Wenger NK. Exercise and physical activity in the prevention and treatment of atherosclerotic cardiovascular disease. A statement from the Council on Clinical Cardiology (Subcommittee on Exercise, Rehabilitation, and Prevention) and the Council on Nutrition, Physical Activity, and Metabolism (Subcommittee on Physical Activity). *Arterioscler Thromb Vasc Biol.* 2003;**23**:e42–e49.

684. Schuler G, Adams V, Goto Y. Role of exercise in the prevention of cardiovascular disease: Results, mechanisms, and new perspectives. *Eur Heart J.* 2013;**34**:1790–1799.

685. Mora S, Cook N, Buring JE, Ridker PM, Lee I-M. Physical activity and reduced risk of cardiovascular events: Potential mediating mechanisms. *Circulation.* 2007;**116**: 2110–2118.

686. Lustig RH. *Fat chance: The hidden truth about sugar, obesity and heart disease.* London: Fourth Estate; 2013.

687. Bravata DM, Smith-Spangler C, Sundaram V, Gienger AL, Lin N, Lewis R, Stave CD, Olkin I, Sirad JR. Using pedometers to increase physical activity and improve health: A systematic review. *JAMA.* 2007;**298**:2296–2304.

688. Lewington S, Clarke R, Qizilbash N, Peto R, Collins R. Age-specific relevance of usual blood pressure to vascular mortality: A meta-analysis of individual data for one million adults in 61 prospective studies. *Lancet.* 2002;**360**:1903–1913.

689. Marshall SJ, Levy SS, Tudor-Locke CE, Kolkhorst FW, Wooten KM, Ji M, Macera CA, Ainsworth BE. Translating physical activity recommendations into a pedometer-based step goal: 3000 steps in 30 minutes. *Am J Prev Med.* 2009;**36**:410–415.

690. Biddiss E, Irwin J. Active video games to promote physical activity in children and youth. *Arch Pediatr Adolesc Med.* 2010;**164**:664–672.

691. Barnett A, Cerin E, Baranowski T. Active video games for youth: A systematic review. *J Phys Act Health.* 2011;**8**:724–737.

692. Peng W, Lin JH, Crouse J. Is playing exergames really exercising? A meta-analysis of energy expenditure in active video games. *Cyberpsychol Behav Soc Netw.* 2011;**14**: 681–688.

693. Graves L, Stratton G, Ridgers ND, Cable NT. Energy expenditure in adolescents play-ing new generation computer games. *Br Med J.* 2007;**335**:1282–1284.

694. Lieberman DA, Chamberlin B, Medina Jr E, Franklin BA, Sanner BM, Vafiadis DK, on behalf of The Power of Play: Innovations in Getting Active Summit Planning Committee. The Power of Play: Innovations in Getting Active Summit 2011: A science panel pro-ceedings report from the American Heart Association. *Circulation.* 2011;**123**:2507–2516.

695. Yankelson L, Sadeh B, Gershovitz L, Werthein J, Heller K, Halpern P, Halkin A, Adler A, Steinvil A, Viskin S. Life-threatening events during endurance sports. Is heat stroke more prevalent than arrhythmic death? *J Am Coll Cardiol.* 2014;**64**:463–469.

696. Rea T, Page RL. Community approaches to improve resuscitation after out-of-hospital cardiac arrest. *Circulation.* 2010;**121**:1134–1140.

697. Lloyd-Jones DM, Hong Y, Labarthe D, Mozaffarian D, Appel LJ, Van Horn L, Greenlund K, Daniels S, Nichol G, Tomaselli GF, Arnett DK, Fonarow GC, Ho PM, Lauer MS, Masoudi FA, Robertson RM, Roger V, Schwamm LH, Sorlie P, Yancy CW, Rosamond WD, American Heart Association Strategic Planning Task Force and Statistics Committee. Defining and setting national goals for cardiovascular health promotion and disease reduction: The American Heart Association's strategic impact goal through 2020 and beyond. *Circulation.* 2010;**121**:586–613.

698. Estes III NAM. Predicting and preventing sudden cardiac death. *Circulation.* 2011;**124**:651–656.

699. Kahn R, Robertson RM, Smith R, Eddy D. The impact of prevention of reducing the burden of cardiovascular disease. *Circulation.* 2008;**118**:576–585.

700. Ravnskov U. *The cholesterol myths: Exposing the fallacy that saturated fat and cholesterol cause heart disease.* Washington, D.C.: NewTrends Publishing, Inc.; 2000.

701. Kendrick M. *The great cholesterol con: The truth about what really causes heart disease and how to avoid it.* London, England: John Blake Publishing Ltd; 2007.

702. Keys A. Coronary heart disease in seven countries. *Circulation.* 1970;**41**(Supp 1):1–211.

703. Keys A, Mienotti A, Karvonen MJ, Aravanis C, Blackburn H, Buzina R, Djordjevic BS, Dontas AS, Fidanza F, Keys MH, Kromhout D, Nedeljkovic S, Punsar S, Seccareccia F, Toshima H. The diet and 15-year death rate in the seven countries study. *Am J Epidemiol.* 1986;**124**:903–915.

704. Sinclair HM. Deficiency of essential fatty acids and atherosclerosis, etcetera. *Lancet.* 1956;**267**:381–383.

705. Bang HO, Dyerberg J, Hjørne N. The composition of food consumed by Greenland Eskimos. *Acta Med Scand.* 1976;**200**:69–73.

706. Bang HO, Dyerberg J, Nielsen A. Plasma lipid and lipoprotein pattern in Greenlandic west-coast Eskimos. *Lancet.* 1971;**297**:1143–1146.

707. Dyerberg J, Bang HO. Haemostatic function and platelet polyunsaturated fatty acids in Eskimos. *Lancet.* 1979;**2**:433–435.

708. Bang HO, Dyerberg J. Personal reflections on the incidence of ischaemic heart dis-ease in Oslo during the Second World War. *Acta Med Scand.* 1981;**210**:245–248.

709. Dyerberg J, Bang HO, Stoffersen E, Moncada S, Vane JR. Eicosapentaenoic acid and prevention of thrombosis and atherosclerosis? *Lancet.* 1978;**312**:117–119.

710. Sinclair HM. Advantages and disadvantages of an Eskimo diet. In: Fumagalli R, Kritchevsky D, Peoletti R, eds. *Drugs affecting lipid metabolism.* Amsterdam: Elsevier/North-Holland Biomedical Press; 1980:363–370.

711. Kromhout D, Bosschieter EB, de Lezenne Coulander C. The inverse relation between fish consumption and 20-year mortality from coronary heart disease. *N Engl J Med.* 1985;**312**:1205–1209.

712. Hu FB, Bronner L, Willett WC, Stampfer MJ, Rexrode KM, Albert CM, Hunter D, Manso JE. Fish and omega-3 fatty acid intake and risk of coronary heart disease in women. *JAMA.* 2002;**287**:1815–1821.

713. Siscovick DS, Raghunathan TE, King I, Weinmann S, Wicklund KG, Albright J, Bovbjerg V, Arbogast P, Smith H, Kushi LH, Retzlaff B, Childs M, Knopp RH. Dietary intake and cell membrane levels of long-chain n-3 polyunsaturated fatty acids and the risk of primary cardiac arrest. *JAMA.* 1995;**274**:1363–1367.

714. Daviglus ML, Stamler J, Orencia AJ, Dyer AR, Liu K, Greenland P, Walsh MK, Morris D, Shekelle RB. Fish consumption and the 30-year risk of fatal myocardial infarction. *N Engl J Med.* 1997;**336**:1046–1053.

715. Bjerregaard LJ, Joensen AM, Dethlefsen C, Jensen MK, Johnsen SP, Tjønneland A, Rasmussen LH, Overvad K, Schmidt EB. Fish intake and acute coronary syndrome. *Eur Heart J.* 2010;**31**:29–34.

716. Burr ML, Gilbert JF, Holliday RM, Elwood PC, Fehily AM, Rogers S, Sweetnam PM, Deadman NM. Effects of changes in fat, fish, and fibre intakes on death and myocardial reinfarction: Diet and Reinfarction Trial (DART). *Lancet.* 1989;**334**:757–761.

717. Yamagishi K, Iso H, Date C, Fukui M, Wakai K, Kikuchi S, Inaba Y, Tanabe N, Tamakoshi A, Japan Collaborative Cohort Study for Evaluation of Cancer Risk Study Group. Fish, omega-3 polyunsaturated fatty acids, and mortality from cardiovascular diseases in a nationwide community-based cohort of Japanese men and women the JACC (Japan Collaborative Cohort Study for Evaluation of Cancer Risk) Study. *J Am Coll Cardiol.* 2008;**52**:988–996.

718. Albert CM, Hennekens CH, O'Donnell CJ, Ajani UA, Carey VJ, Willett WC, Ruskin JN, Manson JE. Fish consumption and risk of sudden cardiac death. *JAMA.* 1998;**279**:23–28.

719. Guallar E, Hennekens CH, Sacks FM, Willett WC, Stampfer MJ. A prospective study of plasma fish oil levels and incidence of myocardial infarction in U.S. male physicians. *J Am Coll Cardiol.* 1995;**25**:387–394.

720. von Lossonczy TO, Ruiter A, Bronsgeest-Schoute HC, van Gent CM, Hermus RJ. The effect of a fish diet on serum lipids in healthy human subjects. *Am J Clin Nutr.* 1978;**31**:1340–1346.

721. Sanders TA, Vickers M, Haines AP. Effect on blood lipids and haemostasis of a supplement of cod-liver oil, rich in eicosapentaenoic and docosahexaenoic acids, in healthy young men. *Clin Sci (Lond).* 1981;**61**:317–324.

722. Saynor R, Verel D, Gillott T. The long-term effect of dietary supplementation with fish lipid concentrate on serum lipids, bleeding time, platelets and angina. *Atherosclerosis.* 1984;**50**:3–10.

723. Harris WS, Connor WE, McMurry MP. The comparative reductions of the plasma lipids and lipoproteins by dietary polyunsaturated fats: Salmon oil versus vegetable oils. *Metabolism.* 1983;**32**:179–184.

724. Smith PJ, Bulmenthal JA, Babyak MA, Georgiades A, Sherwood A, Sketch MH, Watkins LL. Association between n-3 fatty acid consumption and ventricular ectopy after myocardial infarction. *Am J Clin Nutr.* 2009;**89**:1315–1320.

725.   Billman GE, Hallaq H, Leaf A. Prevention of ischemia-induced ventricular fibrillation by *w*3 fatty acids. *Proc Natl Acad Sci USA*. 1994;**91**:4427–4430.

726.   London B, Albert C, Anderson ME, Giles WR, Van Wagoner DR, Balk E, Billman GE, Chung M, Lands W, Leaf A, McAnulty J, Martens JR, Costello RB, Lathrop DA. Omega-3 fatty acids and cardiac arrhythmias: Prior studies and recommendations for future research: A report from the National Heart, Lung, and Blood Institute and Office of Dietary Supplements omega-3 fatty acids and their role in cardiac arrhythmogenesis workshop. *Circulation*. 2007;**116**:e320–e335.

727.   Ebrahimi M, Ghayour-Mobarhan M, Rezaiean S, Hoseini M, Parizade SM, Farhoudi F, Hosseininezhad SJ, Tavallaei S, Vejdani A, Azimi-Nezhad M, Shakeri MT, Rad MA, Mobarra N, Kazemi-Bajestani SM, Ferns GA. Omega-3 fatty acid supplements improve cardiovascular risk profile of subjects with metabolic syndrome, including markers of inflammation and auto-immunity. *Acta Cardiol*. 2009;**64**:321–327.

728.   Zampelas A, Panagiotakos DB, Pitsavos C, Das UN, Chrysohoou C, Skoumas Y, Stefanadis C. Fish consumption among health adults is associated with decreased levels of inflammatory markers related to cardiovascular disease. The ATTICA Study. *J Am Coll Cardiol*. 2005;**46**:120–124.

729.   Dallongeville J, Yarnell J, Ducimetière P, Arveiler D, Ferrières J, Montaye M, Luc G, Evans A, Bingham A, Hass B, Ruidavets J-B, Amouyel P. Fish consumption is associated with lower heart rates. *Circulation*. 2003;**108**:820–825.

730.   Christensen JH, Korup E, Aarøe J, Toft E, Møller J, Rasmussen K, Dyerberg J, Schmidt EB. Fish consumption, n-3 fatty acids in cell membranes, and heart rate variability in survivors of myocardial infarction wtih left ventricular dysfunction. *Am J Cardiol*. 1997;**79**:1670–1673.

731.   Christensen JH, Skou HA, Fog L, Hansen VE, Vesterlund T, Dyerberg J, Toft E, Schmidt EB. Marine n-3 fatty acids, wine intake, and heart rate variability in patients referred for coronary angiography. *Circulation*. 2001;**103**:651–657.

732.   Hartikainen JEK, Malik M, Staunton A, Poloniecki J, Camm AJ. Distinction between arrhythmic and nonarrhythmic death after acute myocardial infarction based on heart rate variability, signal-averaged electrocardiogram, ventricular arrhythmias and left ventricular ejection fraction. *J Am Coll Cardiol*. 1996;**28**:296–304.

733.   Schwellenbach LJ, Olson KL, McConnell KJ, Stolcpart RS, Nash JD, Merenich JA, for the Clinical Pharmacy Cardiac Risk Service Study Group. The triglyceride-lowering effects of a modest dose of docosahexaenoic acid alone versus in combination with low dose eicosapentaenoic acid in patients with coronary artery disease and elevated triglycerides. *J Am Coll Nutr*. 2006;**25**:480–485.

734.   Mori TA, Beilin LJ, Burke V, Morris J, Ritchie J. Interactions between dietary fat, fish, and fish oils and their effects on platelet function in men at risk of cardiovascular disease. *Arterioscler Thromb Vasc Biol*. 1997;**17**:279–286.

735.   Landmark K, Abdelnoor M, Kilhovd B, Dørum HP. Eating fish may reduce infarct size and the occurrence of Q wave infarcts. *Eur J Clin Nutr*. 1998;**52**:40–44.

736.   Thies F, Garry JMC, Yaqoob P, Rerkasem K, Williams J, Shearman CP, Gallagher PJ, Calder PC, Grimble RF. Association of n-3 polyunsaturated fatty acids with stability of atherosclerotic plaques: A randomised controlled trial. *Lancet*. 2003;**361**:477–485.

737.   Kawano H, Yano T, Mizuguchi M, Mochizuki H, Saito Y. Changes in aspects such as the collagenous fiber density and foam cell size of atherosclerotic lesions composed of

foam cells, smooth muscle cells and fibrous components in rabbits caused by all-cis 5, 8, 11, 14, 17-icosapentaenoic acid. *J Atheroscler Thromb*. 2002;**9**:170–177.

738. Terano T, Salmon JA, Moncada S. Effect of orally administered eicosapenaenoic acid (EPA) on the formation of leukotriene B4 and leukotriene B5 by rat leukocytes. *Biochem Pharmacol*. 1984;**33**:3071–3076.

739. Wallace JM, Turley E, Gilmore WS, Strain JJ. Dietary fish oil supplementation alters leukocyte function and cytokine production in healthy women. *Arterioscler Thromb Vasc Biol*. 1995;**15**:185–189.

740. Baumann KH, Hessel F, Larass I, Müller T, Kiefl R, von Schacky C. Dietary omega-3, omega-6, and omega-9 unsaturated fatty acids and growth factor and cytokine gene expression in unstimulated and stimulated monocytes. A randomized volunteer study. *Arterioscler Thromb Vasc Biol*. 1999;**19**:59–66.

741. Miles EA, Wallace FA, Calder PC. Dietary fish oil reduces intercellular adhesion molecule 1 and scavenger receptor expression on murine macrophages. *Atherosclerosis*. 2000;**152**:43–50.

742. Chen H, Li D, Chen J, Robert GJ, Saldeen T, Mehta JL. EPA and DHA attenuate ox-LDL-induced expression of adhesion molecules in human coronary artery endothelial cells via protein kinase B pathway. *J Mol Cell Cardiol*. 2003;**35**:769–775.

743. de Lorgeril M, Renaud S, Salen P, Monjaud I, Mamelle N, Martin JL, Guidollet J, Touboul P, Delaye J. Mediterranean alpha-linolenic acid-rich diet in secondary prevetion of coronary heart disease. *Lancet*. 1994;**343**:1454–1459.

744. de Lorgeril M, Salen P, Martin J-L, Monjaud I, Delaye J, Mamelle N. Mediterranean diet, traditional risk factors, and the rate of cardiovascular complications after myocardial infarction: Final report of the Lyon Diet Heart Study. *Circulation*. 1999;**99**:779–785.

745. Kris-Etherton P, Eckel RH, Howard BV, St Jeor S, Bazzarre TL, for the Nutrition Committee, Population Science Committee, and Clinical Science Committee of the American Heart Association, Lyon Diet Heart Study. Benefits of a Mediterranean-style, National Cholesterol Education Program/American Heart Association step I dietary pattern on cardiovascular disease. *Circulation*. 2001;**103**:1823–1825.

746. Mozaffarian D, Wu JHY. Omega-3 fatty acids and cardiovascular disease: Effects on risk factors, molecular pathways, and clinical events. *J Am Coll Cardiol*. 2011;**58**:2047–2067.

747. Rissanen T, Voutilainen S, Nyyssönen K, Lakka TA, Salonen JT. Fish oil-derived fatty acids, docosahexaenoic acid and docosapentaenoic acid, and the risk of acute coronary events. The Kuopio Ischaemic Heart Disease Risk Factor Study. *Circulation*. 2000;**102**:2677–2679.

748. Salonen J, Seppänen K, Lakka TA, Salonen R, Kaplan GA. Mercury accumulation and accelerated progression of carotid atherosclerosis: A population-based prospective 4-year follow-up study in men in eastern Finland. *Atherosclerosis*. 2000;**148**:265–273.

749. Virtanen JK, Voutilainen S, Rissanen TH, Mursu J, Tuomainen T-P, Korhonen MJ, Valkonen V-P, Seppänen K, Laukkanen JA, Salonen JT. Mercury, fish oils, and risk of acute coronary events and cardiovascular disease, coronary heart disease, and all-cause mortality in men in eastern Finland. *Arterioscler Thromb Vasc Biol*. 2005;**25**:228–233.

750. Guallar E, Sanz-Gallardo MI, van't Veer P, Bode P, Aro A, Gómez-Aracena J, Kark JD, Riemersma RA, Martín-Moreno JM, Kok FJ, Heavy Metals and Myocardial Infarction Study Group. Mercury, fish oils, and the risk of myocardial infarction. *N Engl J Med*. 2002;**347**:1747–1754.

751. Salonen JT, Seppänen K, Nyyssönen K, Korpela H, Kauhanen J, Kantola M, Tuomilehto J, Esterbauer H, Tatzber F, Salonen R. Intake of mercury from fish, lipid peroxidation, and the risk of myocardial infarction and coronary, cardiovascular, and any death in eastern Finnish men. *Circulation.* 1995;**91**:645–655.

752. Mozaffarian D, Shi P, Morris JS, Spiegelman D, Grandjean P, Siscovick DS, Willett WC, Rimm EB. Mercury exposure and risk of cardiovascular disease in two U.S. cohorts. *N Engl J Med.* 2011;**364**:1116–1125.

753. Kromann N, Green A. Epidemiological studies in the Upernavik District, Greenland. *Acta Medica Scandinavica.* 1980;**208**:401–406.

754. Mozaffarian D, Ascherio A, Hu FB, Stampfer MJ, Willett WC, Siscovick DS, Rimm EB. Interplay between different polyunsaturated fatty acids and risk of coronary heart disease in men. *Circulation.* 2005;**111**:157–164.

755. Djoussé L, Arnett DK, Carr JJ, Eckfeldt JH, Hopkins PN, Province MA, Ellison RC. Dietary linolenic acid is inversely associated with calcified atherosclerotic plaque in the coronary arteries. The National Heart, Lung, and Blood Institute Family Heart Study. *Circulation.* 2005;**111**:2921–2926.

756. Singh RB, Niaz MA, Sharma JP, Kumar R, Rastogi V, Moshiri M. Randomized, double-blind, placebo-controlled trial of fish oil and mustard oil in patients with suspected acute myocardial infarction: The Indian experiment of infarct survival-4. *Cardiovasc Drugs Ther.* 1997;**11**:485–491.

757. Oomen CM, Ocké MC, Feskens EJM, Kok FJ, Krombout D. Alpha-linolenic acid intake is not beneficially associated wtih 10-y risk of coronary artery incidence: The Zutphen Elderly Study. *Am J Clin Nutr.* 2001;**74**:457–463.

758. Burdge GC, Jones AE, Wootton SA. Eicosapentaenoic and docosapentaenoic acids are the principal products of alpha-linolenic acid metablism in young men. *Br J Nutr.* 2002;**88**:355–363.

759. Duda MK, O'Shea KMO, Tintinu A, Xu W, Khairallah RJ, Barrows BR, Chess DJ, Azimzadeh AM, Harris WS, Sharov VG, Sabbah HN, Stanley WC. Fish oil, but not flaxseed oil, decreases inflammation and prevents pressure overload-induced cardiac dysfunction. *Cardiovasc Res.* 2009;**81**:319–327.

760. Sanders TAB, Roshania F. The influence of different types of w3 polyunsaturated fatty acids on blood lipids and platelet function in healthy volunteers. *Clin Sci.* 1983;**64**:91–99.

761. Yokoyama M, Origasa H, Matsuzaki M, Matsuzawa Y, Saito Y, Ischikawa Y, Oikawa S, Sasaki J, Hishida H, Itakura H, Kita T, Kitabatake A, Nakaya N, Sakata T, Shimada K, Shirato K, Japan EPA Lipid Intervention Study JELIS) Investigators. Effects of eicosa-pentaenoic acid on major coronary events in hypercholesterolaemic patients (JELIS): A randomised open-label, blinded endpoint analysis. *Lancet.* 2007;**369**:1090–1098.

762. GISSI-Prevenzione Investigators. Dietary supplementation with n-3 polyunsaturated fatty acids and vitamin E after myocardial infarction: Results of the GISSI-Prevenzione trial. *Lancet.* 1999;**354**:447–455.

763. Marchioli R, Barzi F, Bomba E, Chieffo C, Di Gregorio D, Di Mascio R, Franzosi MG, Geraci E, Marfisi RM, Mastrogiuseppe G, Mininni N, Nicolosi GL, Santini M, Schweiger C, Tavazzi L, Tognoni G, Tucci C, Valagussa F, on behalf of the GISSI-Prevenzione Investigators. Early protection against sudden death by n-3 polyunsaturated fatty acids after myocardial infarction. Time-course analysis of the

results of the Gruppo Italiano per lo Studio della Sopravivivenza nell'Infarto Miocardico (GISSI)-Prevenzione. *Circulation.* 2002;**105**:1897–1903.

764. Landmark K, Abdelnoor M, Urdal P, Kilhovd B, Dørum HP, Borge N, Refvem H. Use of fish oils appears to reduce infarct size as estimated from peak creatine kinase and lactate dehydrogenase activities. *Cardiology.* 1998;**89**:94–102.

765. Nilsen DWT, Albrektsen G, Landmark K, Moen S, Aarsland T, Woie L. Effects o a high-dose concentrate of n-3 fatty acids or corn oil introduced early after an acute myocardial infarction on serum triacylglycerol and HDL cholesterol. *Am J Clin Nutr.* 2001;**74**:50–56.

766. Pietinen P, Ascherio A, Korhonen P, Hartman AM, Willett WC, Albanes D, Virtamo J. Intake of fatty acids and risk of coronary heart disease in a cohort of Finnish men. The Alpha-Tocopherol, Beta-Carotene Cancer Prevention Study. *Am J Epidemiol.* 1997;**145**:876–887.

767. Léon H, Shibata MC, Sivakumaran S, Dorgan M, Chatterley T, Tsuyuki RT. Effect of fish oil on arrhythmias and mortality: Systematic review. *Br Med J.* 2008;**337**:a2931.

768. Bucher HC, Hengstler P, Schindler C, Meier G. N3 polyunsaturated fatty acids in coronary heart disease: A meta-analysis of randomized controlled trials. *Am J Med.* 2002;**112**:298–304.

769. The ORIGIN Trial Investigators. n-3 fatty acids and cardiovascular outcomes in patients with dysglycemia. *N Engl J Med.* 2012;**367**:309–318.

770. The Risk and Prevention Study Collaborative Group. n-3 fatty acids in patients with multiple cardiovascular risk factors. *N Engl J Med.* 2013;**368**:1800–1808.

771. Kris-Etherton PM, Harris WS, Appel LJ, for the Nutrition Committee. Fish consumption, fish oil, omega-3 fatty acids, and cardiovascular disease. *Circulation.* 2002;**106**:2747–2757.

772. Foran SE, Flood JG, Lewandrowski KB. Measurement of mercury levels in concentrated over-the-counter fish oil preparations. Is fish oil healthier than fish? *Arch Pathol Lab Med.* 2003;**127**:1603–1605.

773. Hilbert G, Lillemark L, Balchen S, Højskov CS. Reduction of organochlorine contaminants from fish oil during refining. *Chemosphere.* 1998;**37**:1241–1252.

774. Melanson SF, Lewandrowski EL, Flood JG, Lewandrowski KB. Measurement of organochlorines in commerical over-the-counter fish oil preparations. Implications for dietary and therapeutic reccomendations for omega-3 fatty acids and a review of the literature. *Arch Pathol Lab Med.* 2005;**129**:74–77.

775. Jacobs MN, Santillo D, Johnston PA, Wyatt CL, French MC. Organochlorine residues in fish oil dietary supplements: Comparison with industrial grade oils. *Chemosphere.* 1998;**37**:1709–1721.

776. Rawn DF, Breakell K, Verigin V, Nicolidakis H, Sit D, Feeley M, Ryan JJ. Persistent organic pollutants in fish oil supplements on the Canadian market: Polychlorinated dibenzo-p-dioxins, dibenzofurans, and polybrominated diphenyl ethers. *J Food Sci.* 2009;**74**:T31–T36.

777. Marti M, Ortiz X, Gasser M, Marti R, Montaña MJ, Diaz-Ferrero J. Persistent organic pollutants (PCDD/Fs, dioxin-like PCBs, and PBDEs) in health supplements on the Spanish market. *Chemosphere.* 2010;**78**:1256–1262.

778. Burr MI, Ashfield-Watt PA, Dunstan FD, Fehily AM, Breay P, Ashton T, Zotos PC, Haboubi NA, Elwood PC. Lack of benefit of dietary advice to men with angina: Results of a controlled trial. *Eur J Clin Nutr.* 2003;**57**:193–200.

779. Kromhout D, Giltay EJ, Geleijnse JM, For the Alpha Omega Trial Group. n-3 fatty acids and cardiovascular events after myocardial infarction. *N Engl J Med.* 2010;**363**: 2015–2026.

780. Eckel RH. The fish oil story remains fishy. *Circulation.* 2010;**122**:2110–2112.

781. Simopoulos AP. Essential fatty acids in health and chronic disease. *Am J Clin Nutr.* 1999;**70**:560S–569S.

782. Simopoulos A. The importance of the omega-6/omega-3 fatty acid ratio in cardiovascular disease and other chronic diseases. *Exp Biol Med.* 2008;**233**:674–688.

783. Calder PC. n-3 polyunsaturated fatty acids, inflammation, and inflammatory diseases. *Am J Clin Nutr.* 2006;**83**(Suppl):1505S–1519S.

784. Sanders TAB, Oakley FR, Miller GJ, Mitropoulos KA, Crook D, Oliver MF. Influence of n-6 versus n-3 polyunsaturated fatty acids in diets low in saturated fatty acids on plasma lipoproteins and hemostatic factors. *Arterioscler Thromb Vasc Biol.* 1997;**17**: 3449–3460.

785. Hu FB, Stampfer MJ, Manson JE, Rimm EB, Wolk A, Colditz GA, Hennekens CH, Willett WC. Dietary intake of alpha-linolenic acid and riks of fatal ischemic heart disease among women. *Am J Clin Nutr.* 1999;**69**:890–897.

786. Harris WS, Moaffarian D, Rimm E, Kris-Etherton P, Rudel LL, Appel LJ, Engler MM, Engler MB, Sacks F. Omega-6 fatty acids and risk for cardiovascular disease: A Science Advisory from the American Heart Association Nutrition Subcommittee of the Council on Nutrition, Physical Activity, and Metabolism; Council on Cardiovascular Nursing; and Council on Epidemiology and Prevention. *Circulation.* 2009;**119**:902–907.

787. Ramsden CE, Zamora D, Leelarthaepin B, Majchrzak-Hong SF, Faurot KR, Suchindran CM, Ringel A, Davis JM. Use of dietary linoleic acid for secondary prevention of coronary heart disease and death: Evaluation of recovered data from the Sydney Diet Heart Study and updated meta-analysis. *Br Med J.* 2013;**346**:e8707.

788. Louheranta AM, Porkkala-Sarataho EK, Nyyssönen MK, Salonen RM, Salonen JT. Linoleic acid intake and susceptibility of very-low-density and low-density lipoproteins to oxidation in men. *Am J Clin Nutr.* 1996;**63**:698–703.

789. Salonen JT, Nyyssönen K, Salonen R, Porkkala-Sarataho E, Tuomainen T-P, Diczfalusy U, Björkhem I. Lipoprotein oxidation and progression of carotid atherosclerosis. *Circulation.* 1997;**95**:840–845.

790. Lai C-Q, Corella D, Demissie S, Cupples LA, Adiconis X, Zhu Y, Parnell LD, Tucker KL, Ordovas JM. Dietary intake of n-6 fatty acids modulates effect of apolipoprotein A5 gene on plasma fasting triglycerides, remnant lipoprotein concentrations, and lipoprotein particle size. The Framingham Heart Study. *Circulation.* 2006;**113**:2062–2070.

791. Ramsden CE, Ringel A, Feldstein AE, Taha AY, MacIntosh BA, Hibbeln JR, Majchrzak-Hong SF, Faurot KR, Rapoport SI, Cheon Y, Chung YM, Berk M, Mann JD. Lowering dietary linoleic acid reduces bioactive oxidized linoleic acid metabolites in humans. *Prostaglandins Leukot Essent Fatty Acids.* 2012;**87**:135–141.

792. Universal Medical Identification Symbol. *Am J Dis Child.* 1964;**107**:439.

793. Wilcox RA, Whitham EM. The symbol of modern medicne: Why one snake is more than two. *Ann Intern Med.* 2003;**138**:673–677.

794. Arzamendi D, Benito B, Tizon-Marcos H, Flores J, Tanguay JF, Ly H, Doucet S, Leduc L, Leung TK, Campuzano O, Iglesias A, Talajic M, Brugada R. Increase in sudden death from coronary artery disease in young adults. *Am Heart J.* 2011;**161**:574–580.

795. Anderson JL, Rodier HE, Green LS. Comparative effects of beta-adrenergic blocking drugs on experimental ventricular threshold. *Am J Cardiol.* 1983;**51**:1196–1202.

796. Beta-blocker Heart Attack Trial Research Group. A randomized trial of propranolol in patients with acute myocardial infarction, I: Mortality results. *JAMA.* 1982;**247**: 1707–1714.

797. Hansteen V, Møinichen E, Lorentsen E, Andersen A, Strøm O, Søiland K, Dyrbekk D, Refsum A-M, Tromsdal A, Knudsen K, Eika C, Bakken J, Smith P, Hoff PI. One year's treatment with propranolol after myocardial infarction: Preliminary report of Norwegian multicentre trial. *Br Med J.* 1982;**284**:155–160.

798. Hansteen V. Beta blockade after myocardial infarction: The Norwegian propranolol study in high-risk patients. *Circulation.* 1983;**62**:I57-I60.

799. The Norwegian Multicenter Study Group. Timolol-induced reduction in mortality and reinfarction surviving acute myocardial infarction. *N Engl J Med.* 1981;**304**: 801–807.

800. Chadda K, Goldstein S, Byington R, Curb JD. Effect of propranolol after acute myocardial infarction in patients with congestive heart failure. *Circulation.* 1986;**73**:503–510.

801. Al-Gobari M, El Khatib C, Pillon F, Gueyffier F. Beta-blockers for the prevention of sudden cardiac death in heart failure patients: A meta-analysis of randomized controlled trials. *BMC Cardiovascular Disorders.* 2013;**13**:52.

802. Ferreira SH, Bartelt DC, Greene LJ. Isolation of bradykinin-potentiating peptides from *Bothrops jararaca* venom. *Biochemistry.* 1970;**9**:2583–2593.

803. Smith CG, Vane JR. The discovery of captopril. *FASEB J.* 2003;**17**:788–789.

804. Gavras H, Brunner HR, Laragh JH, Sealey JE, Gavras I, Vukovich RA. An angiotensin converting-enzyme inhibitor to identify and treat vasocontrictor and volume factors in hypertensive patients. *N Engl J Med.* 1974;**291**:817–821.

805. Ondetti MA, Rubin B, Cushman DW. Design of specific inhibitors of angiotensin-converting enzyme: New class of orally active antihypertensive agents. *Science.* 1977;**196**:441–444.

806. Domanski MJ, Exner DV, Borkowf CB, Geller NL, Rosenberg Y, Pfeffer MA. Effect of angiotensin converting enzyme inhibition on sudden cardiac death in patients following acute myocardial infarction. A meta-analysis of randomized clinical trials. *J Am Coll Cardiol.* 1999;**33**:598–604.

807. Garg R, Yusuf S, Bussmann WD, Sleight P, Uprichard A, Massie B, McGrath B, Nilsson B, Pitt B, Magnani B, Maskin C, Ambrosioni E, Rucinska W, Kleber FX, Jennings G, Tognoni G, Drexler H, Cleland JGF, Franciosa JA, Remes J, Swedberg K, Joy M, Sharpe N, Desche P, McGarry R, Collins R, Chrysant SG, Cicchetti V. Overview of randomized trials of angiotensin-converting enzyme inhibitors on mortality and morbidity in patients with heart failure. *JAMA.* 1995;**273**:1450–1456.

808. Cohn JN, Johnson G, Ziesche S, Cobb F, Francis G, Tristani F, Smith R, Dunkman WB, Loeb H, Wong M, Bhat G, Goldman S, Fletcher RD, Doherty J, Hughes V, Carson P, Cintron G, Shabetai R, Haakenson C. A comparison of enalapril with hydralazine-isosorbibe dintrate in the treatment of chronic congestive heart failure. *N Engl J Med.* 1991;**325**:303–310.

809. The Heart Outcomes Prevention Evaluation Study Investigators. Effects of an angiotensin-converting-enzyme inhibitor, ramipril, on cardiovascular events in high-risk patients. *N Engl J Med.* 2000;**342**:145–153.

810.   Teo KK, Mitchell LB, Pogue J, Bosch J, Dagenais G, Yusuf S. Effect of ramipril in reducing sudden deaths and nonfatal cardiac arrests in high-risk individuals without heart failure or left ventricular dysfunction. *Circulation.* 2004;**110**:1413–1417.

811.   Cleland JG, Erhart L, Murray G, Hall AS, Ball SG. Effect of ramipril on morbidity and mode of death among survivors of acute myocardial infarction with clinical evidence of heart failure. A report from the AIRE Study Investigators. *Eur Heart J.* 1997;**18**:41–51.

812.   Scholkens BA, Linz W. Local inhibition of angiotensin II formation and bradykinin degradation in isolated hearts. *Clin Exp Hypertens.* 1988;**10**:1259–1270.

813.   Minatoguchi S, Ito H, Koshiji M, Masao K, Hirakawa S, Majewski H. Enalapril decreases plasma noradrenaline levels during the cold pressor test in human hypertensives. *Clin Exp Pharmacol Physiol.* 1992;**19**:279–282.

814.   Pitt B, Segal R, Martinez FA, Meurers G, Cowley AJ, Thomas I, Deedwania PC, Ney DE, Snavely DB, Chang PI, on behalf of the ELITE Study Investigators. Randomised trial of losartan versus captopril in patients over 65 with heart failure (Evaluation of Losartan in the Elderly Study, ELITE). *Lancet.* 1997;**349**:747–752.

815.   Pitt B, Poole-Wilson PA, Segal R, A MF, Dickstein K, Camm AJ, Konstam MA, Riegger G, Klinger GH, Neaton J, Sharman D, Thiyagarajan B, on behalf of the ELITE II Investigators. Effect of losartan compared with captopril on mortality in patients with symptomatic heart failure: Randomised trial — the Losartan Heart Failure Survival Study ELITE II. *Lancet.* 2000;**355**:1582–1587.

816.   Dickstein K, Kjekshus J, the OPTIMAAL Steering Committee for the OPTIMAAL Study Group. Effects of losartan and captopril on mortality and morbidity in high-risk patients after actue myocardial infarction: The OPTIMAAL randomised trial. *Lancet.* 2002;**360**:752–760.

817.   Dahlöf B, Devereux RB, Kjeldsen SE, Julius S, Beevers G, de Faire U, Fyhrquist F, Ibsen H, Kristiansson K, Lederballe-Pedersen O, Lindholm LH, Nieminen MS, Omvik P, Oparil S, Wedel H, for the LIFE Study Group. Cardiovascular morbidity and mortality in the Losartan Intervention For Endpoint reduction in hypertension study (LIFE): A randomised trial against atenolol. *Lancet.* 2002;**359**:995–1003.

818.   Lindholm LH, Ibsen H, Dahlöf B, Devereux RB, Beevers G, de Faire U, Fyhrquist F, Julius S, Kjeldsen SE, Kristiansson K, Lederballe-Pedersen O, Nieminen MS, Omvik P, Oparil S, Wedel H, Aurup P, Edelman J, Snapinn S, for the LIFE study group. Cardiovascular morbidity and mortality in patients with diabetes in the Losartan Intervention For Endpoint reduction in hypertension (LIFE): A randomised trial against atenolol. *Lancet.* 2002;**359**:1004–1010.

819.   Lindholm LH, Dahlöf B, Edelman JM, Ibsen H, Borch-Johnsen K, Olsen MH, Snapinn S, Wachtell K, for the LIFE study group. Effect of losartan on sudden cardiac death in people with diabetes: Data from the LIFE study. *Lancet.* 2003;**362**:619–620.

820   Cohn JN, Tognoni G, For the Valsartan Heart Failure Trial Investigators. A randomized trial of the angiotensin-receptor blocker valsartan in chronic heart failure. *N Engl J Med.* 2001;**345**:1667–1675.

821.   Pfeffer MA, McMurray JJV, Velazquez EJ, Rouleau J-L, Køber L, Maggioni AP, Solomon SD, Swedberg K, Van de Werf F, White H, Leimberger JD, Henis M, Edwards S, Zelenkofske S, Sellers MA, Califf RM, for the Valsartan in Acute Myocardial Infarction Trial Investigators. Valsartan, captopril, or both in myocardial

infarction complicated by heart failure, left ventricular dysfunction, or both. *N Engl J Med.* 2003;**349**:1893–1906.

822. Pfeffer MA, Swedberg K, Granger CB, Held P, McMurray JJV, Michelson EL, Olofsson B, Östergren J, Yusuf S, for the CHARM Investigators and Committees. Effects of candesartan on mortality and morbidity in patients with chronic heart failure: The CHARM-Overall programme. *Lancet.* 2003;**362**:759–766.

823. Solomon SD, Wang D, Finn P, Skali H, Zornoff L, McMurray JJV, Swedberg K, Yusuf S, Granger CB, Michelson EL, Pocock S, Pfeffer MA. Effect of candesartan on cause-specific mortality in heart failure patients. The **C**andesartan in **H**eart failure **A**ssessment of **R**eduction in **M**ortality and morbidity (CHARM) Program. *Circulation.* 2004;**110**:2180–2183.

824. Francia P, Balla C, Uccellini A, Ricotta A, Modestino A, Frattari A, Salvati A, Volpe M. Low-dose angiotensin receptor blockers as an alternate to ACE-inhibitors increase the risk of appropriate ICD interventions in heart failure. *Int J Cardiol.* 2010;**145**:522–524.

825. Konstam MA, Neaton JD, Dickstein K, Drexler H, Komajda M, Martinez FA, Riegger GAJ, Malbecq W, Smith RD, Guptha S, Poole-Wilson PA, for the HEAAL Investigators. Effects of high-dose versus low-dose losartan on clinical outcomes in patients with heart failure (HEAAL study): A randomised, double-blind trial. *Lancet.* 2009;**374**: 1840–1848.

826. Funder JW, Feldman D, Edelman IS. Specific aldosterone binding in rat kidney and parotid. *J Steroid Biochem.* 1972;**3**:309–318.

827. Winer BM, Lubbe WF, Colton T. Antihypertensive actions of diuretics. Comparative study of an aldosterone antagonist and a thiazide, alone and together. *JAMA.* 1968;**204**:775–779.

828. Silvestre J-S, Robert V, Heymes C, Aupetit-Faisant B, Mouas C, Moalic J-M, Swynghedauw B, Delcayre C. Myocardial production of aldosterone and corticosterone in the rat. *J Biol Chem.* 1998;**273**:4883–4891.

829. Oshima N, Onimaru H, Takechi H, Yamamoto K, Watanabe A, Uchida T, Nishida Y, Oda T, Kumagai H. Aldosterone is synthesized in and activates bulbospinal neurons through mineralocorticoid receptors and ENaCs in the RVLM. *Hypertens Res.* 2013;**36**: 504–512.

830. Hatakeyama H, Miyamori I, Fujita T, Takeda Y, Takeda R, Yamamoto H. Vascular aldosterone. Biosynthesis and a link to angiotensin II-induced hypertrophy of vascular smooth muscle cells. *J Biol Chem.* 1994;**269**:24316–24320.

831. Weber KT, Brilla CG. Pathological hypertrophy and cardiac interstitium. Fibrosis and renin-angiotensin-aldosterone system. *Circulation.* 1991;**83**:1849–1865.

832. Rocha R, Chander PN, Khanna K, Zuckerman A, Stier Jr CT. Mineralocorticoid blockade reduces vascular injury in stroke-prone hypertensive rats. *Hypertension.* 1998;**31**: 451–458.

833. Wang W. Chronic administration of aldosterone depresses baroreceptor reflux function in the dog. *Hypertension.* 1994;**24**:571–575.

834. Barr CS, Lang CC, Hanson J, Arnott M, Kennedy N, Struthers AD. Effects of adding spironolactone to an angiotensin-converting enzyme inhibitor in chronic congestive heart failure secondary to coronary artery disease. *Am J Cardiol.* 1995;**76**:1259–1265.

835. Esposito CT, Varahan S, Jeyaraj D, Lu Y, Stambler BS. Spironolactone improves the arrhythmogenic substrate in heart failure by preventing ventricular electrical activation

delays associated with myocardial interstital fibrosis and inflammation. *J Cardiovasc Electrophysiol.* 2013;**24**:806–812.

836. Farquharson CA, Struthers AD. Spironolactone increases nitric oxide bioactivity, improves endothelial vasodilator dysfunction, and suppresses vascular angiotensin I/ angiotensin II conversion in patients with chronic heart failure. *Circulation.* 2000;**101**: 594–597.

837. Jorde UP, Vittorio T, Katz SD, Colombo PC, Latif F, Le Jemtel TH. Elevated plasma aldosterone levels despite complete inhibition of the vascular angiotensin-converting enzyme in chronic heart failure. *Circulation.* 2002;**106**:1055–1057.

838. Pitt B, Zannad F, Remme WJ, Cody R, Castaigne A, Perez A, Palensky J, Wittes J, for the Randomized Aldactone Evaluation Study Investigators. The effects of spironolactone on morbidity and mortality in patients with severe heart failure. *N Engl J Med.* 1999;**341**:709–717.

839. Haynes BA, Mookadam F. Male gynecomastia. *Mayo Clin Proc.* 2009;**84**:672.

840. Pitt B, Remme W, Zannad F, Neaton J, Martinez F, Roniker B, Bittman R, Hurley S, Kleiman J, Gatlin M, for the Eplerenone Post-Acute Myocardial Infarction Heart Failure Efficacy and Survival Study Investigators. Eplerenone, a selective aldosterone blocker, in patients with left ventricular dysfunction after myocardial infarction. *N Engl J Med.* 2003;**348**:1309–1321.

841. Zannad F, McMurray JJV, Krum H, van Veldhuisen DJ, Swedberg K, Shi H, Vincent J, Pocock SJ, Pitt B, for the EMPHASIS-HF Study Group. Eplerenone in patients with systolic heart failure and mild symptoms. *N Engl J Med.* 2011;**364**:11–21.

842. Virchow R. *Cellular pathology based on physiological and pathological histology.* Birmingham, Alabama: Classics of Medicine Library; 1858.

843. Anitschkow N, Chalatow S. Ueber experimentelle cholesterinsteatose und ihre bedeutung fuer die entstehung einiger pathologischer prozesse. *Zentrbl Allg Pathol Anat.* 1913;**24**:1–9.

844. Bullock BC, Lehner NDM, Clarkson TB, Feldner MA, Wagner WD, Lofland HB. Comparative primate atherosclerosis: I. Tissue cholesterol concentration and pathologic anatomy. *Exp Mol Pathol.* 1975;**22**:151–175.

845. Wagner WD, Clarkson TB. Comparative pirmate atherosclerosis: II. A biochemical study of lipids, calcium, and collagen in atherosclerotic arteries. *Exp Mol Pathol.* 1975;**23**:96–121.

846. Lehzen G, Knauss K. Xanthoma multiplex planum, tuberosum, mollusciformis. *Virchows Arch A Pathol Anat Histol.* 1889;**116**:85–104.

847. Rigdon RH, Willeford G. Sudden death during childhood with xanthoma tuberosum. Review of literature and report of a case. *JAMA.* 1950;**142**:1268–1271.

848. Leonard JC. Hereditary hypercholesterolaemic xanthomatosis. *Lancet.* 1956;**268**: 1239–1243.

849. Endo A. A gift from nature: The birth of the statins. *Nat Med.* 2008;**14**:xxiv–xxvi.

850. Cholesterol Treatment Trialist' (CTT) Collaborators. Protocol for a prospective collaborative overview of all current and planned randomized trials of cholesterol treatment regimens. *Am J Cardiol.* 1995;**75**:1130–1134.

851. Cholesterol Treatment Trialists' (CTT) Collaborators. Efficacy and safety of cholesterol-lowering treatment: Prospective meta-analysis of data from 90056 participants in 14 randomised trials of statins. *Lancet.* 2005;**366**:1267–1278.

852. Rahimi K, Majoni W, Merhi A, Emberson J. Effect of statins on ventricular tachyarrhythmia, cardiac arrest, and sudden death: A meta-analysis of published and unpublished evidence from randomized trials. *Eur Heart J.* 2012;**33**:1571–1581.

853. Wanahita N, Chen J, Bangalore S, Shah K, Rachko M, Coleman CI, Schweitzer P. The effect of statin therapy on ventricular tachyarrhythmias: A meta-analysis. *Am J Ther.* 2012;**19**:16–23.

854. Beri A, Contractor T, Khasnis A, Thakur R. Statins and the reduction of sudden cardiac death: Antiarrhythmic or anti-ischemic effect? *Am J Cardiovasc Drugs.* 2010;**10**:155–164.

855. Mitchell LB, Powell JL, Gillis AM, Kehl V, Hallstrom AP, and the AVID Investigators. Are lipid-lowering drugs also antiarrhythmic drugs? An analysis of the Antiarrhythmics Versus Implantable Defibrillators (AVID) Trial. *J Am Coll Cardiol.* 2003;**42**:81–87.

856. Vyas AK, Guo H, Moss AJ, Olshansky B, McNitt SA, Hall WJ, Zareba W, Steinberg J, Fischer A, Ruskin J, Andrews ML, for the MADIT-II Research Group. Reduction in ventricular tachyarrhythmias with statins in the Multicenter Automatic Defibrillation Implantation Trial (MADIT)-II. *J Am Coll Cardiol.* 2006;**47**:69–73.

857. De Sutter J, De Bacquer D, Jordaens I. Intensive lipid-lowering therapy and ventricular arrhythmias in patients with coronary artery disease and internal cardioverter defibrillator implants: The CLARIDI trial. In: *Late-breaking trial, Annual Scientific Meeting of the Heart Rhythm Society.* Boston, MA; 2006.

858. Goldberger JJ, Subacius H, Schaechter A, Howard A, Berger R, Shalaby A, Levine J, Kadish AH, for the DEFINITE Investigators. Effects of statin therapy on arrhythmic events and survival in patients with nonischemic dilated cardiomyopathy. *J Am Coll Cardiol.* 2006;**48**:1228–1233.

859. Buber J, Goldenberg I, Moss AJ, Wang PJ, McNitt S, Hall J, Eldar M, Barsheshet A, Shechter M. Reduction of life-threatening ventricular tachyarrhythmias in statin-treated patients with nonischemic cardiomyopathy enrolled in the MADIT-CRT (Multicenter automatic defibrillator implantation Trial with Cardiac Resynchronization Therapy). *J Am Coll Cardiol.* 2012;**60**:749–755.

860. Rosenson RS, Tangney CC. Antiantherothrombotic properties of statins: Implications for cardiovascular event reduction. *JAMA.* 1998;**279**:1643–1650.

861. Horwich TB, MacLellan WR, Fonarow GC. Statin therapy is associated with improved survival in ischemic and non-ischemic heart failure. *J Am Coll Cardiol.* 2004;**43**:642–648.

862. Furberg CD, Pitt B. Withdrawal of cerivastatin from the world market. *Curr Control Trial Cardiovasc Med.* 2001;**2**:205–207.

863. Hollman A. Quinine and quinidine. *Br Heart J.* 1991;**66**:301.

864. Bowman IA. Jean-Baptiste Sénac and his treatise on the heart. *Tex Heart Inst J.* 1987;**14**:4–11.

865. Wenckehach KF. Cinchona derivatives in the treatment of heart disoders. *JAMA.* 1923;**81**:472–474.

866. The CAPS Investigators. The Cardiac Arrhythmia Pilot Study. *Am J Cardiol.* 1986;**57**:91–96.

867. The Cardiac Arrhythmia Suppression Trial (CAST) Investigators. Preliminary report: Effect of encainide and flecainide on mortality in a randomized trial of arrhythmia supresion after myocardial infarction. *N Engl J Med.* 1989;**321**:406–412.

868. The Cardiac Arrhythmia Suppression Trial II Investigators. Effect of the antiarrhythmic agent moricizine on survival after myocardial infarction. *N Engl J Med.* 1992;**327**: 227–233.

869. Epstein AE, Hallstrom AP, Rogers WJ, Liebson PR, Seals AA, Anderson JL, Cohen JD, Capone RJ, Wyse DG. Mortality following ventricular arrhythmia suppression by encainide, flecainide, and moricizine after myocardial infarction. The original design concept of the Cardiac Arrhythmia Suppression Trial (CAST). *JAMA.* 1993;**270**: 2451–2455.

870. Akhtar M, Breithardt G, Camm AJ, Coumel P, Janse MJ, Lazzara R, Myerburg RJ, Schwartz PJ, Waldo AL, Wellens HJ. CAST and beyond. Implications of the Cardiac Arrhythmia Suppression Trial. Task Force of the Working Group on Arrhythmias of the European Society of Cardiology. *Circulation.* 1990;**81**:1123–1127.

871. Rosenbaum MB, Chaile PA, Halpern MS, Nau GJ, Przbylski J, Levi RJ, Lázzari JO, Elizari MV. Clinical efficacy of amiodarone as an antiarrhythmic agent. *Am J Cardiol.* 1976;**38**:934–944.

872. Rosenbaum MB, Chiale PA, Haedo A, Lázzari JO, Elizari MV. Ten years of experience with amiodarone. *Am Heart J.* 1983;**106**:957–964.

873. Amiodarone Trials Meta-Analysis Investigators. Effect of prophylactic amiodarone on mortality after acute myocardial infarction and in congestive heart failure: Meta-analysis of individual data from 6500 patients in randomised trials. *Lancet.* 1997;**350**:1417–1424.

874. Sim I, McDonald KM, Lavori PW, Norbutas CM, Hlatky MA. Quantitative overview of randomized trials of amiodarone to prevent sudden death. *Circulation.* 1997;**96**: 2823–2829.

875. Torp-Pedersen C, Metra M, Spark P, Lukas MA, Moullet C, Scherhag A, Komajda M, Cleland JG, Remme W, Di Lenarda A, Swedberg K, Poole-Wilson PA, for the COMET Investigators. The safety of amiodarone in patients with heart failure. *J Card Fail.* 2007;**13**:340–345.

876. Thomas KL, Al-Khatib SM, Lokhnygina Y, Solomon SD, Kober L, McMurray JJ, Califf RM, Velazquez EJ. Amiodarone use after acute myocardial infarction complicated by heart failure and/or left ventricular dysfunction may be associated with excess mortality. *Am Heart J.* 2008;**155**:87–93.

877. Piccini JP, Berger JS, M OCC. Amiodarone for the prevention of sudden cardiac death: A meta-analysis of randomized controlled trials. *Eur Heart J.* 2009;**30**: 1245–1253.

878. Travers AH, Rea TD, Bobrow BJ, Edelson DP, Berg RA, Sayre MR, Berg MD, Chameides L, O'Connor RE, Swor RA. Part 4: CPR overview. 2010 American Heart Association Guidelines for Cardiopulmonary Resuscitation and Emergency Cardiovascular Care. *Circulation.* 2010;**122**[Suppl3]:S676–S684.

879. Eisenberg MS, Horwood BT, Cummins RD, Reynolds-Haertle R, Hearne TR. Cardiac arrest and resuscitation: A tale of 29 cities. *Ann Emerg Med.* 1990;**19**:179–186.

880. Cooper JA, Cooper JD, Cooper JM. Cardiopulmonary resuscitation: History, current practice, and future direction. *Circulation.* 2006;**114**:2839–2849.

881. Valenzuela TD, Roe DJ, Cretin S, Spaite DW, Larsen MP. Estimating effectiveness of cardiac arrest interventions: A logistic regression survival model. *Circulation.* 1997;**96**: 3308–3313.

882. Holmberg M, Holmberg S, Herlitz J. Incidence, duration and survival of ventricular fibrillation in out-of-hospital cardiac arrest patients in Sweden. *Resuscitation.* 2000;**44**:7–17.

883. Hoffa M, Ludwig C. Einige neue Versuche uber Herzbewegung. *Zeitschrift Rationelle Medizin.* 1850;**9**:107–144.

884. Vulpian EFA. Notes sur les effets de la faradisation directe des ventricules du coeur chez le chien. *Arch Physiol Norm Path.* 1874;**6**:975–982.

885. McWilliam J. Electrical stimulation of the heart in man. *Br Med J.* 1889;**1**:348–350.

886. McWilliam JA. Fibrillar contraction of the heart. *J Physiol.* 1887;**8**:296–310.

887. Larsen MP, Eisenberg MS, Cummins RO, Hallstrom AP. Predicting survival from out-of-hospital cardiac arrest: A graphic model. *Ann Emerg Med.* 1993;**22**:1652–1658.

888. Sedgwick ML, Dalziel K, Watson J, Carring DJ, Cobbe SM. The causative rhythm in out of hospital cardiac arrests witnessed by the emergency medical services in the Heartstart Scotland Project. *Resuscitation.* 1994;**27**:55–59.

889. Stiell IG, A WG, Field B, Spaite DW, Nesbitt LP, De Maio VJ, Nichol G, Cousineau D, Blackburn J, Munkley D, Luinstra-Toohey L, Campeau T, Dagnone E, Lyver M. Advanced cardiac life support in out-of-hospital cardiac arrest. *N Engl J Med.* 2004;**351**:647–656.

890. Chan PS, Krumholz HM, Nichol G, Nallamothu BK. Delayed time to defibrillation after in-hospital cardiac arrest. *N Engl J Med.* 2008;**358**:9–17.

891. Cobb LA, Fahrenbruch CE, Walsh TR, Copass MK, Olsufka M, Breskin M, Hallstrom AP. Influence of cardiopulmonary resuscitation prior to defibrillation in patients with out-of-hospital ventricular fibrillation. *JAMA.* 1999;**281**:1182–1188.

892. Sasson C, Rogers MAM, Dahl J, Kellerman AL. Predictors of survival from out-of-hospital cardiac arrest: A systematic review and meta-analysis. *Circ Cardiovasc Qual Outcomes.* 2010;**3**:63–81.

893. Abildgaard PC. Tentamina electrica in animalibus insituta. *Societas Medical Havniensis Collectanea.* 1775;**2**:157.

894. Prevost JL, Battelli F. Le mort par les descharges electrique. *J Physiol.* 1899;**1**: 1085–1100.

895. Hooker DR, Kouwenhoven WB, Langworthy OR. The effect of alternating electrical currents on the heart. *Am J Physiol.* 1933;**103**:444–454.

896. Kouwenhoven WHD. Resuscitation by countershock. *Electrical Eng.* 1933;**52**:475–477.

897. Beck CS, Pritchard WH, Feil HS. Ventricular fibrillation of long duration abolished by electric shock. *JAMA.* 1947;**135**:985–986.

898. Gurvich NL. Restoration of vital functions of the organism following fatal electric shock. *Klin Med (Mosk).* 1952;**30**:66–70.

899. Zoll PM, Linenthal AJ, Gibson W, Paul MH, Norman LR. Termination of ventricular fibrillation in man by externally applied electric countershock. *N Engl J Med.* 1956;**254**:727–732.

900. Weaver WD, Cobb LA, Hallstrom AP, Fahrenbruch C, Copass MK, Ray R. Factors influencing survival after out-of-hospital cardiac arrest. *J Am Coll Cardiol.* 1986;**7**: 752–757.

901. Swor RA, Jackson RE, Cynar M, Sadler E, Basse E, Boji B, Rivera-Rivera EJ, Maher A, Grubb W, Jacobson R, Dalbec DL. Bystander CPR, ventricular fibrillation, and survival in witnessed, unmonitored out-of-hospital cardiac arrest. *Ann Emerg Med.* 1995;**25**: 780–784.

902. Chen P-S, Wu T-J, Ting C-T, Karagueuzian HS, Garfinkel A, Lin S-F, Weiss JN. A tale of two fibrillations. *Circulation.* 2003;**108**:2298–2303.

903. Sakai T, Iwami T, Tasaki O, Kawamura T, Hayashi Y, Rinka H, Ohishi Y, Mohri T, Kishimoto M, Nishiuchi T, Kajino K, Matsumoto H, Uejima T, Nitta M, Shiokawa C, Ikeuchi H, Hiraide A, Sugimoto H, Kuwagata Y. Incidence and outcomes of out-of-hospital cardiac arrest with shock-resistant ventricular fibrillation: Data from a large population-based cohort. *Resuscitation.* 2010;**81**:956–961.

904. Effert S. Automatic monitoring equipment and indication for implantation of electrical pacemakers. *Thoraxchir Vask Chir.* 1963;**11**:158–166.

905. Diack AW, Welborn WS, Rullman RG. Cardiac resuscitator and monitoring apparatus. In: *United States Patent Office.* United States of America: Cardiac Resuscitator Corporation, Portland, OR; 9 May 1978: #4,088,138.

906. Diack AW, Welborn WS, Rullman RG, Walter CW, Wayne MA. An automatic cardiac resuscitator for emergency treatment of cardiac arrest. *Med Instrum.* 1979;**13**:78–83.

907. Jaggarao NS, Heber M, Grainger R, Vincent R, Chamberlain DA, Aronson AL. Use of an automated external defibrillator-pacemaker by ambulance staff. *Lancet.* 1982;**320**:73–75.

908. Morgan CB, Yerkovich D, Lyster TH, Roberts DH. Interactive portable defibrillator. In: *United States Patent Office.* United States of America: Physio-Control Corporation; 9 Sep 1986: #4,610,254.

909. Cummins RO, Bergner L, Eisenberg M, Murray JA. Sensitivity, accuracy, and safety of an automated external defibrillator. *Lancet.* 1984;**324**:318–320.

910. Cummins RO, Stults KR, Haggar B, Berber RE, Schaeffer S, Brown DD. A new rhythm library for testing automatic external defibrillators: Performance of three devices. *J Am Coll Cardiol.* 1988;**11**:597–602.

911. Weaver WD, Hill DL, Fahrenbruch C, Cobb LA, Copass MK, Hallstrom AP, Martin J. Automatic external defibrillators: Importance of field testing to evaluate performance. *J Am Coll Cardiol.* 1987;**10**:1259–1264.

912. Weaver WD, Hill D, Fahrenbruch CE, Copass MK, Martin JS, Cobb LA, Hallstrom AP. Use of the automatic external defibrillator in the management of out-of-hospital cardiac arrest. *N Engl J Med.* 1988;**319**:661–666.

913. Weaver WD, Copass MK, Bufi D, Ray R, Hallstrom AP, Cobb LA. Improved neurologic recovery and survival after early defibrillation. *Circulation.* 1984;**69**:943–948.

914. Emergency Care Research Institute. ECRI responds to FDA Safety Alert on Laerdal automated external defibrillators. *Health Devices.* 1994;**23**:254–256.

915. Cummins RO, White RD, Pepe PE. Ventricular fibrillation, automatic external defibrillators, and the United States Food and Drug Administration: Confrontation without comprehension. *Ann Emerg Med.* 1995;**26**:621–631.

916. Auble TE, Menegazzi JJ, Paris PM. Effect of out-of-hsopital defibrillaton by basic life support providers on cardiac arrest mortality: A metaanalysis. *Ann Emerg Med.* 1995;**25**:642–648.

917. Kerber RE, Becker LB, Bourland JD, Cummins RO, Hallstrom AP, Michos MB, Nichol G, Ornato JP, Thies WH, White RD, Zuckerman BD, and Members endorsed by the Board of Trustees of the American College of Cardiology. Automatic external defibrillators for public access defibrillaton: Recommendations for specifying and reporting arrhythmia analysis algorithm performance, incorporating new waveforms, and enhancing safety: A statement for health professionals from the American Heart

Association Task Force on Automatic External Defibrillation, Subcommittee on AED Safety and Efficacy. *Circulation.* 1997;**95**:1677–1682.

918. White RD, Hankins DG, Bugliosi TF. Seven year' experience with early defibrillation by police and paramedics in an emergency medical services system. *Resuscitation.* 1998;**39**:145–151.

919. Mosesso VNJ, Davis EA, Auble TE, Paris PM, Yealy DM. Use of automated external defibrillators by police officers for treatment of out-of-hospital cardiac arrest. *Ann Emerg Med.* 1998;**32**:200–207.

920. McDaniel CM, Berry VA, Haines DE, DiMarco JP. Automatic external defibrillation of patients after myocardial infarction by family members: Practical aspects and psychological impact of training. *Pacing Clin Electrophysiol.* 1988;**11** (Pt 2):2029–2034.

921. Chamberlain D, Smith A, Woollard M, Colquhoun M, Handley AJ, Leaves S, Kern KB. Trials of teaching methods in basic life support (3): Comparison of simulated CPR performance after first training and at 6 months, with a note on the value of re-training. *Resuscitation.* 2002;**53**:179–187.

922. Bardy GH, Lee KL, Mark DB, Poole JE, Toff WD, Tonkin AM, Smith W, Dorian P, Packer DL, White RD, Longstreth Jr WT, Anderson J, Johnson G, Bischoff E, Yallop JJ, McNulty S, Ray LD, Clapp-Channing NE, Rosenberg Y, Schron EB, for the HAT Investigators. Home use of automated external defibrillators for sudden cardiac death. *N Engl J Med.* 2008;**358**:1793–1804.

923. Christenson J, Nafziger S, Compton S, Vijayaraghavan K, Slater B, Ledingham R, Powell J, McBurnie MA, PAD Investigators. The effect of time on CPR and automated external defibrillator skills in the Public Access Defibrillation Trial. *Resuscitation.* 2007;**74**:52–62.

924. Valenzuela TD, Roe DJ, Nichol G, Clark LL, Spaite DW, Hardman RG. Outcomes of rapid defibrillation by security officers after cardiac arrest in casinos. *N Engl J Med.* 2000;**343**:1206–1209.

925. Aldrette JA, Aldrette LE. Oxygen concentrations in commercial aircraft flights. *South Med J.* 1983;**76**:12–14.

926. Hampson NB, Kregenow DA, Mahoney AM, Kirtland SH, Horan KL, Holm JR, Gerbino AJ. Altitude exposures during commercial flight: A reappraisal. *Aviat Space Environ Med.* 2013;**84**:27–31.

927. Crewdson J. Special Report: Code blue: Survival in the sky. In: *Chicago Tribune.* Chicago; 1996.

928. O'Rourke MF, Donaldson E, Geddes JS. An airline cardiac arrest program. *Circulation.* 1997;**96**:2849–2853.

929. Crewdson J. 1st airline in US adds heart rescue equipment: Defibrillators could save scores of lives. In: *Chicago Tribune.* Chicago; 1996.

930. McKenas DK. First, do no harm: The role of defibrillators and advanced medical care in commercial aviation. *Aviat Space Environ Med.* 1997;**68**:365–367.

931. O'Rourke RA. Saving lives in the sky. *Circulation.* 1997;**96**:2775–2777.

932. Page RL, Joglar JA, Kowal RC, Zagrodzky JD, Nelson LL, Ramaswamy K, Barbera SJ, Hamdan MH, McKenas DK. Use of automated external defibrillators by a U.S. airline. *N Engl J Med.* 2000;**343**:1210–1216.

933. U.S. Federal Aviation Administration (FAA). Emergency Medical Equipment. *Federal Register.* 2004;**66**:19028.

934.   Emergency Cardiac Care Committee and Subcommittees AHA. Guidelines for cardio-pulmonary resuscitation and emergency care. *JAMA.* 1992;**268**:2171–2183.

935.   Pell JP, Sirel JM, Marsden AK, Ford I, Walker NL, Cobbe SM. Potential impact of public access defibrillators on survival after out of hospital cardiopulmonary arrest: Retrospective cohort study. *Br Med J.* 2002;**325**:515.

936.   Secretary of State for Health. Saving lives: Our healthier nation. In: *London: Department of Health*; 1999:3.37–3.40.

937.   Sasaki M, Iwami T, Kitamura T, Nomoto S, Nishiyama C, Sakai T, Tanigawa K, Kajino K, Irisawa T, Nishiuchi T, Hayashida S, Hiraide A, Kawamura T. Incidence and out-come of out-of-hospital cardiac arrest with public-access defibrillation. A descriptive epidemiological study in a large urban community. *Circ J.* 2011;**75**:2821–2826.

938.   Weisfeldt ML, Sitlani CM, Ornato JP, Rea T, Aufderheide TP, Davis D, Dreyer J, Hess EP, Jui J, Maloney J, Sopko G, Powell J, Nichol G, Morrison LJ, for the ROC Investigators. Survival after application of automatic external defibrillators before arrival of the emer-gency medical system. Evaluation in the Resuscitation Outcomes Consortium population of 21 million. *J Am Coll Cardiol.* 2010;**55**:1713–1720.

939.   Cobb LA, Fahrenbruch CE, Olsufka M, Copass MK. Changing incidence of out-of-hospital ventricular fibrillation, 1980–2000. *JAMA.* 2002;**288**:3008–3013.

940.   Ko PC, Ma MH, Yen ZS, Shih CL, Chen WJ, Lin FY. Impact of community-wide deploy-ment of biphasic waveform automated external defibrillators on out-of-hopsital cardiac arrest in Taipei. *Resuscitation.* 2004;**63**:167–174.

941.   Gallagher EJ, Lombardi G, Gennis P. Effectiveness of bystander cardio-pulmonary resus-citation and survival following out-of-hospital cardiac arrest. *JAMA.* 1995;**274**:1922–1925.

942.   Bobrow BJ, Clark LL, Ewy GA, Chikani V, Sanders AB, Berg RA, Richman PB, Kern KB. Minimally interrupted cardiac resuscitation by emergency medical services for out-of-hospital cardiac arrest. *JAMA.* 2008;**299**:1158–1165.

943.   Drezner JA, Chun JS, Harmon KG, Derminer L. Survival trends in the United States following exercise-related sudden cardiac arrest in the youth: 2000–2006. *Heart Rhythm.* 2008;**5**:794–799.

944.   Drezner JA, Rao AL, Heistand J, Bloomingdale MK, Harmon KG. Effectiveness of emergency response planning for sudden cardiac arrest in United States high schools with automated external defibrillators. *Circulation.* 2009;**120**:518–525.

945.   Hallstrom AP, Ornato JP, Weisfeldt M, Travers A, Christenson J, McBurnie MA, Zalenski R, Becker LB, Schron EB, Proschan M. Public access defibrillation and sur-vival after out-of-hospital cardiac arrest. *N Engl J Med.* 2004;**351**:637–646.

946.   Handley AJ, Koster R, Monsieurs K, Perkins GD, Davies S, Bossaert L. European Resuscitation Council Guidelines for Resuscitation 2005. Section 2. Adult basic life support and use of automated external defibrillators. *Resuscitation.* 2005;**67**:S7–S23.

947.   Aufderheide T, Hazinski MF, Nichol G, Steffens SS, Buroker A, McCune R, Stapleton E, Nadkarni V, Potts J, Ramirez RR, Eigel B, Epstein A, Sayre M, Halperin H, Cummins RO. Community lay rescuer automated external defibrillation programs: Key state legislative components and implementation strategies: A summary of a decade of experience for healthcare providers, policymakers, legislators, employers, and com-munity leaders from the American Heart Association Emergency Cardiovascular Care Committee, Council on Clinical Cardiology, and Office of State Advocacy. *Circulation.* 2006;**113**:1260–1270.

948. Folke F, Lippert FK, Nielsen SL, Gislason GH, Hansen ML, Schramm TK, Sørensen R, Fosbøl EL, Andersen SS, Rasmussen S, Køber L, Torp-Pedersen C. Location of cardiac arrest in a city center: Strategic placement of automated external defibrillators in public locations. *Circulation.* 2009;**120**:510–517.

949. Koster RW, Baubin MA, Bossaert LL, Caballero A, Cassan P, Castrén M, Granja C, Handley AJ, Monsieurs KG, Perkins GD, Raffay V, Sandroni C. European Resuscitation Council Guidelines for Resuscitation 2010. Section 2. Adult basic life support and use of automated external defibrillators. *Resuscitation.* 2010;**81**:1277–1292.

950. Meaney PA, Bobrow BJ, Mancini ME, Christenson J, de Caen AR, Bhanji F, Abella BS, Kleinman ME, Edelson DP, Berg RA, Aufderheide TP, Menon V, Leary M, on behalf of the CPR Quality Summit Investigators, the American Heart Association Emergency Cardiovascular Care Committee, and the Council on Cardiopulmonary, Critical Care, Perioperative and Resuscitation, Cardiopulmonary resuscitation quality: Improving cardiac resuscitation outcomes both inside and outside the hospital. A consensus statement from the American Heart Association endorsed by the American College of Emergency Physicians. *Circulation.* 2013;**128**:417–435.

951. ECC Committee S, and Task Forces for the American Heart Association, 2005 American Heart Association guidelines for cardiopulmonary resuscitation and emergency cardiovascular care. Part 3: Overview of CPR. *Circulation.* 2005;**112**:IV-12–IV-18.

952. Bahr J, Klingler H, Panzer W, Rode H, Kettler D. Skills of lay people in checking the carotid pulse. *Resuscitation.* 1997;**35**:23–26.

953. Eberle B, Dick WF, Schneider T, Wisser G, Doetsch S, Tzanova I. Check-ing the carotid pulse check: Diagnostic accuracy of first responders in patients with and without a pulse. *Resuscitation.* 1996;**33**:107–116.

954. Lapostolle F, Le Toumelin P, Agostinucci JM, Catineau J, Adnet F. Basic cardiac life support providers checking the carotid pulse: Performance, degree of conviction, and influencing factors. *Acad Emerg Med.* 2004;**11**:878–880.

955. Moule P. Checking the carotid pulse: Diagnostic accuracy in students of the health-care professions. *Resuscitation.* 2000;**44**:195–201.

956. Mirowski M, Mower MM, Gott VL, Brawley RK. Feasibility and effectiveness of low-energy catheter defibrillation in man. *Circulation.* 1973;**47**:79–85.

957. Mirowski M, Mower MM, Langer A, Heilman MS, Schreibman J. A chronically implanted system for automatic defibrillation in active conscious dogs. Experimental model for treatment of sudden death from ventricular fibrillation. *Circulation.* 1978;**58**:90–94.

958. Mirowski M, Reid PR, Mower MM, Watkins L, Gott VL, Schauble JF, Langer A, Heilman MS, Kolenik SA, Fischell RE, Weisfeldt ML. Termination of malignant ventricular arrhythmias with an implanted automatic defibrillator in human beings. *N Engl J Med.* 1980;**303**:322–324.

959. Mirowski M, Reid PR, Winkle RA, Mower MM, Watkins Jr L, Stinson EB, Griffith LSC, Kallman CH, Weisfeldt ML. Mortality in patients with implanted automatic defibrillators. *Ann Intern Med.* 1983;**95** (Part 1):585–588.

960. Cohen TJ, Reid PR, Mower MM, Mirowski M, Aarons D, Juanteguy J, Veltri EP. The automatic implantable cardioverter-defibrillator. Long-term clinical experience and outcome at a hospital without an open-heart surgery program. *Arch Intern Med.* 1992;**152**:65–69.

961. Caldwell J, Moreton N, Khan N, Kerzin-Storrar L, Metcalfe K, Newman W, Garratt CJ. The clinical management of relatives of young sudden unexplained death victims; implantable defibrillators are rarely indicated. *Heart.* 2012;**98**:631–636.

962. Ezekowitz JA, Armstrong PW, McAlister FA. Implantable cardioverter defibrillators in primary and secondary prevention: A systematic review of randomized, controlled trials. *Ann Intern Med.* 2003;**138**:445–452.

963. Wyse DG, Friedman PL, Brodsky MA, Beckman KJ, Carlson MD, Curtis AB, Hallstrom AP, Raitt MH, Wilkoff BL, Greene HL, for the AVID Investigators. Life-threatening ventricular arrhythmias due to transient or correctable causes: High risk for death in follow-up. *J Am Coll Cardiol.* 2001;**38**:1718–1724.

964. Connolly SJ, Hallstrom AP, Cappato R, Schron EB, Kuck K-H, Zipes DP, Greene HL, Boczor S, Domanski M, Follmann D, Gent M, Roberts RS, on behalf of the investigators of AVID CaCs. Meta-analysis of implantable cardioverter defibrillator secondary prevention trials. *Eur Heart J.* 2000;**21**:2071–2078.

965. The Antiarrhythmics versus Implantable Defibrillators (AVID) Investigators. A comparison of antiarrhythmic-drug therapy with implantable defibrillators in patients resuscitated from near-fatal ventricular arrhythmias. *N Engl J Med.* 1997;**337**:1576–1583.

966. Connolly SJ, Gent M, Roberts RS, Dorian P, Roy D, Sheldon RS, Mitchell LB, Green MS, Klein GJ, O'Brien B. Canadian implantable defibrillator study (CIDS): A randomized trial of the implantable cardioverter defibrillator against amiodarone. *Circulation.* 2000;**101**:1297–1302.

967. Kuck KH, Cappato R, Siebels J, Rüppel R. Randomized comparison of antiarrhythmic drug therapy with implantable defibrillators in patients resuscitated from cardiac arrest: The Cardiac Arrest Study Hamburg (CASH). *Circulation.* 2000;**102**:748–854.

968. Begley DA, Mohiddin SA, Tripodi D, Winkler JB, Fananapazir L. Efficacy of implantable cardioverter defibrillator therapy for primary and secondary prevention of sudden cardiac death in hypertrophic cardiomyopathy. *Pacing Clin Electrophysiol.* 2003;**26**:1887–1896.

969. Goldenberg I, Vyas AK, Hall WJ, Moss AJ, Wang H, He H, Zareba W, Mcnitt S, Andrews ML. Risk stratification for primary implantation of a cardioverter-defibrillator in patients with ischemic left ventricular dysfunction. *J Am Coll Cardiol.* 2008;**51**:288–296.

970. Dunbar SB, Dougherty CM, Sears SF, Carroll DL, Goldstein NE, Mark DB, McDaniel G, Pressler SJ, Schron E, Wang P, Zeigler VL, on behalf of the American Heart Association Council on Cardiovascular Nursing Council on Clinical Cardiology, and Council on Cardiovascular Disease in the Young, Educational and psychological interventions to improve outcomes for recipients of implantable cardioverter defibrillators and their families. Endorsed by the Heart Rhythm Society and the American Association of Critical Care Nurses. *Circulation.* 2012;**126**:2146–2172.

971. Davids JS, McPherson CA, Earley C, Batsford WP, Lampert R. Benefits of cardiac rehabilitation in patients with implantable cardioverter-defibrillators: A patient survey. *Arch Phys Med Rehabil.* 2005;**86**:1924–1928.

972. Steinke EE. Sexual concerns of patients and partners after implantable cardioverter defibrillator. *Dimens Crit Care Nurs.* 2003;**22**:447–453.

973. Berg SK, Elleman-Jensen L, Zwisler AD, Winkel P, Svendsen JH, Pedersen PU, Moons P. Sexual concerns and practices after ICD implantation: Findings of the COPE-ICD rehabilitation trial. *Eur J Cardiovasc Nurs.* 2013;**12**:468–474.

974. Cook SC, Valente AM, Maul TM, Dew MA, Hickey J, Burger JP, Harmon A, Clair M, Webster G, Cecchin F, Khairy P, Alliance for Adult Research in Congenital Cardiology. Shock-related anxiety and sexual function in adults with congenital heart disease and implantable cardioverter-defibrillators. *Heart Rhythm.* 2013;**10**:805–810.

975. Sears SF, Hauf JD, Kirian K, Hazelton G, Conti JB. Posttraumatic stress and the implantable cardioverter-defibrillator patient: What the electrophysiologist needs to know. *Circ Arrhythm Electrophysiol.* 2011;**4**:242–250.

976. Sears Jr SF, Conti JB, Curtis AB, Saia TL, Foote R, Wen F. Affective distress and implantable cardioverter defibrillators: Cases for psychological and behavioral interventions. *Pacing Clin Electrophysiol.* 1999;**22**:1831–1834.

977. Sears Jr SF, Conti JB. Quality of life and psychological functioning of ICD patients. *Heart.* 2002;**87**:488–493.

978. Burke JL, Hallas CN, Clark-Carter D, White D, Connelly D. The psychosocial impact of the implantable cardioverter defibrillator: A meta-analytic review. *Br J Health Psychol.* 2003;**8**:165–178.

979. Redhead AP, Turkington D, Rao S, Tynan MM, Bourke JP. Psychopathology in postinfarction patients implanted with cardioverter-defibrillators for secondary prevention: A cross-sectional, case-controlled study. *J Psychosom Res.* 2010;**69**:555–563.

980. Pedersen SS, den Broek KC, Theuns DA, Erdman RA, Alings M, Meijer A, Jordaens L, Denollet J. Risk of chronic anxiety in implantable defibrillator patients: A multi-center study. *Int J Cardiol.* 2011;**147**:420–423.

981. Bilge AK, Ozben B, Demirgan S, Cinar M, Yilmaz E, Adalet K. Depression and anxiety status of patients with implantable cardioverter defibrillator and precipitating factors. *Pacing Clin Electrophysiol.* 2006;**29**:619–626.

982. Kapa S, Rotondi-Trevisan D, Mariano Z, Aves T, Irvine J, Dorian P, Hayes DL. Psychopathology in patients with ICDs over time: Results of a prospective study. *Pacing Clin Electrophysiol.* 2010;**33**:198–208.

983. Pedersen SS, Hoogwegt MT, Jordaens L, Theuns DA. Relation of symptomatic heart failure and psychological status to persistent depression in patients with implantable cardioverter-defibrillator. *Am J Cardiol.* 2010;**108**:69–74.

984. Magyar-Russell G, Thombs BD, Cai JX, Baveja T, Kuhl EA, Singh PP, Montenegro Braga Barroso M, Arthurs E, Roseman M, Amin N, Marine JE, Ziegelstein RC. The prevalence of anxiety and depression in adults with implantable cardioverter defibrillators: A systematic review. *J Psychosom Res.* 2011;**71**:223–231.

985. Dougherty CM. Longitudinal recovery following sudden cardiac arrest and internal cardioverter defibrillator implantation: Survivors and their families. *Am J Crit Care.* 1994;**3**:145–154.

986. Doolittle ND, Sauvé MJ. Impact of aborted sudden cardiac death on survivors and their spouses: The phenomenon of different reference points. *Am J Crit Care.* 1995;**4**:389–396.

987. Schron EB, Exner DV, Yao Q, Jenkins LS, Steinberg JS, Cook JR, Kutalek SP, Friedman PL, Bubien RS, Page RL, Powell J. Quality of life in the Antiarrhythmics Versus Implantable Defibrillators trial: Impact of therapy and influence of adverse symptoms and defibrillator shocks. *Circulation.* 2002;**105**:589–594.

988. Irvine J, Dorian P, Baker B, O'Brien BJ, Roberts R, Gent M, Newman D, Connolly SJ. Quality of life in the Canadian Implantable Defibrillator Study (CIDS). *Am Heart J.* 2002;**144**:282–289.

989.   Mark DB, Anstrom KJ, Sun JL, Clapp-Channing NE, Tsiatis AA, L D-R, Lee KL, Bardy GH, Sudden Cardiac Death in Heart Failure Trial Investigators. Quality of life with defibrillator therapy or amiodarone in heart failure. *N Engl J Med.* 2008;**359**:999–1008.

990.   Kamphuis HC, de Leeuw JR, Derksen R, Hauer RN, Winnubst JA. Implantable cardioverter defibrillator recipients: Quality of life in recipients with and without ICD shock delivery: A prospective study. *Europace.* 2003;**5**:381–389.

991.   Newall EG, Lever NA, Prasad S, Hornabrook C, Larsen PD. Psychological implications of ICD implantation in a New Zealand population. *Europace.* 2007;**9**:20–24.

992.   Passman R, Subacius H, Ruo B, Schaechter A, Howard A, Sears SF, Kadish A. Implantable cardioverter defibrillators and quality of life: Results from the Defibrillators in Nonischemic Cardiomyopathy Treatment Evaluation study. *Arch Intern Med.* 2007;**167**:2226–2232.

993.   Myerburg RJ, Kessler KM, Castellanos A. Sudden cardiac death. Structure, function, and time-dependence of risk. *Circulation.* 1992;**85** (Suppl):I2–I20.

994.   Chiuve SE, Fung TT, Rexrode KM, Spiegelman D, Manson JE, Stampfer MJ, Albert CM. Adherence to a low-risk, healthy lifestyle and risk of sudden cardiac death among women. *JAMA.* 2011;**306**:62–69.

995.   Fung TT, Rexrode KM, Mantzoros CS, Manson JE, Willett WC, Hu FB. Mediterranean diet and incidence of and mortality from coronary heart disease and stroke in women. *Circulation.* 2009;**119**:1093–1100.

996.   Reddy PR, Reinier K, Singh T, Mariani R, Gunson K, Jui J, Chugh SS. Physical activity as a trigger of sudden cardiac arrest: The Oregon Sudden Unexpected Death Study. *Int J Cardiol.* 2009;**131**:345–349.

997.   Thompson PD, Funk EJ, Carleton RA, Sturner WQ. Incidence of death during jogging in Rhode Island from 1975 through 1980. *JAMA.* 1982;**247**:2535–2538.

998.   Behr E, Wood DA, Wright M, Syrris P, Sheppard MN, Casey A, Davies MJ, McKenna W, Sudden Arrhythmic Death Syndrome Steering Group. Cardiological assessment of first-degree relatives in sudden arrhythmic death syndrome. *Lancet.* 2003;**362**: 1457–1459.

999.   Semsarian C, Hamilton RM. Key role of the molecular autopsy in sudden unexpected death. *Heart Rhythm.* 2012;**9**:145–150.

1000.   Meder B, Haas J, Keller A, Heid C, Just S, Borries A, Boisguerin V, Scharfenberger-Schmeer M, Stähler P, Beier M, Weichenhan D, Strom TM, Pfeufer A, Korn B, Katus HA, Rottbauer W. Targeted next-generation sequencing for molecular genetic diagnostics of cardiomyopathies. *Circ Cardiovasc Genet.* 2011;**4**:110–112.

Index